EDITORIAL COMMITTEE

Senior Editor
Richard J. Schanler, MD, FAAP

Editors
Sharon Dooley, MD, MPH, FACOG
Lawrence M. Gartner, MD, FAAP
Nancy F. Krebs, MD, FAAP
Sharon B. Mass, MD, FACOG

Staff
AAP
  Laura D. Aird, MS
  Diane Beausoleil
  Betty L. Crase, IBCLC, RLC
  Holly Kaminski
  Cyndy Rouse
  Thomas F. Tonniges, MD, FAAP
ACOG
  Janet Chapin, RN, MPH
  Luella Klein, MD, FACOG
  Elaine Locke, MPA

AAP WORK GROUP/TASK FORCE ON BREASTFEEDING

Members, 1994–2000
  Lawrence M. Gartner, MD, FAAP (Chair)
  Linda S. Black, MD, FAAP
  Antoinette Parisi Eaton, MD, FAAP
  Michael Georgieff, MD, FAAP
  Ruth A. Lawrence, MD, FAAP
  Audrey J. Naylor, MD, DrPH, FAAP
  Marianne E. Neifert, MD, FAAP
  Donna O'Hare, MD, FAAP
  Yvette Piovanetti, MD, FAAP
  Richard J. Schanler, MD, FAAP
Liaison Representatives
  Nancy F. Krebs, MD, FAAP
  Alice Lenihan, MPH, RD
  John T. Queenan, MD, FACOG

AAP SECTION ON BREASTFEEDING EXECUTIVE COMMITTEE

2000–2003

Lawrence M. Gartner, MD, FAAP (Chair)
Linda S. Black, MD, FAAP
Ruth A. Lawrence, MD, FAAP
Audrey J. Naylor, MD, DrPH, FAAP
Donna O'Hare, MD, FAAP
Richard J. Schanler, MD, FAAP

Liaison Representatives

Nancy F. Krebs, MD, FAAP
Alice Lenihan, MPH, RD
John T. Queenan, MD, FACOG

2003–2005

Lawrence M. Gartner, MD, FAAP (Chair)
Ruth A. Lawrence, MD, FAAP
Jane Morton, MD, FAAP
Audrey J. Naylor, MD, DrPH, FAAP
Donna O'Hare, MD, FAAP
Richard J. Schanler, MD, FAAP

Liaison Representatives

Laura Dean, MD, FACOG
Nancy F. Krebs, MD, FAAP
Alice Lenihan, MPH, RD
Sharon B. Mass, MD, FACOG
Denise Sofka, MPH, RD
Julie Wood, MD, FAAFP

CONTRIBUTORS

Every attempt has been made to recognize all these who contributed to this handbook; we regret any omissions that may have occurred.

Pamela D. Berens, MD, FACOG, FABM, University of Texas Health Sciences Center at Houston, Houston, TX

Lori Berkowitz, MD, FACOG, Massachusetts General Hospital, Boston, MA

Cheston M. Berlin, Jr, MD, FAAP, Pennsylvania State University College of Medicine, Hershey, PA

Breastfeeding Handbook for Physicians

American Academy of Pediatrics

DEDICATED TO THE HEALTH OF ALL CHILDREN™

The American College of Obstetricians and Gynecologists

Women's Health Care Physicians

ISBN 1-58110-090-6 AAP
ISBN 1-932328-17-3 ACOG
MA 0206
LOC 2002103911

American Academy of Pediatrics
141 Northwest Point Blvd
Elk Grove Village, IL 60007-1098

The American College of Obstetricians and Gynecologists
409 12th St, SW
PO Box 96920
Washington, DC 20090-6920

Illustrations by Anthony Alex LeTourneau

The recommendations in this publication do not indicate an exclusive
course of treatment or serve as a standard of care. Variations, taking
into account individual circumstances, may be appropriate.

Development of this handbook was supported in part by Project 4U93
MC00022 from the Maternal and Child Health Bureau (Title V, SSA),
Health Resources and Services Administration, US Department of
Health and Human Services.

4-18/0705

Linda S. Black, MD, FAAP, Emory University, Atlanta, GA

Keith R. Brill, MD, FACOG, FACS, Spring Valley Hospital, Las Vegas, NV

Margarett K. Davis, MD, MPH, Centers for Disease Control and Prevention, Atlanta, GA

Sharon L. Dooley, MD, MPH, FACOG, Northwestern University's Feinberg School of Medicine, Chicago, IL

Arthur I. Eidelman, MD, FAAP, Shaare Zedek Medical Center, Jerusalem, Israel

Lori Feldman-Winter, MD, MPH, FAAP, FABM, Children's Regional Hospital at Cooper-University of Medicine and Dentistry New Jersey-RWJMS, Camden, NJ

Lawrence M. Gartner, MD, FAAP, University of Chicago, Chicago, IL

Madeline H. Gartner, MD, FACS, North Memorial Hospital, Robbinsdale, MN, and University of Minnesota, Minneapolis, MN

M. Jane Heinig, PhD, University of California at Davis, Davis, CA

Nancy F. Krebs, MD, MS, FAAP, University of Colorado Health Sciences Center, Denver, CO

Susan Landers, MD, FAAP, FABM, Pediatrix Medical Group of Texas, Austin, TX

Ruth A. Lawrence, MD, FAAP, FABM, FAACT, University of Rochester School of Medicine, Rochester, NY

Sharon B. Mass, MD, FACOG, Morristown Memorial Hospital, Morristown, NJ

Joan Y. Meek, MD, MS, RD, FAAP, FABM, Florida State University, Orlando, FL

Margaret C. (Peggy) Neville, PhD, University of Colorado Health Sciences Center, Aurora, CO

Edward R. Newton, MD, FACOG, FABM, East Carolina University, Greenville, NC

Victoria Nichols-Johnson, MD, FACOG, Southern Illinois University, Springfield, IL

Barbara L. Philipp, MD, FAAP, FABM, Boston University School of Medicine, Boston, MA

Larry Pickering, MD, FAAP, Centers for Disease Control and Prevention, Atlanta, GA

Nancy G. Powers, MD, FAAP, FABM, Wesley Medical Center, Wichita, KS

Richard J. Schanler, MD, FAAP, Schneider Children's Hospital at North Shore, Manhasset, NY, and Albert Einstein College of Medicine, Bronx, NY

Wendelin Slusser, MD, MS, FAAP, UCLA Schools of Medicine and Public Health, Los Angeles, CA

Carol L. Wagner, MD, FAAP, FABM, FASCN, Medical University of South Carolina, Charleston, SC

Nancy E. Wight, MD, FAAP, FABM, Children's Hospital & Health Center and Sharp Mary Birch Hospital for Women, San Diego, CA

CONSULTANTS
Raul Artal, MD, FACOG
Susan S. Baker, MD, PhD, FAAP
Gene Burkett, MD, FACOG
Harold E. Fox, MD, FACOG
Michael F. Greene, MD, FACOG
Frank Greer, MD, FAAP
Joyce Haas, AAFP
Ann Koontz, DrPH, CNM
Michael K. Lindsay, MD, MPH, FACOG
Charles J. Lockwood, MD, FACOG
Nancy F. Petit, MD, FACOG, CDR, MC, USNR
John T. Queenan, MD, FACOG
Laura E. Riley, MD, FACOG
Deborah M. Smith, MD, FACOG
Sharon S. Sweede, MD, FAAFP
Isabelle A. Wilkins, MD, FACOG
John Williams III, MD, FACOG
Julie Wood, MD, FAAFP

Table of Contents

Contents

Contents

Contents

Preface

Breastfeeding Handbook for Physicians was written to provide health care professionals in all specialties with a concise and inexpensive teaching and reference aid on breastfeeding and human lactation. The overall goal of the handbook is to enhance physicians' knowledge of breastfeeding physiology and clinical practice so that they become comfortable encouraging and supporting breastfeeding.

Breastfeeding Handbook for Physicians can be used as a guide to teaching breastfeeding and lactation theory and practice to medical students, residents, and fellows. Similarly, postgraduate continuing medical education programs can be built around its contents. It is hoped that this handbook will encourage physicians to become teachers of breastfeeding and lactation medicine.

This handbook represents the collaborative efforts of the American Academy of Pediatrics (AAP) and the American College of Obstetricians and Gynecologists (ACOG), with additional critical review by the American Academy of Family Physicians (AAFP). As befits a book written jointly by different specialties, it addresses collaboration among physicians and between physicians and other health care professionals, especially lactation specialists. To recognize the physician as the coordinator of health care that is often provided by a large number of other professionals, the handbook stresses the concept of a medical home for both infant and mother, namely the infant's primary physician and the mother's primary physician. It also helps to provide a framework on which to build hospital and office policies.

While the book is designed primarily for physicians, use by other health professionals, including nurses, dietitians, and lactation specialists, is welcomed; its use may serve as a bridge between these health professionals and physicians in achieving coordinated and optimal care.

The publication of this handbook comes at an important time for breastfeeding awareness as part of the national agenda for health care in the United States. The US Surgeon General released *HHS Blueprint for Action on Breastfeeding* to support and promote breastfeeding in the health care system, workplace, family, and community, as well as in research. The publication provides guidance in meeting the US Department of Health and Human Services broad goals contained in the Healthy People 2010 campaign, which strive to eliminate disparities among different segments of the population, increase breastfeeding initiation rates to 75%, and increase the proportion of mothers who breastfeed their infants at 6 months to 50% and at 12 months to 25%. The goals of the national agenda also are highlighted by the efforts of the US Breastfeeding Committee, which has produced a strategic plan for protecting, promoting, and supporting breastfeeding in the United States. The use of this handbook, therefore, is expected to contribute substantially to meeting these national health care goals.

After introductory chapters on epidemiology, the importance of breastfeeding, and anatomy and physiology, the handbook is organized in a life-cycle format to allow for quick reference. *Breastfeeding Handbook for Physicians* is the product of numerous experts in the field of breastfeeding and human lactation. We hope you will find the reference useful for breastfeeding education.

The Editors

Chapter 1

The Scope of Breastfeeding

Knowledge of the biology of human milk and the physiology of its production, secretion, and delivery is helpful for all physicians regardless of their specialty. But for those who care for the mother and the child, such knowledge is particularly important and should be accompanied by an understanding of the process of breastfeeding in its normal and abnormal states.

Breastfeeding may be thought of as a natural function that every mother would be able to do without preparation or support. Unfortunately, this is not the case for many women in our modern culture. Successful breastfeeding requires education, support, and an environment that values and understands breastfeeding. This need for support may derive from the fact that our modern culture has evolved a series of messages that inhibit these automatic and natural behaviors. Because children and adults rarely observe breastfeeding, health care professionals must supply the appropriate education, support, and encouragement necessary to enable human milk to be provided to the child.

I. Definitions of Breastfeeding

Common definitions of breastfeeding have developed over time to facilitate teaching, research, and clinical evaluation. (See Table 1-1.) These definitions of breastfeeding should be combined with delineation of the *duration* of breastfeeding to fully describe the experience of the mother and infant. Other factors that help define breastfeeding are the number of breastfeeds in a 24-hour period, the duration of breastfeeding at each breast, and the length of time between breastfeeds.

TABLE 1-1. BREASTFEEDING DEFINITIONS

Exclusive: Human milk is the only food provided. Medicines, minerals, and vitamins may also be given under this definition, but no water, juice, or other preparations. Infants fed expressed human milk from their own mothers or from a milk bank by gavage tube, cup, or bottle also can be included in this definition if they have had no non-human milk or foods.

Almost Exclusive: Human milk is the predominant food provided with very rare feedings of other milk or food. The infant may have been given 1 or 2 formula bottles during the first few days of life, but none after that.

Partial or Mixed: This may vary from mostly human milk with small amounts or infrequent feedings of non-human milk or food (*high partial*) to infants receiving significant amounts of non-human milk or food as well as human milk (*medium partial*) to infants receiving predominantly non-human milk or food with some human milk (*low partial*).

Token: The infant is fed almost entirely with non-human milk and food, but either had some breastfeeds shortly after birth or continues to have occasional ⁀astfeeds. This type of breastfeeding may be seen late in the weaning process.

ɪy Breastfeeding: This definition includes all of the above.

ᴊever Breastfed: This infant has *never* received *any* human milk, either by direct breastfeeding or expressed milk with artificial means of delivery.

II. Breastfeeding Rates in the United States

Until recently the only published breastfeeding surveillance system in the United States was a yearly marketing survey, originating in 1955 by Ross Products Division of Abbott Laboratories (Columbus, OH), that collected data from responses to a mailed questionnaire. In 1999, following a Congressional mandate, the US Centers for Disease Control and Prevention (CDC) began to develop an independent surveillance system as part of the National Immunization Survey to provide more comprehensive data (www.cdc.gov/ breastfeeding/NIS_data/index.htm).

In 2003 70.9% of all US women initiated breastfeeding, which is close to the Healthy People 2010 objective of 75% initiation (Table 1-2). Although this has been the highest rate in recent years (Figure 1-1), only 41% were *exclusively* breastfeeding at 3 months (Figure 1-2). At 6 months, only 36% of infants were receiving any human milk, well below the Healthy People 2010 goal of 50%, and only 14% were exclusively breastfeeding (Table 1-3). Considerable

TABLE 1-2. HEALTHY PEOPLE 2010 GOALS

Initiation	75%
6 months	50%
1 year	25%

FIGURE 1-1. BREASTFEEDING RATES IN THE US 1967–2001

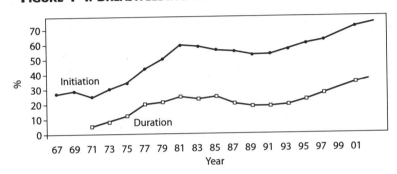

Initiation refers to any breastfeeding in the hospital and duration refers to any breastfeeding at 6 months. Adapted with permission from Wright (2001) and Ryan (2002).

FIGURE 1-2. BREASTFEEDING RATES BY AGE

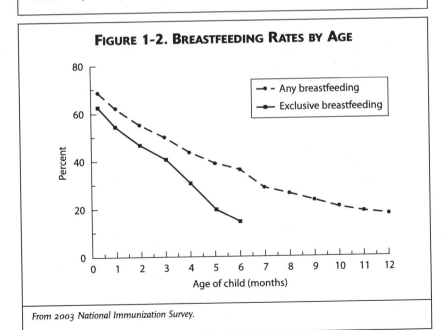

From 2003 National Immunization Survey.

3

TABLE 1-3. BREASTFEEDING RATES BY SOCIODEMOGRAPHIC FACTORS (PERCENT ± HALF 95% CONFIDENCE INTERVAL)

Sociodemographic Factors	Ever Breastfeeding	Breastfeeding at 6 Months	Breastfeeding at 12 Months	Exclusive Breastfeeding* at 3 Months	Exclusive Breastfeeding* at 6 Months
US National	70.9 ± 0.8	36.2 ± 0.8	17.2 ± 0.7	41.1 ± 0.9	14.2 ± 0.6
Gender					
Male	70.7 ± 1.2	35.6 ± 1.2	16.3 ± 0.9	40.3 ± 1.2	13.7 ± 0.8
Female	71.0 ± 1.2	36.8 ± 1.2	18.2 ± 1.0	41.9 ± 1.2	14.8 ± 0.9
Birth Order					
First born	69.9 ± 1.1	37.5 ± 1.1	18.5 ± 0.9	42.6 ± 1.1	14.6 ± 0.8
Not first born	72.5 ± 1.3	34.1 ± 1.3	15.2 ± 1.0	38.6 ± 1.3	13.6 ± 0.9
Race/ethnicity					
American Indian or Alaskan Native	68.6 ± 4.8	32.0 ± 4.5	14.9 ± 3.2	43.7 ± 5.2	13.1 ± 3.2
Asian or Pacific Islander	79.3 ± 3.3	44.1 ± 44.1	22.5 ± 3.4	47.8 ± 4.2	16.7 ± 2.8
Asian	79.3 ± 43.6	44.0 ± 44.5	22.0 ± 3.7	46.7 ± 4.7	15.9 ± 3.0
Native Hawaiian and other Pacific Islander	80.9 ± 45.6	50.2 ± 48.3	28.4 ± 7.7	58.9 ± 7.8	25.4 ± 8.0
Black or African American	54.9 ± 42.2	23.9 ± 1.8	9.8 ± 1.3	29.2 ± 2.0	9.8 ± 1.3
White	73.8 ± 40.9	38.6 ± 1.0	18.7 ± 0.8	43.2 ± 1.0	15.2 ± 0.7
Hispanic or Latino	77.8 ± 41.7	38.2 ± 1.9	20.0 ± 1.6	48.6 ± 1.9	13.4 ± 1.3
Not Hispanic or Latino	68.4 ± 40.9	35.4 ± 0.9	16.3 ± 0.7	38.4 ± 1.0	14.5 ± 0.7
Black or African American	51.1 ± 42.4	21.9 ± 1.9	8.9 ± 1.3	26.2 ± 2.1	9.7 ± 1.4
White	72.2 ± 41.0	38.5 ± 1.1	17.7 ± 0.8	41.1 ± 1.1	15.8 ± 0.8
Receiving WIC†					
Yes	64.2 ± 41.2	28.5 ± 1.1	13.5 ± 0.9	35.6 ± 1.2	11.1 ± 0.8

	Col 1	Col 2	Col 3	Col 4	Col 5
No but eligible	75.6 ± 43.4	44.8 ± 3.8	25.7 ± 3.3	49.8 ± 3.9	19.4 ± 3.0
No and ineligible	79.9 ± 41.1	46.4 ± 1.3	21.5 ± 1.1	48.0 ± 1.4	18.0 ± 1.0
Maternal Age, Year					
<=19	54.5 ± 45.6	14.9 ± 44.2	6.9 ± 2.8	25.1 ± 4.9	6.1 ± 2.4
20–<30	67.6 ± 41.3	30.6 ± 1.2	14.2 ± 0.9	37.5 ± 1.3	12.5 ± 0.9
>=30	74.9 ± 41.1	42.6 ± 1.2	20.7 ± 0.9	45.4 ± 1.2	16.4 ± 0.8
Maternal Education					
<High school	63.4 ± 42.3	28.6 ± 2.1	15.2 ± 1.7	36.8 ± 2.2	10.5 ± 1.3
High school	63.5 ± 41.5	28.3 ± 1.5	13.0 ± 1.1	34.3 ± 1.6	11.8 ± 1.1
Some college	74.4 ± 41.7	37.5 ± 1.8	17.0 ± 1.4	43.0 ± 1.9	15.1 ± 1.3
College graduate	84.0 ± 0.9	51.9 ± 1.3	24.8 ± 1.1	52.1 ± 1.3	19.9 ± 1.0
Maternal Marital Status					
Married	76.8 ± 0.9	42.2 ± 1.0	20.6 ± 0.8	46.2 ± 1.0	16.5 ± 0.7
Unmarried‡	57.8 ± 1.7	22.8 ± 1.4	9.8 ± 1.0	29.9 ± 1.6	9.2 ± 0.9
Residence					
MSA§, central city	69.8 ± 1.4	35.4 ± 1.4	17.2 ± 1.1	40.6 ± 1.4	14.0 ± 1.0
MSA, non-central city	74.6 ± 1.2	39.6 ± 1.3	18.7 ± 1.1	44.1 ± 1.4	14.9 ± 0.9
Non-MSA	63.8 ± 1.9	29.2 ± 1.7	13.6 ± 1.2	34.6 ± 1.8	13.0 ± 1.3
Poverty Income Ratio‖, %					
<100%	62.7 ± 2.0	27.9 ± 1.8	14.2 ± 1.4	36.0 ± 2.0	11.5 ± 1.2
100%–<185%	67.9 ± 2.0	33.0 ± 2.0	16.8 ± 1.6	39.1 ± 2.1	12.9 ± 1.4
185%–<350%	74.0 ± 1.6	38.8 ± 1.7	18.6 ± 1.3	41.8 ± 1.7	15.0 ± 1.2
>=350%	79.7 ± 1.4	46.2 ± 1.6	19.5 ± 1.3	47.5 ± 1.7	17.8 ± 1.2

*Exclusive breastfeeding is defined in this study as only breastmilk and water—no solids or other liquids.

†WIC = Special Supplemental Nutrition Program for Women, Infants, and Children.

‡Unmarried includes never married, widowed, separated, divorced, and deceased.

§MSA = Metropolitan statistical area defined by the Census Bureau.

‖Poverty income ratio = Ratio of self-reported family income to the federal poverty threshold value depending on the number of people in the household.

Source: 2003 National Immunization Survey, Centers for Disease Control and Prevention, Department of Health and Human Services.

disparity occurs among racial and ethnic groups. Although African American breastfeeding initiation rates in 2003 were only 54.9% and at 6 months were only 23.9%, this group has had the most rapid gains in breastfeeding rates in recent years (30% increase from 1996 to 2001). Breastfeeding rates for Latino/Hispanic mothers are very close to that of the total US population. Significant increases in breastfeeding rates also have been reported for young mothers (≤20 years of age), primiparous women, participants in the Special Supplemental Nutrition Program for Women, Infants, and Children (WIC), and mothers of low birth weight infants.

Data on breastfeeding rates at 1 year of age have only recently been collected (Table 1-4). Whereas the Healthy People 2010 goal for 1 year is 25%, the total US rate in 2003 was only 17.2%, and the African American rate was 9.8%. In all populations, married, older, and more highly educated women not working outside the home were more likely to initiate and sustain breastfeeding for longer durations.

There is still considerable need to overcome obstacles and continue breastfeeding support efforts to reach and maintain the modest goals set by the United States in its Healthy People 2010 program. This effort is of particular importance for infant and maternal health because the populations at highest risk are the ones with the lowest breastfeeding rates and stand to gain the greatest health and developmental benefits from breastfeeding. The WIC program has addressed this population and has made significant strides in increasing successful breastfeeding. Returning to employment or schooling outside the home by the mother is a major negative influence on initiation and continuation of breastfeeding. Efforts have been made to develop breastfeeding support programs in many work locations, often with great success. (See Chapter 10.)

In a nation with as diverse a population as the United States, cultural practices vary widely. Traditional knowledge and beliefs can influence the way breastfeeding is practiced and how families respond to promotional and educational efforts as well as to medical advice. Health care professionals will be most successful in supporting breastfeeding if they learn and understand the basis of these traditional practices.

TABLE 1-4. ANY AND EXCLUSIVE BREASTFEEDING RATES BY AGE (PERCENT ± HALF 95% CONFIDENCE INTERVAL)

US National Breastfeeding Rates

Ever breastfeeding	70.9 ± 0.8		
Breastfeeding at 7 days	68.9 ± 0.8	Exclusive breastfeeding* at 7 days	62.5 ± 0.9
Breastfeeding at 14 days	67.2 ± 0.8	Exclusive breastfeeding at 14 days	57.9 ± 0.9
Breastfeeding at 21 days	64.1 ± 0.9	Exclusive breastfeeding at 21 days	56.9 ± 0.9
Breastfeeding at 28 days	62.8 ± 0.9	Exclusive breastfeeding at 28 days	55.4 ± 0.9
Breastfeeding at 42 days	57.9 ± 0.9	Exclusive breastfeeding at 42 days	49.4 ± 0.9
Breastfeeding at 1 month	62.3 ± 0.9	Exclusive breastfeeding at 1 month	54.7 ± 0.9
Breastfeeding at 2 months	55.2 ± 0.9	Exclusive breastfeeding at 2 months	47.0 ± 0.9
Breastfeeding at 3 months	50.2 ± 0.9	Exclusive breastfeeding at 3 months	41.1 ± 0.9
Breastfeeding at 4 months	43.2 ± 0.9	Exclusive breastfeeding at 4 months	30.7 ± 0.8
Breastfeeding at 5 months	38.7 ± 0.9	Exclusive breastfeeding at 5 months	19.6 ± 0.7
Breastfeeding at 6 months	36.2 ± 0.8	Exclusive breastfeeding at 6 months	14.2 ± 0.6
Breastfeeding at 9 months	23.5 ± 0.7		
Breastfeeding at 12 months	17.2 ± 0.7		
Breastfeeding at 18 months	5.7 ± 0.4		

*Exclusive breastfeeding is defined in this study as only breastmilk and water—no solids or other liquids.

Source: 2003 National Immunization Survey, Centers for Disease Control and Prevention, Department of Health and Human Services.

III. Breastfeeding Education

Educating health care professionals, parents, and the general public about the importance and practice of breastfeeding is needed because in many modern countries this knowledge was part of the social fabric in the past, but has now been lost. Until recently breastfeeding management was not taught in medical and nursing schools and was certainly not included in general education curricula of secondary schools or colleges. Recognition of this deficiency has led to the development of new curricula including breastfeeding education in schools from kindergarten to medical school.

A. Specific Audiences

1. *Physicians.* Over the past decade, breastfeeding theory and practice have been introduced into the curricula of many, but not all, medical schools. Residency training programs in obstetrics, pediatrics, and family medicine are now increasingly including formal teaching and supervised practice in breastfeeding. Residency review committees are beginning to require inclusion of breastfeeding education in the programs they accredit. All 3 primary care board examinations include questions on breastfeeding and lactation. Continuing education for physicians in breastfeeding is available through many medical organizations.

2. *Parents.* Because it is no longer assumed that parents have a basic knowledge of breastfeeding, it is incumbent on all health care systems to provide prenatal and continuing education to parents about the benefits and practice of breastfeeding. The education should be culturally sensitive and conducted, whenever possible, in relation to the understandings and misunderstandings that individuals bring with them. Every health care contact, prenatal and postnatal, is an opportunity to educate parents about breastfeeding.

    One of the most important people to influence the mother's decision to breastfeed is the baby's father. Breastfeeding education programs, especially during the prenatal period, are most effective when they include the father to provide critical encouragement and emotional support. Furthermore, the knowledgeable father can often provide direct assistance in the breastfeeding process by helping with positioning, evaluating latch and milk transfer, and taking responsibility for baby and household duties, freeing the mother to give more attention to breastfeeding. While fathers may fear their exclusion from baby care when the mother is breastfeeding, physicians can encourage the father to be an active partner in the nurturing of the baby.

3. *Legislators, Business Leaders, and the Public.* Government officials, legislators, judges, and public administrators have responsibilities for health and general welfare of the population and are in a position to influence support for breastfeeding through laws and their enforcement, funding of programs, and education. Employers should provide safe and appropriate locations for mothers to pump milk, sufficient break time and frequency to maintain milk production, and a generally supportive atmosphere that sees breastfeeding as a resource to be preserved. (See Chapter 10.)

4. *Medical Offices.* Physicians have a unique opportunity to encourage and support breastfeeding through the design and operation of their medical office or clinic. (See Chapter 15.) A strong message to the families is given when images of breastfeeding mothers and infants are presented in waiting and examining rooms.

5. *Hospitals.* Hospital policies; the education of physicians, nurses, and staff in breastfeeding; and an environment supportive of breastfeeding are all essential in conveying the message that breastfeeding is important and providing help and support to every new mother. Hospitals and their staff can design their own programs for breastfeeding support or they can follow the guidance of the Baby Friendly Hospital Initiative and become accredited as a Baby Friendly Hospital. (See Chapter 6.) A broad-based hospital breastfeeding task force and a supportive administration are essential in establishing an institutional culture and policies that support breastfeeding.

6. *Midwives.* Nurse-midwives have become increasingly effective members of the perinatal health care team, practicing either within an obstetric group or hospital, or independently. Most modern midwives are knowledgeable about

lactation and breastfeeding and provide excellent support for the breastfeeding mother. Some are lactation specialists. Within an obstetric group, the midwife can often provide the specialized help that a breastfeeding mother may need.

7. ***Managed Care Organizations.*** Breastfeeding has been shown in several studies to reduce child health costs in the first year of life, and some managed care organizations have adopted extensive programs to promote and support breastfeeding for their enrollees. Physicians in managed care organizations are in a position to encourage development of strong breastfeeding programs for health and economic reasons. (See Chapter 2.)

8. ***Federal and State Governments.*** Congress has given a mandate to the US Department of Agriculture to provide breastfeeding education and support for clients in their WIC program nationwide. Breastfeeding mothers who participate in the WIC program are given additional food allocations in lieu of the formula coupons that other mothers receive. In many parts of the country, WIC has significantly increased breastfeeding initiation, duration, and overall success for more economically deprived families.

    The Surgeon General's office and the Department of Health and Human Services have had a significant influence on breastfeeding promotion for many years using national conferences and, most recently, with the publication of *HHS Blueprint for Action on Breastfeeding.* This publication contains a plan for federal efforts in breastfeeding "education, training, awareness, support and research." The Maternal and Child Health Bureau of the Health Resources and Services Administration has been a major funder of research and program development in breastfeeding for many years. The National Institutes of Health and the CDC also have supported basic research and epidemiologic studies in breastfeeding, greatly raising the level of knowledge in the field. Many states also have developed programs in support of breastfeeding, including educational publications, Web sites, conferences, and direct services.

9. ***Non-governmental Organizations.*** The US Breastfeeding Committee is an advisory organization to the government

with membership from the major breastfeeding organizations in the United States. Its national agenda for breastfeeding provides detailed guidance to needs for future research, program development, and education in breastfeeding.

The World Health Organization (WHO) and UNICEF have been among the most effective organizations worldwide in supporting breastfeeding through education, direct service, and development of special programs, such as the Baby Friendly Hospital Initiative of UNICEF.

Professional organizations providing and/or advocating breastfeeding support and education include the AAP, ACOG, AAFP, American Dietetic Association, and Academy of Breastfeeding Medicine (ABM), an international physician organization dedicated to professional breastfeeding education and translation of research into practice. The ABM recognizes physicians who distinguish themselves in lactation as Fellows (FABM). An important aspect in the scientific documentation of the effects of breastfeeding on the infant, mother, and society has been the formation of the multidisciplinary International Society for Research in Human Milk and Lactation.

Wellstart International has been providing physician education in breastfeeding and lactation worldwide and has developed a major physician education curriculum that can be adapted to various levels of training from medical school through residency, and into postgraduate education. La Leche League International, an organization of mothers, provides peer counseling and support groups, educational materials, and professional education programs. The International Lactation Consultant Association, which includes some physician members, serves lactation specialists, most of whom are certified by the International Board of Lactation Consultant Examiners (IBLCE).

IV. Ethics

As with all medical care, ethical issues must be considered in the field of breastfeeding promotion and management. These include informed choice, medical care responsibilities, custody rights in parental separation and divorce, workplace rights, breastfeeding in public places, duration of breastfeeding, and formula marketing. For many of these ethical concerns, there are no simple answers.

A. **Informed Choice.** It is incumbent on the physician and all health care professionals to inform the pregnant woman and new mother of all of the differences between breastfeeding and formula feeding in health outcomes for herself and her child. With this knowledge, the mother can then make a choice appropriate to her own circumstances. (See Chapter 2.)

B. **Medical Home.** The management of breastfeeding is often a shared responsibility with participation by the obstetric and pediatric care professionals and lactation specialists. To provide this coordination, it is important for the mother and the infant to have an identified medical home. The medical home is defined as an approach to providing health care services that are accessible, continuous, comprehensive, family-centered, coordinated, compassionate, and culturally effective. Health care professionals and families act as partners in a medical home to identify and access the medical and nonmedical services needed. Through this structure, communication among all involved is conveyed effectively.

C. **Workplace Rights.** The right of the mother who is returning to work to maintain her breastfeeding has been the subject of much recent discussion and legislative efforts. Only a few states have enacted laws that give mothers the right to pump their breasts while on the employment site. Child care policies at work also have been addressed. (See Chapter 10.)

D. **Breastfeeding in Public Places.** The right of the mother to breastfeed in a public location in which she is legally entitled to be has been ensured by legislation in most of the states and at US federal sites. These laws either exclude breastfeeding from indecent exposure restrictions or provide a specific right of the mother to breastfeed in public.

E. **Duration of Breastfeeding.** The question of whether there is an upper limit to the duration of breastfeeding has been asked. Data on the scientific foundation for an age above which it is inappropriate or harmful to the child to continue breastfeeding do not exist.

F. **Formula Marketing.** Physicians and other health care professionals should recognize marketing practices that have been shown to adversely affect the choice of breastfeeding or continuation of breastfeeding. No subject in the ethical realm of breastfeeding has received as much attention as the issues related to the marketing of human milk substitutes. The *International Code of Marketing of Breast-milk Substitutes* (www.who. int/nut/documents/code_english.pdf) and a subsequent WHO resolution provide detailed guidelines on formula marketing to ensure that it does not diminish breastfeeding initiation or continuation. Although virtually all countries in the world (including the United States) have endorsed the WHO code, many (including the United States) have not enacted legislation to give the force of law to these guidelines. Despite this absence of legal authority, the principles of the code provide a sound ethical basis for examination of marketing practices by manufacturers and distributors of infant formulas. Physicians should work toward eliminating policies and practices that discourage breastfeeding in the hospital and office. (See Chapters 6 and 15.)

G. **Custody Rights.** Some of the most difficult and intense ethical controversies occur in the course of marital separation and divorce proceedings when a breastfeeding child is involved. Separate visitation with the father is the issue that leads to confrontation over breastfeeding, particularly when the child is older than 1 year. The health and welfare of the child should be given highest priority, including the maintenance of breastfeeding. Determining whether breastfeeding is a legitimate need or is being used inappropriately to deny visitation rights is extremely difficult, with experts supporting both sides.

V. Recommended Practices

Table 1-5 provides comments on some of the obstacles to breastfeeding. Table 1-6 summarizes how the health care professional can affect breastfeeding rates in the community. Several of these points will be the subject of discussion in the cited chapters.

TABLE 1-5. SOME OF THE OBSTACLES TO INITIATION AND CONTINUATION OF BREASTFEEDING

1. Insufficient prenatal education about breastfeeding
2. Disruptive hospital policies and practices
3. Inappropriate interruption of breastfeeding
4. Early hospital discharge in some populations
5. Lack of timely routine follow-up care and postpartum home health visits
6. Maternal employment (especially in the absence of workplace facilities and support for breastfeeding)
7. Lack of family and broad societal support
8. Media portrayal of bottle-feeding as normative
9. Commercial promotion of infant formula
10. Misinformation and lack of health care professional concern and involvement

---

TABLE 1-6. RECOMMENDED BREASTFEEDING PRACTICES

1. Health care professionals should recommend human milk for all infants in whom breastfeeding is not specifically contraindicated and provide parents with complete, current information on the benefits and techniques of breastfeeding to ensure that their feeding decision is a fully informed one (Chapter 2).
2. Encourage peripartum policies and practices that optimize breastfeeding implementation and maintenance (Chapter 6).
3. Healthy infants should be placed and remain in direct skin-to-skin contact with their mothers immediately after delivery until the first feeding is accomplished (Chapter 6).
4. Supplements (water, glucose water, formula, and other fluids) should not be given to breastfeeding newborns and infants unless ordered by a physician when a medical indication exists (Chapter 6).
5. Pacifier use is best avoided during initiation of breastfeeding and used only after breastfeeding is well established (Chapters 6 and 7).
6. During the early weeks of breastfeeding, mothers should be encouraged to have 8 to 12 feedings at the breast every 24 hours, offering a breast whenever the infant shows early signs of hunger, such as increased alertness, physical activity, mouthing, or rooting (Chapters 6 and 7).

TABLE 1-6. RECOMMENDED BREASTFEEDING PRACTICES (CONTINUED)

7. Formal evaluation of breastfeeding, including observation of position, latch, and milk transfer, should be undertaken by trained caregivers at least twice daily and fully documented in the record during each day in the hospital (Chapter 7).

8. All breastfeeding newborns should be seen by a pediatrician or other knowledgeable and experienced health care professional at 3 to 5 days of age as described in the AAP "Recommendations for Preventative Pediatric Health Care" (Chapters 7 and 8).

9. Breastfeeding infants should have a second ambulatory visit at 2 to 3 weeks of age to monitor weight gain and provide additional support and encouragement to the mother during this critical period (Chapter 8).

10. Exclusive breastfeeding is sufficient to support optimal growth and development for approximately the first 6 months of life and provides continuing protection against diarrhea and respiratory tract infection. The ACOG indicates that a longer breastfeeding experience is, of course, beneficial. The professional objectives, therefore, are to encourage and enable as many women as possible to breastfeed and to help them continue as long as possible. The AAP states that breastfeeding should be continued for at least the first year and beyond for as long as mutually desired by mother and child (Chapter 8). The AAP Committee on Nutrition supports introduction of complementary foods between 4 and 6 months of age when safe and nutritious complementary foods are available.

11. All infants should receive vitamin K intramuscularly *after* the first feed is completed and within the first 6 hours of life (Chapter 8).

12. All breastfed infants should receive 200 IU of oral vitamin D drops daily beginning during the first 2 months of life and continuing until daily consumption of vitamin D-fortified formula or milk is 500 mL (Chapter 8).

13. Supplementary fluoride should not be provided during the first 6 months of life (Chapter 8).

14. Breastfeeding is facilitated when the mother and infant sleep in close proximity to each other (Chapter 8).

15. Should hospitalization of the breastfeeding mother or infant be necessary, every effort should be made to maintain breastfeeding, preferably directly, or by pumping the breasts and feeding expressed human milk, if necessary (Chapters 8 and 11).

16. Hospitals and physicians should recommend mother's own milk for premature and other high-risk infants either by direct breastfeeding and/or using expressed own mother's milk (Chapter 14).

Selected References

American Academy of Family Physicians, Commission on Public Health, Family Physicians Supporting Breastfeeding. AAFP Policy on Breastfeeding. AAFP Position Statement on Breastfeeding. Fall 2001. Available at: http://www. aafp.org/x6633.xml

American Academy of Pediatrics Medical Home Initiatives for Children With Special Needs Project Advisory Committee. The medical home. *Pediatrics.* 2002;110:184–186

American Academy of Pediatrics Section on Breastfeeding. Breastfeeding and the use of human milk. *Pediatrics.* 2005;115:496–506

American Academy of Pediatrics Work Group on Breastfeeding. Breastfeeding and the use of human milk. *Pediatrics.* 1997;100:1035–1039

American College of Obstetricians and Gynecologists. Breastfeeding: maternal and infant aspects. *ACOG Educ Bull.* 2000;258:1–16

American Dietetic Association. Position of the American Dietetic Association: breaking the barriers to breastfeeding. *J Am Diet Assoc.* 2001;101:1213–1220

Centers for Disease Control and Prevention. Breastfeeding practices: results from the 2003 National Immunization Survey. Available at: www.cdc.gov/ breastfeeding/NIS_data/index.htm

Coffin CJ, Labbok MH, Belsey M. Breastfeeding definitions. *Contraception.* 1997; 55:323–325

Freed GL, Clark SJ, Sorenson J, Lohr JA, Cefalo R, Curtis P. National assessment of physicians' breast-feeding knowledge, attitudes, training, and experience. *JAMA.* 1995;273:472–476

Howard CR, Howard FM, Weitzman ML. Infant formula distribution and advertising in pregnancy: a hospital survey. *Birth.* 1994;21:14–19

Howard FM, Howard CR, Weitzman ML. The physician as advertiser: the unintentional discouragement of breast-feeding. *Obstet Gynecol.* 1993;81:1048–1051

Li R, Zhao Z, Mokdad A, Barker L, Grummer-Strawn L. Prevalence of breastfeeding in the United States: the 2001 National Immunization Survey. *Pediatrics.* 2003;111(suppl):1198–1201

New York State Department of Health. Breastfeeding: first step to good health. Breastfeeding education activity package for grades K–12. Available at: http://www.health.state.ny.us/nysdoh/b_feed/index.htm

Power ML, Locke E, Chapin J, Klein L, Schulkin J. The effort to increase breastfeeding: do obstetricians, in the forefront, need help? *J Reprod Med.* 2003;48: 72–78

Ryan AS, Wenjun Z, Acosta A. Breastfeeding continues to increase into the new millennium. *Pediatrics.* 2002;110:1103–1109

Spisak S, Gross SS. *Second Followup Report: The Surgeon General's Workshop on Breastfeeding and Human Lactation.* Washington, DC: National Center for Education in Maternal and Child Health; 1991

US Breastfeeding Committee. *Breastfeeding in the United States: A National Agenda.* Rockville, MD: US Department of Health and Human Services, Health Resources and Services Administration, Maternal and Child Health Bureau; 2001

US Department of Health and Human Services. *HHS Blueprint for Action on Breastfeeding.* Washington, DC: US Department of Health and Human Services, Office on Women's Health; 2000

US Department of Health and Human Services. *Healthy People 2010: Conference Edition.* Vols 1 & 2. Washington, DC: US Department of Health and Human Services, Public Health Service, Office of the Assistant Secretary for Health; 2000:2, 47–48. Available at http://www.healthypeople.gov/document/html/volume2/16MICH.htm#_toc494699668

Wolf JH. Low breastfeeding rates and public health in the United States. *Am J Public Health.* 2003;93:2000–2010

World Health Assembly. *International Code of Marketing of Breast-milk Substitutes.* Geneva, Switzerland: World Health Organization; 1981

World Health Organization. *Protecting, Promoting and Supporting Breast-Feeding: The Special Role of Maternity Services.* Geneva, Switzerland: World Health Organization; 1989:13–18

Wright AL, Schanler RJ. The resurgence of breastfeeding at the end of the second millennium. *J Nutr.* 2001;131:421S–425S

Chapter 2

15·

The Importance of Breastfeeding for Infants, Mothers, and Society

A woman's decision to breastfeed is one that has far-reaching benefits that include the infant's and her own health as well as socioeconomic benefits to society. This chapter outlines the unique nutritional and non-nutritional components in human milk, preventive benefits for acute and chronic illness in infant and mother, and economic effects of breastfeeding.

I. Milk Composition

A. **Nutritional Components.** Human milk has a dynamic nutrient composition that may vary through lactation, over the course of a day, within a feeding, and from woman to woman. The variable composition of human milk provides nutrients specifically adapted to the changing needs of the infant, and also provides an array of flavors and tastes to stimulate sensory integration. It is important to understand that human milk has unique specificity for our species. Many components in human milk serve dual roles; a single component may enhance nutrition and host defense, or nutrition and neurodevelopment. The milk produced in the first few days is colostrum, a relatively denser milk characterized by high concentrations of protein and antibodies. The transition to mature milk begins around days 3 to 5, with mature milk appearing by about day 10 postpartum. Table 2-1 lists representative values for the constituents of mature human milk.

1. *Nitrogen* is provided by protein (80%) and by non-protein nitrogen (NPN)–containing compounds (20%). In the first few weeks postpartum, the total nitrogen content of milk

TABLE 2-1. REPRESENTATIVE VALUES FOR CONSTITUENTS OF HUMAN MILK

Constituent (per liter)	Mature Milk (after 2 weeks' lactation)
Energy (kcal)	650–700
Macronutrients	
Lactose (g)	67–70
Oligosaccharides (g)	12–14
Total nitrogen (g)	1.9
Non-protein nitrogen (% total nitrogen)	23
Protein nitrogen (% total nitrogen)	77
Total protein (g)	9
Total lipids (g)	35
Triglyceride (% total lipids)	97–98
Cholesterol (% total lipids)	0.4–0.5
Phospholipids (% total lipids)	0.6–0.8
Water-Soluble Vitamins	
Ascorbic acid (mg)	100
Thiamin (μg)	200
Riboflavin (μg)	400–600
Niacin (mg)	1.8–6.0
Vitamin B_6 (mg)	0.09–0.31
Folate (μg)	80–140
Vitamin B_{12} (μg)	0.5–1.0
Pantothenic acid (mg)	2–2.5
Biotin (μg)	5–9

TABLE 2-1. REPRESENTATIVE VALUES FOR CONSTITUENTS OF HUMAN MILK (CONTINUED)

Constituent (per liter)	Mature Milk (after 2 weeks' lactation)
Fat-Soluble Vitamins	
Retinol (mg)	0.3–0.6
Carotenoids (mg)	0.2–0.6
Vitamin K (μg)	2–3
Vitamin D (μg)	0.33
Vitamin E (mg)	3–8
Minerals	
Calcium (mg)	200–250
Magnesium (mg)	30–35
Phosphorus (mg)	120–140
Sodium (mg)	120–250
Potassium (mg)	400–550
Chloride (mg)	400–450
Trace Elements	
Iron (mg)	0.3–0.9
Zinc (mg)	1–3
Copper (mg)	0.2–0.4
Manganese (μg)	3
Selenium (μg)	7–33
Iodine (μg)	150
Fluoride (μg)	4–15

Adapted from Pediatric Clinics of North America, *Volume 48, Picciano MF, Representative values for constituents of human milk, page 263, copyright 2001, with permission from Elsevier.*

from mothers who have premature infants (preterm milk) is greater than the milk of women who have term infants (term milk). The content of protein nitrogen declines until 2 to 4 weeks postpartum and then remains relatively constant until weaning. The content of NPN, such as free amino acids and urea, remains relatively constant throughout lactation and accounts for a larger fraction of total nitrogen (20%) than in bovine milk (5%).

a. *Whey and Casein.* The protein quality (proportion of whey [70%] and casein [30%]) of human milk differs from that in bovine milk (18% whey, 82% casein). The caseins are proteins with low solubility in acid media. Whey proteins are soluble and remain in solution after acidification. Generally, the whey fraction is more easily digested and associated with more rapid gastric emptying.

The plasma amino acid pattern in breastfed infants serves as the model on which enteral and parenteral amino acid solutions are based. The whey protein fraction provides lower concentrations of phenylalanine, tyrosine, and methionine.

Different proteins comprise the whey fraction of human milk when compared with those of bovine milk. The major human whey protein is α-lactalbumin. Lactoferrin, lysozyme, and secretory immunoglobulin A (sIgA) are specific human whey proteins involved in host defense. Because these host defense proteins resist proteolytic digestion, they serve as a first line of defense by lining the gastrointestinal tract. The 3 proteins are present only in human milk. The major whey protein in bovine milk is β-lactoglobulin.

2. *Carbohydrates.* The major carbohydrate in human milk is the disaccharide lactose, which increases in content from colostrum to mature milk. The lactose content of mature milk remains relatively constant. A small proportion of the lactose is not absorbed. This unabsorbed lactose promotes a softer stool consistency, reduced pathogenic bacterial fecal flora, and improved absorption of minerals. Oligo-

saccharides are carbohydrate polymers that comprise approximately 5% to 10% of total carbohydrates in human milk. In addition to their role in nutrition, oligosaccharides exert a protective role in the infant.

3. **Lipids**

   a. *Components of the Lipid System.* The lipid system in human milk is composed of an organized milk fat globule; a bile salt-stimulated lipase; and an abundance of essential fatty acids (linoleic [C18:2 ω6] and linolenic [C18:3 ω3] acids). Most fatty acids exist as triglycerides and together the human milk lipids represent approximately 50% of the calories in the milk.

   b. *Fat Absorption.* The resulting products of lipase action on the triglyceride molecule in the proximal small intestine are free fatty acids and 2-monoglycerides. Palmitic acid is the predominant fatty acid esterified in the 2-position of the triglyceride molecule. As such, after hydrolysis it is prevented from interacting with minerals to form soaps. Fat and mineral absorption from human milk are superior to bovine milk in part because of this interaction. Furthermore, because the lipase is heat labile, the superior fat absorption from human milk is reported only when unprocessed human milk is fed.

   c. *Fatty Acids.* The fat blend in infant formula contains a greater quantity of medium- and intermediate-chain fatty acids in an attempt to simulate the overall fat absorption in human milk. The pattern of fatty acids in human milk also is unique in its composition of long-chain polyunsaturated fatty acids (LCPUFAs). Arachidonic acid (C20:4 ω6) and docosahexaenoic acid (DHA) (C22:6 ω3), derivatives of the essential fatty acids linoleic and linolenic acids, respectively, are found in human but not bovine milk. Arachidonic acid and DHA are constituents of retinal and brain phospholipid membranes and have been associated with improved visual function and neurodevelopmental outcome.

d. *Variability of Fat Content.* Of all the components of human milk, the total fat content is the most variable. The fat content of milk rises slightly throughout lactation, changes over the course of 1 day, increases during a feed (foremilk to hindmilk), and varies from mother to mother. During a feeding, the lipid content of milk rises 2- to 3-fold from beginning to end (foremilk to hindmilk). (See Chapter 14.) On standing in a container, the fat in human milk may separate from the other components because it is not homogenized. The non-homogeneity in human milk has implications for the collection and storage of milk. (See Chapter 11.)

4. *Minerals and Trace Elements.* Although relatively constant through lactation, the human milk content of calcium and phosphorus is significantly lower than in bovine milk and infant formula. The macrominerals in human milk are more bioavailable (absorbable) than those in infant formula because they are bound to digestible proteins and are present in complexes and in ionized states, which are more readily absorbed. Despite lower mineral intake, the bone mineral content of breastfed infants is considered the norm on which bone mineralization in formula-fed infants is based.

   The concentrations of iron, zinc, and copper decline through lactation. The concentration of copper, despite its decline, seems adequate to meet the infant's nutritional needs. The concentration of iron and zinc, however, may not meet the infant's needs beyond 6 months of age. At that time, intake of these nutrients from complementary foods is indicated to prevent deficiencies.

5. *Vitamins*

   a. *Vitamin K* deficiency with resulting hypoprothrombinemia and hemorrhage can occur in the young infant without supplementation. The content of vitamin K in human milk is low. Therefore, to ensure adequate vitamin K, all infants receive a single intramuscular dose (0.5–1.0 mg) of vitamin K at birth. (See Chapter 8.)

b. *The content of vitamin D in human milk is low,* so all breastfed infants should receive daily oral doses (200 IU) of vitamin D starting before 2 months of age. (See Chapter 8.)

B. **Non-nutritional Components in Human Milk**

1. *Bioactive Proteins* (Table 2-2). Specific factors such as lactoferrin, lysozyme, and sIgA reside in the whey fraction of human milk. Lactoferrin exhibits antimicrobial activity when not conjugated to iron (apolactoferrin). By binding

---

TABLE 2-2. SELECTED BIOACTIVE FACTORS IN HUMAN MILK

Secretory IgA	Specific antigen-targeted anti-infective action
Lactoferrin	Immunomodulation, iron chelation, anti-adhesive, trophic for intestinal growth
Lysozyme	Bacterial lysis, immunomodulation
κ-casein	Anti-adhesive, bacterial flora
Oligosaccharides	Blocks bacterial attachment
Cytokines	Anti-inflammatory, epithelial barrier function
Growth factors	
Epidermal growth factor	Luminal surveillance, repair of intestine
Transforming growth factor	Promotes epithelial cell growth Suppresses lymphocyte function
Nerve growth factor	Growth
Enzymes	
PAF-acetylhydrolase	Blocks action of platelet-activating factor
Glutathione peroxidase	Prevents lipid oxidation
Nucleotides	Enhance antibody responses, bacterial flora
Vitamin A, E, C	Antioxidants
Amino acids	
Glutamine	Intestinal cell fuel, immune responses
Lipids	Anti-infective properties

Adapted from Pediatric Clinics of North America, *Volume 48, Hamosh M, Bioactive factors in human milk, pages 69–89, copyright 2001, with permission from Elsevier.*

excess iron, it prevents bacterial iron uptake and bacterial growth. Lactoferrin also functions with other host defense proteins to kill bacteria and viruses. A growth-promoting effect on intestinal epithelium also has been attributed to lactoferrin. Lysozyme is active against bacteria by cleaving cell walls.

SIgA is the most common immunoglobulin in human milk. SIgA is synthesized by maternal intestinal lymphoid tissue in response to challenge by specific antigens and rapidly transfers into milk. It acts to neutralize foreign antigens. The concentration of sIgA is greatest in colostrum and declines in the first 4 weeks postpartum. The lowest content is observed at 6 months, and thereafter the values rise slightly to levels that remain relatively constant through 2 years of lactation. IgM, IgG, IgD, and IgE also are present in human milk.

Cytokines are proteins that are produced by immune cells and affect the function and development of the immune system. Pro-inflammatory cytokines are IL-6 and IL-8. Anti-inflammatory cytokines include IL-10.

Free amino acids may exert dual roles in infants. Taurine is trophic for intestinal growth and glutamine is a fuel for the enterocyte. Glutamine also affects the gut immune system.

2. *Bioactive Lipids and Carbohydrates* (Table 2-2). The products of lipid hydrolysis, free fatty acids and monoglycerides, exhibit antimicrobial activity against a variety of pathogens by preventing their attachment and subsequent infection. Oligosaccharides and glycoproteins mimic bacterial epithelial receptors in the respiratory and gastrointestinal tracts and, in doing so, prevent attachment of pathogenic agents to the epithelial lining of mucosal surfaces. The predominant bacteria found in the gastrointestinal tract of breastfed infants is *Lactobacillus bifidus*. A nitrogen-containing carbohydrate factor in human milk (bifidus factor), not found in other mammalian milks, supports the growth of the nonpathogenic *Lactobacillus,* which results in an inhibition of the growth of pathogenic bacteria.

3. *Cellular Elements.* Human milk contains living cells, including macrophages, lymphocytes, neutrophils, and epithelial cells. Colostrum contains the most cells, predominantly neutrophils. As milk matures, the number of cells decreases and the type of cells changes to mononuclear cells such as macrophages (90%) and lymphocytes (10%). The neutrophils in colostrum promote bacterial killing, phagocytosis, and chemotaxis. Some investigators view the neutrophil as a protector of the mammary gland in defense of inflammation with little role in the infant. The macrophage in human milk functions in phagocytosis, secretion of lysozyme, bacterial killing, and interactions with lymphocytes to aid in host defense.

4. *Nucleotides* are immediate precursors for RNA and DNA synthesis. Dietary nucleotides have been reported to affect immune function, iron absorption, intestinal flora, lipoprotein metabolism, and cellular growth of intestinal and hepatic tissues.

5. *Hormones and Growth Factors.* Many hormones (eg, cortisol, somatomedin-C, insulin-like growth factors, insulin, thyroid hormone), growth factors (eg, epidermal growth factor [EGF], nerve growth factor), and gastrointestinal mediators (eg, neurotensin, motilin) that may affect gastrointestinal function and/or body composition are present in human milk. The EGF, for example, is a polypeptide that stimulates DNA synthesis, protein synthesis, and cellular proliferation in intestinal cells. The EGF resists proteolytic digestion, and one of its functions is intestinal lumen surveillance, repairing any disruptions in intestinal integrity. Nerve growth factor may play a role in the innervation of the intestinal tract. The hormonal components in milk may affect intestinal growth and mucosal function.

6. *Enteromammary and bronchomammary immune systems* of the mother produce sIgA antibody when exposed to foreign antigens either via her gastrointestinal or respiratory tracts. The plasma cells traverse the lymphatic system and are secreted at mucosal surfaces, including the mammary gland. Ingestion of human milk, therefore, provides the

infant with passive sIgA antibodies against a variety of antigens. This response is quite rapid; within 3 to 4 days after maternal exposure to a foreign antigen, antibodies appear in the milk. The intimate contact of the breastfeeding mother and infant allows for such a system to operate. Skin-to-skin protocols for hospitalized premature infants facilitate this biological intimacy.

II. Benefits of Breastfeeding for the Infant

Breastfeeding provides a number of physical and biochemical barriers against infectious agents to enhance the infant's host defenses (Table 2-3).

A. **Acute Illness.** Not only is the illness rate lower in breastfed infants, but the duration and severity of illness seem to be shortened as well. Breastfed infants experience the same infections but generally are asymptomatic or have milder symptoms than formula-fed infants. These effects are observed in developing and industrialized countries. In addition, breastfeeding limits infants' exposure to environmental pathogens (microorganisms, chemicals) that may be introduced through contaminated foods, fluids, or feeding devices. Breastfed infants also have significantly higher responses to BCG (bacille Calmette–Guerin), *Haemophilus influenzae* type b, polio, tetanus, and diphtheria toxoid immunizations.

1. *Gastrointestinal infection* is prevented and the severity is attenuated in breastfed infants, with specific effects against enteric pathogens such as rotavirus, *Giardia, Shigella, Campylobacter,* and enterotoxigenic *Escherichia coli.* Breastfeeding may not prevent colonization of *Vibro cholerae,* but it will protect against disease.

2. *Respiratory illnesses,* including wheezing and lower respiratory tract disease, are reduced in frequency and/or duration in breastfed infants. Breastfeeding prevents a major portion of disease from *H influenzae* type b and *Streptococcus pneumoniae.*

3. *Otitis Media.* Large prospective studies of otitis media show a protective effect of breastfeeding. Infants exclusively breastfed for at least 4 months may experience as few as

TABLE 2-3. HUMAN MILK MAY PROTECT AGAINST MANY DISEASES IN CHILDHOOD

Acute disorders

    Diarrhea

    Otitis media

    Recurrent otitis media

    Respiratory infections

    Urinary tract infection

    Necrotizing enterocolitis

    Septicemia

    Bacterial meningitis

    Infant botulism

Hospitalizations

Postneonatal infant mortality

Sudden infant death syndrome

Chronic disorders

    Insulin-dependent diabetes mellitus (type 1)

    Non–insulin-dependent diabetes mellitus (type 2)

    Celiac disease

    Crohn disease

    Childhood cancer

        Lymphoma

        Leukemia

        Hodgkin disease

Allergy

Asthma

Obesity and overweight

Hypercholesterolemia

half the number of episodes of otitis media as formula-fed infants and also half as many episodes of recurrent otitis media. These associations remained significant after controlling for a number of confounders, including socioeconomic status, sibling factors, and maternal smoking. In many of these studies not only is the incidence of disease diminished with breastfeeding, but also the duration of individual episodes is reduced.

4. *Necrotizing Enterocolitis.* Human milk protects the premature infant from infection and necrotizing enterocolitis (NEC). Several of the factors in human milk, such as sIgA, acetylhydrolase, EGF, and cytokines, have been identified as potential factors associated with the prevention of NEC.

5. *Urinary tract infections* are more frequent among formula-fed infants than among breastfed infants. Reduced adhesion by pathogens to uroepithelial cells, as mediated by oligosaccharides, sIgA, or lactoferrin, has been hypothesized as a protective mechanism.

6. *Infant Botulism.* In a study of infant botulism and its role in sudden infant death, onset of the disease occurred at an earlier age in formula-fed infants compared with breastfed infants. Formula-fed infants were more likely to experience severe illness, while those who were hospitalized and survived the disease were more likely to be breastfed. Possible reasons why breastfed infants with botulism have fared better than formula-fed infants include differences in intestinal microflora between breastfed and formula-fed infants and earlier detection of illness by breastfeeding mothers because of perceived changes in infant suck. The intestinal tract pH of breastfed infants is lower than in formula-fed infants. Proliferation of *Clostridium botulinum* declines as pH declines.

7. *Sepsis and Meningitis.* Prior to the availability of vaccine, the risk of developing sepsis and meningitis due to *H influenzae* was reduced among breastfed infants (particularly among those breastfed for at least 6–9 months) compared with formula-fed infants. One of these studies indicated that protection lasted beyond the period of

breastfeeding. A lower incidence of late-onset sepsis and a reduction in the number of positive blood cultures also has been associated with feeding human milk to premature infants.

B. **Chronic Diseases of Childhood.** Some studies suggest that chronic pediatric disorders such as Crohn disease, leukemia, lymphoma, diabetes mellitus, obesity, hypercholesterolemia, sudden infant death syndrome, asthma, and certain allergic conditions occur less frequently among children who were breastfed as infants.

1. *Diabetes.* Breastfeeding offers several potential mechanisms for protection against type 1 diabetes, including protection against infections, effects on maturation of the gut-associated lymphoid tissue, and modulation of immune response to insulin. Alternatively, short duration (<3 months) of exclusive breastfeeding and early exposure (<4 months) to bovine milk and/or complementary foods also have been implicated in increased risk of diabetes. Elevated concentrations of specific IgG antibodies to bovine serum albumin that cross-react with β-cell–specific surface protein have been identified in children with insulin-dependent diabetes mellitus. Currently available data are inconclusive regarding the precise relationship between breastfeeding and development of β-cell autoantibodies, and this remains an area of active research.

2. *Obesity.* Data are emerging to suggest that adolescent obesity is inversely related to the duration of breastfeeding in infancy. Postulated mechanisms for this association relate to how food intake is regulated and to metabolic effects of human milk. Hypercholesterolemia in adolescence also is less if there is a history of breastfeeding.

3. *Allergy.* There are conflicting data regarding the protection against allergy afforded by breastfeeding, possibly because in some studies maternal diet did not exclude the potentially offending antigens, particularly bovine milk proteins. Breastfeeding, however, seems to be protective against some food allergies. Atopic dermatitis may be lessened in infants whose mothers follow a restricted diet. A lower

incidence of atopic conditions is reported in breastfed infants with a family history of atopy. A lower incidence of asthma has been reported in breastfed children.

C. **Neurobehavioral Benefits.** Maternal-infant bonding is enhanced during breastfeeding. Breastfeeding has been associated with slightly enhanced performance on tests of cognitive development. Improved long-term cognitive development in premature infants also has been correlated with being fed human milk, including pasteurized, banked donor human milk during hospitalization. A meta-analysis of studies where a multitude of confounding factors (including maternal education and intelligence) were considered concluded that breastfeeding conferred a small but significant benefit to cognitive function well beyond the period of actual breastfeeding. The positive effects of breastfeeding on subsequent school performance have been reported into adolescence.

Visual acuity, particularly in premature infants, seems to be enhanced by breastfeeding compared with formula feeding. The LCPUFAs have been implicated as factors associated with better visual acuity in breastfed infants. The visual acuity of the breastfed infant is the model for studies of LCPUFA supplementation. Breastfeeding also provides analgesia to infants during painful procedures.

III. Benefits of Breastfeeding for the Mother

There is a tendency to assume that only infants and children benefit from breastfeeding. There are, however, positive effects of breastfeeding for the mother.

A. **Immediate Health Benefits**

1. *Prevention of Hemorrhage.* Women who breastfeed have uterine contractions similar to those stimulated by the administration of oxytocin. Breastfeeding in the first hour after delivery increases uterine contractility. Increased uterine activity from oxytocin release during milk let-down reduces maternal blood loss, supporting the World Health Organization recommendation to decrease postpartum hemorrhage by nipple stimulation and/or breastfeeding in areas where oxytocics are not readily available. Breast-

feeding also causes the uterus to shrink to pre-pregnancy size more rapidly.

2. ***Weight loss*** postpartum may be facilitated in breastfeeding women. Several studies indicate that the greatest effect on weight loss occurs when the duration of breastfeeding exceeds 6 months.

3. ***Bonding and Stress Reduction.*** Psychological advantages to breastfeeding are obvious because it creates a quiet time for the nursing mother and fosters bonding. Human data show decreased levels of steroid hormones in lactating women. The blunted response of stress hormones is thought to be an adaptive mechanism for negotiating the stressful time of the puerperium. In addition to decreasing the stress response, oxytocin also may play a role in blunting the perception of pain via the dopaminergic pathway.

B. Long-term Health Benefits

1. ***Amenorrhea/Birth Spacing.*** Exclusive breastfeeding delays the resumption of normal ovarian cycles and the return of fertility in most mothers. As such, the contraceptive effects of breastfeeding contribute globally to increased child spacing. (See Chapter 13.) Amenorrhea is most likely to occur in women exclusively breastfeeding, particularly in the first 6 months postpartum. This allows for repletion of maternal iron stores and correction of anemia. World epidemiologic data indicate that prolonged breastfeeding into the second year, but not exclusively beyond 6 months, prolongs the interpregnancy interval to 1 year, resulting in the birth of the next infant 20 to 24 months after the previous infant. This longer interval may be a factor in reducing infant mortality.

2. ***Cancer Prevention.*** Breastfeeding has been shown to decrease the risk of breast cancer. The relative risk of premenopausal breast cancer was significantly reduced in women who, when younger than 20 years, breastfed their infants for at least 6 months. A reduced risk of breast cancer also was observed in women who, when older than 20 years, breastfed from 3 to 6 months compared with

women who did not breastfeed. The anovulation associated with lactation also may protect against ovarian cancer, which has been shown to increase with greater frequency of ovulation.

3. ***Effect on Bone Density.*** Losses in bone density (approximately 5%) are seen during lactation, with remineralization occurring during weaning. Increased calcium supplementation beyond the normal intake does not prevent bone mineral loss. Calcium needs during this time may be compensated for by decreased urinary excretion. Epidemiologic studies suggest that breastfeeding does not increase the risk of postmenopausal osteoporosis. In fact, one study showed that the incidence of hip fracture was decreased with longer duration of lactation. It has been suggested that the repeated cycles of demineralization-remineralization may strengthen bone.

IV. Economic Impact of Breastfeeding

The economic advantages of breastfeeding can be calculated at the personal and national levels. The obvious personal advantage is in the savings accrued by not purchasing infant formula, a figure conservatively estimated to range from $750 to $1,200 per year.

From the perspective of the national economy, the expected savings for infants in the US Special Supplemental Nutrition Program for Women, Infants, and Children (WIC) who were breastfed exclusively for 6 months would be estimated to be more than $950 million annually in 1997 compared with not breastfeeding for 6 months. These savings would come from a combined reduction in household expenditure for formula, as well as reductions in health care expenditures.

Studies conducted by managed care organizations indicate that breastfeeding for 3 months significantly reduces the costs of medical care compared with no breastfeeding. In addition, reduction in incidence of one or more cases of chronic diseases in children or mothers would provide formidable health care savings and allow continued productivity.

In summary, breastfeeding results in reduced annual health care costs, reduced public health and WIC costs, reduced parental employee absenteeism and associated loss of family income, more time for attention to siblings and other family matters due to reduced infant illness, reduced environmental burden for disposal of formula cans and bottles, and reduced energy demands for production and transport of artificial feeding products. It is estimated these savings potentially are $3.6 billion in the United States.

Selected References

Ball TM, Wright AL. Health care cost of formula-feeding in the first year of life. *Pediatrics.* 1999;103:870–876

Carver JD, Walker WA. The role of nucleotides in human nutrition. *Nutr Biochem.* 1995;6:58–72

Glass RI, Stoll BJ. The protective effect of human milk against diarrhea. A review of studies from Bangladesh. *Acta Paediatr Scand Suppl.* 1989;351:131–136

Goldman AS, Frawley S. Bioactive components of milk. *J Mammary Gland Biol Neoplasia.* 1996;1:241–242

Greer FR. Do breastfed infants need supplemental vitamins? *Pediatr Clin North Am.* 2001;48:415–423

Hamosh M. Bioactive factors in human milk. *Pediatr Clin North Am.* 2001;48:69–86

Hanson LA, Adlerberth I, Carlsson B, et al. Host defense of the neonate and the intestinal flora. *Acta Paediatr Scand Suppl.* 1989;351:122–125

Heinig MJ. Host defense benefits of breastfeeding for the infant. Effect of breastfeeding duration and exclusivity. *Pediatr Clin North Am.* 2001;48:105–123

Ivarsson A, Hernell O, Stenlund H, Persson LA. Breast-feeding protects against celiac disease. *Am J Clin Nutr.* 2002;75:914–921

Jensen RG, Jensen GL. Specialty lipids for infant nutrition. I. Milks and formulas. *J Pediatr Gastroenterol Nutr.* 1992;15:232–245

Kreiter SR, Schwartz RP, Kirkman HN Jr, Charlton PA, Calikoglu AS, Davenport ML. Nutritional rickets in African American breast-fed infants. *J Pediatr.* 2000;137:153–157

Labbok MH. Effects of breastfeeding on the mother. *Pediatr Clin North Am.* 2001;48:143–158

Lawrence R. Host resistance factors and immunologic significance of human milk. In: Lawrence RL, Lawrence R, eds. *Breastfeeding: A Guide for the Medical Profession.* 5th ed. St Louis, MO: Mosby; 1999:159–195

Montgomery DL, Splett PL. Economic benefit of breast-feeding infants enrolled in WIC. *J Am Diet Assoc.* 1997;97:379–385

Neville MC, Keller RP, Seacat J, Casey CE, Allen JC, Archer P. Studies on human lactation. I. Within-feed and between-breast variation in selected components of human milk. *Am J Clin Nutr.* 1984;40:635–646

Picciano MF. Representative values for constituents of human milk. *Pediatr Clin North Am.* 2001;48:263–264

Rogan WJ, Gladen BC. Breast-feeding and cognitive development. *Early Hum Dev.* 1993;31:181–193

Schanler RJ. The use of human milk for premature infants. *Pediatr Clin North Am.* 2001;48:207–219

United Kingdom Cancer Study Investigators. Breastfeeding and childhood cancer. *Br J Cancer.* 2001;85:1685–1694

Victora CG, Smith PG, Vaughan JP, et al. Evidence for protection by breast-feeding against infant deaths from infectious diseases in Brazil. *Lancet.* 1987;2:319–322

Weimer J. *The Economic Benefits of Breast Feeding: A Review and Analysis.* Food Assistance and Nutrition Research Report No. 13. Washington, DC: Food and Rural Economics Division, Economic Research Service, US Department of Agriculture; 2001

Chapter 3

Who Can and Who Cannot Breastfeed?

It is estimated that most women are able to establish and sustain breastfeeding for an extended period if they are motivated and if they have support from their families, employer, community, and the medical system. Despite motivation and support, however, women with certain medical and psychosocial conditions may not meet their breastfeeding goals. In rare situations, an infant should not be breastfed.

I. Physical Conditions of the Breast That May Inhibit Breastfeeding

A. **Breast size** is not an indicator of breastfeeding success. Small breast size does not indicate a woman cannot breastfeed because most breast mass is fat tissue, not glandular tissue. Thus even small breasts may have enough glandular tissue to produce sufficient milk. Small breast size, however, may limit the volume of milk that can be stored and may necessitate more frequent feeding to provide the infant with sufficient milk intake.

B. **Hypoplastic/Tubular Breasts.** Breast maldevelopment, sometimes characterized by a tubular shape, although uncommon, has been associated with a high risk for insufficient milk production.

C. **Breast enlargement during pregnancy** is an important factor in lactation success. If breasts do not enlarge during pregnancy, milk production may not occur and exclusive breastfeeding may not succeed. Hormonal or anatomic factors may be the cause. Regardless of the cause, breastfeeding, and especially measures of adequate milk intake, should be monitored closely. (See Chapter 8.)

D. Breast injury and breast surgery, whether for reduction mammoplasty, implantation, removal of a mass, or as a result of trauma, may be a cause for breastfeeding difficulties. Generally, breastfeeding should be encouraged and attempted if the mother so desires. Additional assistance, monitoring, and encouragement should be provided during the first few days and beyond to ensure sustained, successful milk production. The possibility of difficulty in establishing lactation should be discussed with the mother, and she should receive continuous encouragement and support.

1. ***Reduction Mammoplasty.*** Women who have had reduction mammoplasty with repositioning of the areolae and nipples are likely to have difficulty producing adequate milk. Periareolar incisions are likely to interrupt the ducts and block the flow of milk into the nipple ducts. Because there may be some recannulization, the mother may produce some milk. Exclusive breastfeeding is rare. If the nipple and areola are left on a pedicle during surgery, the prognosis for successful lactation is improved.

2. ***Augmentation mammoplasty*** is compatible with successful breastfeeding, especially if the implant was placed behind the pectoral muscles. Excessively large implants may impinge on the capacity of the breast to enlarge during lactation, and thereby limit the volume of milk that the mother can store. Excessively large implants also may restrict blood flow to the mammary gland tissue, restricting milk production. The rationale for breast augmentation may need clarification. For example, augmentation may have been performed for abnormal shape or breast asymmetry, which may indicate inadequate breast tissue to support breastfeeding. Changes in the breast during pregnancy, and milk production during the immediate postpartum period, should be monitored closely.

3. ***Lumpectomy,*** or removal of a mass in the breast, may affect breastfeeding if significant nerves and ducts have been severed or removed. Of greatest concern are incisions around the periphery of the areola. Milk production and infant weight gain should be monitored closely.

4. *Previous Treatment for Breast Cancer.* Pregnancy after breast cancer treatment has not been shown to increase the recurrence and may confer a survival benefit. It has been recommended that women wait 5 years after treatment for breast cancer to conceive. If a woman does become pregnant sooner, she usually is able to breastfeed on the unaffected breast and, in some cases, on both breasts if surgery and/or radiation therapy did not interfere. Radiation therapy after lumpectomy may lead to insufficient lactation on the affected side.

5. *Trauma and Burns.* The effect of breast tissue trauma and burns on lactational performance varies depending on how much direct injury to the ducts and mammary gland tissue occurred. Even women who suffered severe burns to the chest in childhood requiring extensive grafting have been able to breastfeed successfully.

6. *Pierced Nipples.* A history of pierced nipples has not been associated with breastfeeding difficulties unless there is infection or scarring. Nipple devices should be removed before feeding to avoid the risk of infant choking.

II. Absolute and Relative Maternal Contraindications to Breastfeeding

A. **Infection Risk.** Transmission of microorganisms from mother to milk has been shown to occur. The degree of infant risk varies.

1. *HIV and HTLV.* Women in the United States who are infected with human immunodeficiency virus (HIV) and women with human T-cell lymphotropic virus 1 (HTLV, type I or type II) should not breastfeed because of the risk of transmission to the nursing infant. In developing countries where infectious diseases and malnutrition are the predominant causes of infant mortality, the health risks of not breastfeeding must be balanced with the risk of HIV acquisition.

2. *Tuberculosis.* Because of concern that the disease could be transmitted by close contact with the mother, women with

active pulmonary tuberculosis should not feed their infant themselves until they have received appropriate antibiotic treatment for approximately 2 weeks and are no longer contagious, as determined by their physician or public health official. It is not clear whether the tubercle bacillus actually passes into the milk.

3. *Varicella-Zoster Virus.* Neonates should be given varicella-zoster immune globulin if their mothers develop varicella between the period beginning 5 days before delivery through 2 days after delivery. Varicella vaccine may be given to susceptible breastfeeding mothers if the risk of exposure to natural varicella is high. It is not known if varicella virus is excreted in milk. Some clinicians recommend breastfeeding only after the exposed infant receives immune globulin. The infant should not have direct contact with lesions that have not crusted over.

4. *Herpes Simplex Virus.* Women with herpetic breast lesions should not breastfeed from the affected breast and should cover the lesions to prevent infant contact. Women with genital herpes, however, can breastfeed. Proper handwashing procedures should be stressed.

5. *Cytomegalovirus (CMV)* may be found in the milk of seropositive mothers. In healthy term infants, symptomatic CMV disease from transmission through human milk is uncommon. There is some concern that premature infants may be at greater risk of symptomatic disease manifest as sepsis-like syndromes. Freezing at -20°C may decrease CMV infectivity. Clinicians should consider the benefits of human milk versus the risk of CMV transmission in premature infants whose mothers are known to be CMV positive or seroconvert during lactation.

6. *Hepatitis B.* Infants born to women who are hepatitis B surface antigen (HbsAg) positive routinely receive hepatitis B immune globulin and hepatitis B vaccine, eliminating concerns of transmission through breastfeeding. There is no need to delay initiation of breastfeeding until after the infant is immunized because breastfeeding was not contraindicated, even before these measures were initiated.

7. *Hepatitis C.* Hepatitis C virus and hepatitis C antibody have been detected in human milk. There are no reports of infant acquisition of the virus through breastfeeding. Maternal hepatitis C infection is not a contraindication to breastfeeding.

B. **Substance Abuse.** Women ingesting drugs of abuse need counseling and should not breastfeed until they are free of the abused drugs that may harm the infant. (See Chapter 12.)

C. **Alcohol.** Changes in infant feeding patterns have been reported in infants soon after mothers have ingested large amounts of alcohol quickly. Mothers should be advised to limit alcohol consumption during lactation. Alcohol is one of the few substances ingested by the mother that achieves high concentrations in human milk. The Institute of Medicine recommends lactating women limit alcohol intake to 0.5 g or less of alcohol per kilogram maternal body weight per day. For a 60-kg woman, this represents the equivalent of 2 cans of beer, 2 glasses of table wine, or 2 oz of liquor. (See Chapter 12.)

D. **Cigarette Smoking.** Metabolites of cigarette smoke have been found in infants who live in an environment in which tobacco is smoked. Mothers should be discouraged from smoking during lactation. If they persist in smoking, breastfeeding should be encouraged for the protective effects in the infant, especially with respect to respiratory illnesses. Mothers and all others should be advised not to smoke in the presence of infants and children. (See Chapter 12.)

E. **Medications.** Most medications are compatible with breast-feeding or, if not compatible, a substitute medication may exist and should be sought. (See Chapter 12.)

F. **Cancer Therapy.** Women with breast cancer should not delay treatment so they can breastfeed. Depending on the therapy, women receiving antimetabolite chemotherapy may be able to breastfeed by pumping and discarding their milk after each treatment until the chemical has been cleared. Radiation therapy generally is compatible with breastfeeding. Radiation treatment of the breast, however, may significantly damage sensitive breast tissue and be detrimental to future lactation performance of the affected breast. (See No. 4 on page 39.)

G. **Radiopharmaceuticals.** Mothers receiving diagnostic or therapeutic radioactive isotopes or who have had accidental exposure to radioactive materials should not breastfeed for as long as there is radioactivity in the milk. (See Chapter 12.)

III. Infant Contraindications to Breastfeeding

A. **Galactosemia.** Infants with classic galactosemia (galactose 1-phosphate uridyltransferase deficiency) cannot ingest lactose-containing milk. Therefore, because lactose is the principal carbohydrate in human and bovine milk, infants with classic galactosemia should not breastfeed or receive formula containing lactose. However, in some of the genetically milder forms of galactosemia, partial breastfeeding may be possible.

B. **Inborn Errors of Metabolism.** Infants with other inborn errors of metabolism may ingest some human milk, but this recommendation would depend on the desired protein intake and other factors. Phenylketonuria has been managed with a combination of partial breastfeeding and phenylalanine-free formula. Human milk contains relatively low levels of phenylalanine compared with formula.

C. **Hyperbilirubinemia.** For most newborns with jaundice and hyperbilirubinemia, breastfeeding can and should be continued without interruption. In rare circumstances of severe hyperbilirubinemia, breastfeeding may need to be interrupted for a brief period. (See Chapter 8.)

IV. Primary Insufficient Milk Syndrome

Approximately 5% of women will not produce adequate milk. A history of breast changes during pregnancy may be an important early sign of potential insufficient milk syndrome. A history of breast surgery or trauma also should alert caregivers to potential problems. (See Chapter 8.)

Selected References

American Academy of Pediatrics. *Red Book®: 2003 Report of the Committee on Infectious Diseases.* Pickering LK, ed. 25th ed. Elk Grove Village, IL: American Academy of Pediatrics; 2003

Institute of Medicine Subcommittee on Nutrition During Lactation. *Nutrition During Lactation.* Washington, DC: National Academy Press; 1991

Lawrence RM, Lawrence RA. Given the benefits of breastfeeding, what contraindications exist? *Pediatr Clin North Am.* 2001;48:235–251

Neifert MR. Prevention of breastfeeding tragedies. *Pediatr Clin North Am.* 2001;48:273–297

Chapter 4

Anatomy and Physiology of Lactation

The defining characteristic of mammals is the provision of milk, a fluid whose composition exactly mirrors the needs of the young of the species. In the human breast, milk is produced and stored in differentiated alveolar units, often called lobules. These lobules contain small ducts, which coalesce into 15 to 25 main ducts that drain sectors of the gland. The main ducts dilate into small sinuses as they near the areola, where they open directly on the nipple. The amount of milk produced is regulated by prolactin and local factors. Removal of the milk from the breast is accomplished by a process called milk ejection brought about by a neuroendocrine reflex. Afferent stimuli lead to the secretion of oxytocin from the posterior pituitary into the bloodstream, where it is carried to the myoepithelial cells that surround the ducts and alveoli. Contraction of these cells leads to milk ejection.

I. Anatomy of the Breast

The breast contains a tubuloalveolar parenchyma embedded in a connective and adipose tissue stroma. In the mature breast of the non-pregnant, non-lactating woman, 6 to 10 branching ducts form a tree-like pattern that extends from the nipple to the edges of a specialized fat pad on the anterior wall of the thorax. Lobules of varying complexity extend from these ducts. These lobules form the acinar structures that will become the milk-secreting organ. The milk-secreting unit is composed of a single layer of epithelial cells with surrounding supporting structures that include myoepithelial cells, contractile cells responsible for milk ejection, and a connective tissue stroma containing a large number of adipocytes and a copious blood supply.

A. **Stages in Breast Development.** The breast, or mammary gland, like most reproductive organs, is not fully developed until sexual maturity. Development of the mammary gland can be divided into 5 major stages: embryogenesis, pubertal development, development in pregnancy, lactation, and involution.

 1. *Embryogenesis* begins in the 18- to 19-week fetus when a bulb-shaped mammary bud can be discerned extending from the epidermis into the dense subepidermal mesenchyme. At the same time, a loose condensation of mesenchyme extends subdermally to form the fat pad precursor. The ducts elongate to form a mammary sprout, invade the fat pad precursor, branch, and canalize to form the rudimentary mammary ductal system that is present at birth in the connective tissue just below the nipple. Limited milk secretion may take place at birth under the influence of changes in maternal hormones. After birth the gland remains as a set of small branching ducts that grow in parallel with the child. The breast then remains inactive until puberty.

 2. *Mammogenesis During Puberty.* Thelarche, which indicates the beginning of puberty, is the period during which breast development occurs. The initial stages are increase in size and pigmentation of the areola and development of a mass of tissue underneath the areola (breast bud). Thelarche typically begins at a mean age of 9.6 years, but may begin as early as 8 years of age, with ethnic and environmental factors accounting for the variation. Normal breast development takes an average of 3 to 3½ years. Thelarche typically occurs approximately 2½ to 3 years prior to the onset of menstruation (menarche).

    At puberty, estrogen and a pituitary factor that is probably growth hormone stimulate the growth of the mammary ducts into the preexisting mammary fat pad. In early puberty, bare ducts course through the fat. With the onset of the menses and ovulatory cycles, the progesterone secreted by the ovary during the luteal phase brings about some lobulo-alveolar development. The alveolar clusters are dynamic structures that increase in size and complexity during each luteal phase but tend to regress with the onset of the menses and the loss of hormonal support. However, there is a gradual accretion of epithelial tissue with each successive cycle.

3. ***The mature mammary gland*** comprises 6 to 10 lobes, each of which has a single opening (galactophore) in the nipple. Each mammary acinus consists of epithelial-lined ductules that form a round alveolus. Myoepithelial cells surround the cuboidal cells of the alveolus and contract under the influence of oxytocin during milk ejection. Multiple alveoli are clustered into lobules, which are then connected via lactiferous ducts to form a distinct mammary lobe. Each lobe is anatomically separate from all other lobes. This is important to remember when examining the breast for abnormal nipple discharge. Each mammary duct connects to a separate lactiferous sinus or ampulla and terminates at the galactophore at the nipple (Figure 4-1).

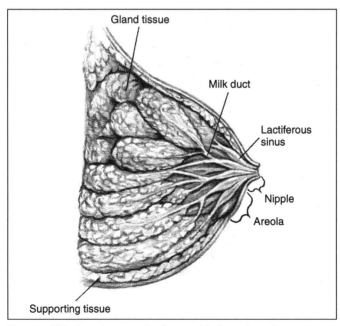

Gland tissue

Milk duct

Lactiferous sinus

Nipple

Areola

Supporting tissue

Figure 4-1. This schematic cross-section diagram of the breast shows that as pregnancy progresses, the fatty and supportive tissues that normally make up most of the breast volume are replaced by glandular tissue necessary to produce milk.

The areola contains numerous small sebaceous glands, Montgomery tubercles, which usually are not visible prior to pregnancy and lactation. Their function is to secrete a cleansing and lubricating fluid that is bacteriostatic.

B. **Breast Development in Pregnancy.** The breast undergoes marked changes during pregnancy. Physically, the breasts experience a doubling of weight, an increase in blood flow, lobular and alveolar growth, and increased secretory activity. Pregnancy hormones bring about full alveolar development. In addition to increasing levels of progesterone, a lactogenic hormone, either prolactin or human placental lactogen, is thought to be essential for the final stages of mammary growth and differentiation. By midpregnancy the gland has developed extensive lobular clusters and, indeed, small amounts of secretion product are formed and lactose can be detected in the blood and urine. This maturation process is sometimes referred to as lactogenesis stage 1. Some women will notice a slight leakage of colostrum in the second half of the pregnancy, which is normal. Furthermore, patients will begin to notice superficial veins as their breasts enlarge, as well as enlargement and darkening in pigmentation of the areola; the Montgomery tubercles will begin to protrude from the areola. The gland continues to develop until parturition, with the secretory process being held in check by the high circulating concentrations of progesterone.

C. **What Is Lactogenesis Stage 2?** The initiation of lactation is defined as the process by which the mammary gland develops the capacity to secrete milk. This process, sometimes called lactogenesis stage 2, starts at parturition and consists of a set of patterned changes that lead over about 4 days to full lactation. A major volume increase around 40 hours postpartum often is referred to as the "coming in" of the milk. For most women, this change in the volume of the breasts is noticeable between the second and fifth postpartum day, with the process occurring later in primiparous women than in multiparous women. Because the phrase "milk coming in" might contribute to the maternal perception that milk production is inadequate in the first few days postpartum, it is best to avoid using this term. Although milk volume is low during the first 2 days postpartum, the amount of colostrum is usually sufficient to meet the needs of the term infant.

Lactation is initiated whether the newborn breastfeeds or not, so even non-breastfeeding mothers experience breast fullness and leaking of milk. The process is marked by an increase in blood flow to the breasts, an increase in milk volume, and a change in composition so that the milk appears somewhat creamy in color and consistency, compared with the thick, yellow colostrum. Some women experience engorgement, or extreme fullness of the breasts, during this stage, especially if the newborn is not feeding frequently. During this stage and after, continued milk production becomes dependent on regular milk removal.

D. **Lactation** is the process of milk secretion, which continues as long as milk is removed from the gland on a regular basis. Prolactin is required to maintain milk secretion and oxytocin to produce let-down, to allow the infant to extract milk from the gland.

E. **Involution takes place at weaning** (ie, when regular extraction of milk from the gland ceases or in many, but not all species, when prolactin is withdrawn). Like the initiation of lactation, this stage involves an orderly sequence of events to bring the mammary gland back nearly to the pre-pregnant state.

II. Physiology of Lactation

A. **Regulation of Milk Synthesis, Secretion, and Ejection.** Milk is synthesized continuously and secreted into the alveolar lumen, where it is stored until milk removal from the breast is initiated. This means that 2 levels of regulation must exist: regulation of the rate of synthesis and secretion and regulation of milk ejection. Although both processes ultimately depend on sucking by the infant or other stimulation of the nipple, the mechanisms involved, central and local, are very different. Prolactin is necessary for milk secretion, and its secretion is directly linked to suckling stimulation at the breast, the intensity of suckling being related to the height of the prolactin peak. However, as described below, the level of plasma prolactin is not

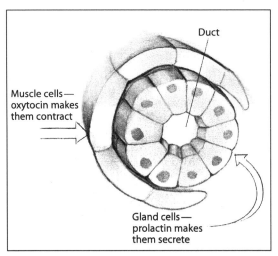

Figure 4-2. Breastfeeding stimulates the increase of hormones oxytocin and prolactin.

directly related to the amount of milk produced, which is a function of poorly understood local factors that depend on milk removal from the breast. Oxytocin participates in a neuroendocrine reflex that results in stimulation of the myoepithelial cells that surround the alveoli and ducts (Figures 4-2 and 4-3). When these cells contract, milk is forced out of the alveoli to the nipple (the letdown reflex). Only then does it become available to the suckling infant. If the let-down reflex is inhibited, milk cannot be removed from the breast, and local mechanisms bring about an inhibition of milk secretion. With partial removal of milk on a consistent basis, these local factors adjust milk secretion to a new steady-state level. If milk removal ceases altogether, involution sets in and the gland loses its competency to secrete milk.

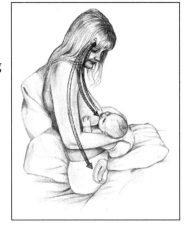

Figure 4-3. An infant's mouth on the mother's nipple signals the brain to release oxytocin, which causes the milk ducts to contract and expel milk, and the uterus to contract.

1. *Milk production* in lactating women is regulated by infant demand. When the milk has a lower caloric density, increased suckling by the infant is thought to result in increased emptying of the breast, in turn bringing about an increase in milk secretion. Mothers of twins, and occasionally even triplets, are able to produce volumes of milk sufficient for complete nutrition of their multiple infants. However, if infants are supplemented with foods other than human milk, milk secretion is proportionately reduced.

2. *Prolactin secretion* occurs episodically with peaks of up to 75 minutes in duration that occur 7 to 20 times a day. The prolactin peaks seem to be superimposed on a continuous background level of secretion whose magnitude depends on the physiologic condition. During pregnancy, serum prolactin levels increase steadily from about 10 ng/mL in the pre-pregnant state to about 200 ng/mL at term. After parturition the basal prolactin levels decrease, returning to pre-pregnancy values at 2 to 3 weeks in the woman who is not breastfeeding. In the lactating woman, suckling usually leads to a rapid rise in prolactin secretion. If the activity of the nerves to the nipple is inhibited, the prolactin rise is abolished. Increases in prolactin also can be achieved in non-lactating women by tactile stimulation of the nipples. Although prolactin levels are consistently above basal values for the duration of lactation, they are not proportional to milk volume secretion. Thus, while prolactin is necessary for milk secretion in women, plasma prolactin concentrations do not directly regulate milk synthesis and secretion.

3. *Local Regulation of Milk Production.* Two local mechanisms have been implicated in the regulation of milk volume production. An inhibitor of milk secretion, the protein called Feedback Inhibitor of Lactation builds up as milk accumulates in the lumen of the mammary gland. Thus the actual volume of milk secreted may be reduced if the breast is not drained adequately. Distention or stretch of the alveoli also may regulate milk synthesis and secretion.

B. Oxytocin Stimulation of Milk Ejection. Milk removal from the breast is accomplished by the contraction of myoepithelial cells, whose processes form a basket-like network around the alveoli where milk is stored, in concert with sucking by the infant. When the infant is suckled, afferent impulses from sensory stimulation of nerve terminals in the areolae travel to the central nervous system where they promote the release of oxytocin from the posterior pituitary. Oxytocin release often is associated with such stimuli as the sight or sound, or even the thought, of the infant indicating a significant psychological component in this neuroendocrine reflex. Oxytocin is transported systemically to the mammary gland where it interacts with specific receptors on myoepithelial cells, initiating their contraction and expelling milk from the alveoli into the ducts and subareolar sinuses. The process by which milk is forcibly moved out of the alveoli is called milk ejection or let-down and is essential to milk removal from the lactating breast. Clinically, there is a great deal of individual variation in women's perception of let-down. In the first few days after delivery, uterine contractions or "after pains" associated with suckling indicate oxytocin release, which probably aids in uterine involution. Some women experience leaking of milk, some feel sensations in the breast, and some have none of these physical sensations in the presence of let-down. If present, the sensations are confirmatory; if absent, no specific conclusions can be drawn without further investigation into the feeding process.

1. *Effect of Suckling.* During correct suckling, the nipple and much of the areola are drawn well into the mouth. The mammary sinuses are drawn into the mouth. Milk is removed not so much by suction as by the stripping motion of the tongue against the hard palate. The sinuses refill as the continued action of oxytocin forces milk from the alveoli into the ducts (Figure 4-4).

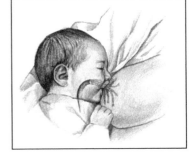

Figure 4-4. An example of an infant latched on properly and compressing the milk sinuses.

2. ***Effect of Emotional State and Drugs.*** Psychological stress, pain, or fatigue can decrease milk output due to inhibition of oxytocin release. Oxytocin release begins with the onset of suckling in relaxed, undisturbed mothers, but may occur prior to suckling if the infant cries or becomes restless. Although lower doses of alcohol may enhance milk letdown by decreasing stress, higher doses of alcohol inhibit oxytocin release. Opioids also may affect oxytocin release.

Selected References

Arthur PG, Kent JC, Potter JM, Hartmann PE. Lactose in blood in nonpregnant, pregnant, and lactating women. *J Pediatr Gastroenterol Nutr.* 1991;13:254–259

Chiodera P, Salvarani C, Bacchi-Modena A, et al. Relationship between plasma profiles of oxytocin and adrenocorticotropic hormone during suckling or breast stimulation in women. *Horm Res.* 1991;35:119–123

Crowley WR, Armstrong WE. Neurochemical regulation of oxytocin secretion in lactation. *Endocr Rev.* 1992;13:33–65

Giraldi A, Enevoldsen AS, Wagner G. Oxytocin and the initiation of parturition. A review. *Dan Med Bull.* 1990;37:377–383

Kleinberg DL. Early mammary development: growth hormone and IGF-1. *J Mammary Gland Biol Neoplasia.* 1997;2:49–57

Neville MC. Volume and caloric density of human milk. In: Jensen RG, ed. *Handbook of Milk Composition.* San Diego, CA: Academic Press, Inc; 1995: 101–113

Neville MC. Anatomy and physiology of lactation. *Pediatr Clin North Am.* 2001; 48:13–34

Neville MC, Morton J, Umemura S. Lactogenesis. The transition from pregnancy to lactation. *Pediatr Clin North Am.* 2001;48:35–52

Peaker M, Wilde CJ. Feedback control of milk secretion from milk. *J Mammary Gland Biol Neoplasia.* 1996;1:307–315

Ueda T, Yokoyama Y, Irahara M, Aono T. Influence of psychological stress on suckling-induced pulsatile oxytocin release. *Obstet Gynecol.* 1994;84:259–262

Chapter 5

Breastfeeding: Management Before and After Conception

Annual office encounters and preconception visits offer the practitioner an opportunity to discuss the benefits of breastfeeding and allow patients to ask questions and seek resources that will maximize the chances for successful breastfeeding. To further optimize breastfeeding, the practitioner can assess the patient's specific history, perform a breast examination to identify any problems, or suggest lifestyle or medication changes. Furthermore, cancer detection is easier before pregnancy or lactation, so this opportunity should not be missed.

I. Initial Prenatal Meeting

Once a patient presents for prenatal care, the initial and subsequent prenatal visits are excellent opportunities for the obstetric care professional to introduce and encourage breastfeeding. Most women make their feeding choice early; in fact, one study reported that 78% of women made their feeding decision before the pregnancy or during the first trimester. Early intervention by the obstetric care professional positively affects initiation and continuation of breastfeeding. The initial input from the obstetric care professional may give the mother confidence to pursue her goal of breastfeeding. Ideally, the patient and practitioner will discuss breastfeeding and decide on a plan well before the patient presents in labor. If the advantages and benefits of breastfeeding are reinforced at multiple visits, patients may be more likely to succeed.

II. History

Whether a woman presents for a preconception visit or a prenatal visit, a database should be compiled that would form the basis for her future care and aid in detecting any concerns that may arise with respect to future breastfeeding. In addition to an obstetric history, a complete medical history, including tabulation of chronic conditions, medications, diet and dietary supplements, smoking, alcohol use and substance use/abuse, should be included. These data can be revisited at the first obstetric visit. Table 5-1 lists factors that can be identified before delivery, or even pregnancy, which potentially may affect the success of lactation.

A. **Medical History**

   1. *Medical conditions* that may affect breastfeeding should be discussed, including a history of human immunodeficiency virus infection or herpetic breast lesions.

   2. *Medications* known to be problematic during lactation can be identified and alternative medications may be suggested. (See Chapter 12.)

   3. *Prior breast surgery,* breast disease, or trauma should be explored, especially that involving the areolar area, because

---

TABLE 5-1. RISK FACTORS FOR LACTATION PROBLEMS THAT CAN BE IDENTIFIED BEFORE DELIVERY

History/Social Factors

Early intention to breastfeed and bottle-feed

History of previous breastfeeding problems or breastfed infant with slow weight gain

History of hormone-related infertility; intended use of oral contraceptives

Significant medical problems (eg, untreated hypothyroidism, diabetes, cystic fibrosis)

Maternal age (eg, adolescent mother)

Psychosocial problems, especially depression

Anatomic/Physiologic Factors

Flat or inverted nipples

Variation in breast appearance (marked asymmetry, hypoplastic, tubular)

Previous breast surgery that severed milk ducts or nipple afferent nerves

Previous breast surgery to correct abnormal appearance or developmental variants

Previous breast abscess

Neifert MR. Ped Clin North Am. 2001;48:285. See Table 7-1 for additional factors identified after delivery.

periareolar incisions are most likely to interrupt the ducts and innervation. Breast reduction surgery may be more disruptive to adequate milk supply than other breast surgeries. (See Chapter 3.)

B. **Nutritional Assessment.** Adequate dietary intake should be assessed, and proper dietary habits should be encouraged. Even prior to conception, patients should begin taking a prenatal multivitamin (including folic acid, iron, and vitamin D) and have the adequacy of their diet assessed.

C. **Social History.** Substance use/abuse and other potentially harmful habits should be discussed. Discontinuation prior to conception is recommended, and appropriate support services should be provided.

D. **Prior breastfeeding history** should be documented. This allows an excellent opportunity to broach the topic of future breastfeeding and help the patient address barriers to breastfeeding she may have experienced, as well as concerns the patient and her family and friends have expressed regarding breastfeeding.

III. Physical Examination

A breast examination should be performed at an annual or preconception visit. If a recent breast examination is not documented, at the first prenatal visit one should be performed gently, yet thoroughly, because breasts are generally more tender in early pregnancy. *The examination offers an ideal opportunity to reassure the patient that she is physically capable of providing nutrition to her infant.* It may be appropriate to describe the stage of breast development in the medical record. (Figure 5-1, A–E).

A. **The ideal timing for breast examination** when a patient is not pregnant is in the early follicular phase, after completion of the menses and prior to the midcycle increases in edema, mastalgia, and cutaneous tactile sensitivity.

B. **Structural evaluation of the breast** should include identification of scars or lesions, as well as the maturational stage and symmetry of the breasts. Inverted nipples and tubular or hypoplastic breasts can also be identified.

1. *Breast Symmetry.* Patients with hypoplastic or inadequately developed breasts should be evaluated further for prior hormonal deficiencies in the developmental process. Many

Figure 5-1A. Breast Stage 1.There is no devel-opment. Only the papilla is elevated.

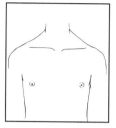 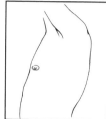

Figure 5-1B. Breast Stage 2. The "breast bud" stage. The areola widens, darkens slightly, and elevates from the rest of the breast as a small mound. A bud of breast tissue is palpable below the nipple.

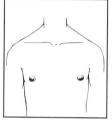 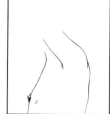

Figure 5-1C. Breast Stage 3. The breast and areola further enlarge and present a rounded contour. There is no separation of contour between the nipple and areola. Note that lack of separation of contour between the areola and the rest of the breast also is a feature of Stage 5. These stages may be distinguished from one another by the greater diameter of breast tissue in Stage 5. At Stage 3 the breast tissue creates a small cone as opposed to the wider cone in Stage 5.

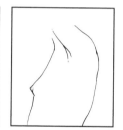

Figure 5-1D. Breast Stage 4. The breast con-tinues to expand. The papilla and areola pro-ject to form a secondary mound above the rest of the breast tissue. Approximate median age is 12 years.

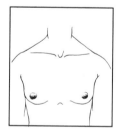 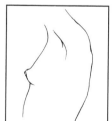

Figure 5-1E. Breast Stage 5. The mature adult stage. The secondary mound made by the nipple and areola present in Stage 4 dis-appears. Only the papilla projects. Even in a small-breasted individual, the diameter of the breast tissue (as opposed to the height) has extended to cover most of the area between the sternum and lateral chest wall.

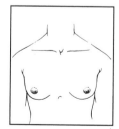 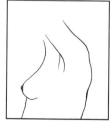

patients will present with slight breast asymmetry, which is normal. Significant asymmetry between breasts warrants further consideration, especially if the asymmetry is a recent occurrence.

2. **Inverted Nipples.** Nipple size and shape generally do not affect the ability to breast-feed (Figure 5-2). Patients may complain of inverted (turned in) nipples (Figure 5-3) and question the effect on future breastfeeding. A woman who has flat (Figure 5-4) or inverted nipples is able to breastfeed if her nipples can become erect. The use of breast shells for inverted nipples, however, has not been shown to be effective in the limited research done to date. Similarly, stretching or rolling the nipples during pregnancy has not been found to be beneficial. Indeed, nipple rolling may result in oxytocin release, which might induce uterine contractions.

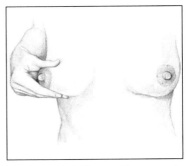

Figure 5-2. A normally protruding, or everted nipple, becomes erect when you press the areola between 2 fingers.

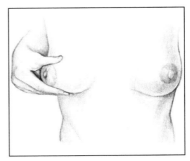

Figure 5-3. Inverted nipples retract toward the breast when pressure is applied to the areola.

3. **Breast Size.** Patients with small breasts should be reassured that their breastfeeding potential is not affected by breast size.

4. **Suspicious lumps** should be managed appropriately, with surgical consultation as appropriate. (See Chapter 9.)

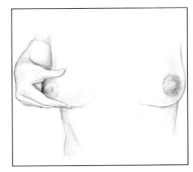

Figure 5-4. Flat nipples neither retract nor protrude.

IV. Education

The history and physical examination of a patient allow ample opportunity to initiate discussion and encouragement for breast-feeding. Anatomic considerations, practical concerns, and fears can be addressed. It is important to provide complete information on human milk, breastfeeding, and other infant feeding in relation to the health of women and their infants, and to offer resources and support for breastfeeding. The clinician's recommendations and reassurance to the patient are essential and should not be under-estimated. The timing of implementing various breastfeeding-related interventions is summarized in Table 5-2.

TABLE 5-2. GUIDE FOR PRENATAL BREASTFEEDING SUPPORT DURING OBSTETRIC VISITS

Obstetric Visit	Discussion	Examination
Initial visit	• Breastfeeding plans: Re-inforce and/or explore reasoning, education, correction of myths. • Note prior breast surgical history. • Note breast growth during pregnancy. • Note prior breastfeeding experience. • Review impact of medical conditions and applicable drugs on pregnancy and lactation.	• Palpate for masses or adenopathy. • Evaluate for inverted nipples and prior surgical scars.
14–20 weeks	• Discuss breast growth (if not previously noted). • Discuss feeding plans.	
24–28 weeks	• Recommend birthing classes. • Reinforce breastfeeding decision.	• Repeat breast examination with patient-voiced breast complaints at ANY subsequent visit.

Obstetric Visit	Discussion	Examination
	TABLE 5-2. GUIDE FOR PRENATAL BREASTFEEDING SUPPORT DURING OBSTETRIC VISITS (CONTINUED)	
32 weeks	• Readdress prior breast surgeries if applicable.	• Consider routine examination around this time.
34–36 weeks	• Discuss potential obstacles placed by hospital practices and strategies to overcome (eg, separation of mother and infant).	
	• Encourage breastfeeding during first hour after delivery, rooming-in, avoiding supplementation unless medical indication, avoiding bottle nipples, pacifiers, etc.	
	• Discuss return to work, breast pumps, child care choices, etc.	
	• Review pertinent medical conditions and medications and potential changes after delivery and during breastfeeding.	
	• Reexplore prior breastfeeding experiences if relevant.	
	• Discuss pediatric care professional visit.	
36+ weeks	• Review patient knowledge and pertinent questions.	
	• Discuss pediatric care professional visit.	
	• Discuss plans for additional childbearing/family planning.	

A. **Educating the Individual**

1. *Patient Education Resources.* The importance of early and continuing discussion about the decision to breastfeed cannot be overemphasized. Individual and group discussions between health care professionals and mothers-to-be have been shown to be effective. Contact information from pediatric health care professionals, nurses, and lactation specialists, as well as breastfeeding support groups, can augment the education efforts of the woman's health care professional. Finally, Internet-based resources allow the patient to explore the many benefits of breastfeeding. (See the Appendix.)

2. *Planning and Expectations.* Proper planning during antepartum care can help ensure successful breastfeeding. More than 60% of all new mothers will be returning to school or work, and these women often do not breastfeed. Patients should be assured that successful breastfeeding is possible even if the mother will be apart from the child at times. Early discussions of practical issues and plans, including breast pumps and milk storage, can help mothers continue breastfeeding when separated from their infants. (See Chapter 10.) It is helpful to suggest that the patient discuss breastfeeding and pumping locations and timing with her school administrator or employer prior to delivery.

3. *Family and friends'* experiences with breastfeeding may be helpful in predicting the type of support the mother will receive. Negative experiences and attitudes can be discussed to allay the patient's fears and suggest solutions to any problems encountered. The father and other significant family members should be included in breastfeeding discussions, if feasible and culturally appropriate. The father can be the mother's most important support person. (See Chapters 1 and 15.)

4. *A visit to the pediatric care professional* in the third trimester should be encouraged to discuss plans for infant nutrition. The patient should select a pediatric care professional who meets her needs, especially one who is a knowledgeable supporter of breastfeeding (Table 5-3).

TABLE 5-3. THE PRENATAL VISIT: MEETING WITH A POTENTIAL PEDIATRIC CARE PROFESSIONAL

Gathering Information/Anticipatory Guidance

- Discuss the family's thoughts and feelings about breastfeeding.

- Acknowledge the family's concerns.

- Provide accurate information on the topics that concern the family.

- State your support for breastfeeding.

- Review the benefits of breastfeeding.

- Obtain information about previous breastfeeding experiences.

- Review medical history about breast-related conditions, including surgery or injury.

- Discuss importance of prenatal breast examination to prepare for breastfeeding. Pediatrician may perform the examination or refer to mother's physician.

- Review important aspects of management of breastfeeding immediately after birth.

- Discuss available breastfeeding classes in the community.

- Have appropriate videotapes and books for parents to purchase or borrow.

Closing the Visit

- Ask parents if they have any other questions about breastfeeding.

- Encourage parents to call with questions.

- Encourage patients with phrases such as, "Well, from all we discussed, it seems you are going to do very well at breastfeeding."

Adapted from Breastfeeding Health Supervision Checklist. *Elk Grove Village, IL: American Academy of Pediatrics; 1999.*

B. Educating the Public

1. *Mass media* provides an opportunity to impact many potential current and future mothers and their supporting families. More focus should be provided by the media in portraying breastfeeding as the standard or normative form of infant nutrition. It is important that accurate information, in content and in portrayal, be provided. Subtle marketing strategies may undermine breastfeeding; health care professionals should recognize the risk these strategies represent, help their patients understand these risks, and work to minimize their influence.

2. *Legislative initiatives* have been undertaken and are being undertaken to ensure women's ability to breastfeed. Legislation exists in much of the United States to protect various concerns related to breastfeeding. State laws fall into 3 categories: 1) protecting the right to breastfeed, 2) breastfeeding in the workplace, and 3) exempting breastfeeding mothers from jury duty. In some states, companies providing specific features that promote and support breastfeeding for their employees are designated as breastfeeding-friendly work sites. (See Chapter 10.) Businesses meeting certain criteria can then advertise this benefit to their employees. Currently legislation is underway to require minimum standards for breast pumps and potential tax-free status for breastfeeding devices.

Selected References

American Academy of Pediatrics. *New Mother's Guide to Breastfeeding.* Meek JY, ed. New York, NY: Bantam Books; 2002

American Academy of Pediatrics Committee on Psychosocial Aspects of Child and Family Health. The prenatal visit. *Pediatrics.* 2001;107:1456–1458

American Academy of Pediatrics Section on Breastfeeding. *Ten Steps to Support Parents' Choice to Breastfeed Their Baby* [brochure]. Elk Grove Village, IL: American Academy of Pediatrics; 2003

American Academy of Pediatrics Work Group on Breastfeeding. *Checklists for Breastfeeding Health Supervision.* Elk Grove Village, IL: American Academy of Pediatrics; 1999

American College of Obstetricians and Gynecologists. *Breastfeeding Your Baby* [pamphlet]. Washington, DC: American College of Obstetricians and Gynecologists; 2001

American College of Obstetricians and Gynecologists. *Planning Your Pregnancy and Birth.* 3rd ed. Washington, DC: American College of Obstetricians and Gynecologists; 2000

Gartner LM, Newton ER. Breastfeeding: role of the obstetrician. *ACOG Clin Rev.* 1998;3:1–2, 14–15

Michels DL. *Breastfeeding Annual International 2001.* Washington, DC: Platypus Media LLC; 2001

Neifert MR. Clinical aspects of lactation. Promoting breastfeeding success. *Clin Perinatol.* 1999;26:281–306

Speroff L, Glass RH, Kase NG. *Clinical Gynecologic Endocrinology and Infertility.* 6th ed. Baltimore, MD: Lippincott Williams & Wilkins; 1999

Chapter 6

Peripartum Care:
The Transition to Lactation

The labor and delivery period represent a vulnerable time for the success of breastfeeding. Some clinicians estimate that 15% to 20% of women who state at the onset of labor that they wish to exclusively breastfeed are discharged from the hospital either supplementing breastfeeding or not breastfeeding at all. The obstetric care professional should have the knowledge and resources to support a woman who chooses to breastfeed. Immediate management issues are discussed in this chapter, while issues dealing with the entire hospital stay are described in Chapter 7.

I. Labor and Delivery Management

Hospital policies and practices, including those in the obstetric suite, can make a critical difference in the successful establishment of breastfeeding (Table 6-1).

A. Early initiation of breastfeeding within the first hour after birth should be practiced unless the medical condition of the mother or infant indicates otherwise. Infants who are placed on their mother's abdomen after birth and who attach to the breast within 1 hour of birth have better breastfeeding outcomes than infants who do not self-attach early. Indeed, early nursing in the delivery room is associated with a marked increase in the percentage of mothers who continue breastfeeding at 2 to 4 months postpartum compared with initiation of nursing 2 hours after birth. Successful lactation management includes encouraging nursing in the delivery room and avoiding maternal-infant separation in the first hours.

TABLE 6-1. HOSPITAL PRACTICES THAT INFLUENCE BREASTFEEDING

Strongly Encouraging	Encouraging	Discouraging	Strongly Discouraging
Physical Contact			
■ Baby put to breast immediately in delivery room ■ Baby not taken from mother after delivery ■ Mother helped by staff to suckle baby in recovery room ■ Rooming-in; staff help with baby care in room, not only in nursery	■ Staff sensitivity to cultural norms and expectations of mother	■ Scheduled feedings regardless of mother's breastfeeding wishes	■ Mother-infant separation at birth ■ Mother-infant housed on separate floors in postpartum period ■ Mother separated from baby due to bilirubin problem ■ No rooming-in policy
Verbal Communication			
■ Staff initiates discussion re: mother's intention to breastfeed pre- and intrapartum ■ Staff encourages and reinforces breastfeeding immediately on labor and delivery ■ Staff discusses use of breast pump and realities of separation from baby, re: breastfeeding	■ Appropriate language skills of staff, teaching how to handle breast engorgement and nipple problem ■ Staff's own skills and comfort re: art of breastfeeding and time to teach mother on one-to-one basis	■ Staff instructs woman to "get a good night's rest and miss the feed" ■ Strict times allotted for breastfeeding regardless of mother/baby's feeding "cycle"	■ Mother told to "take it easy," "get your rest" . . . impression that breastfeeding is effortful/tiring ■ Mother told she doesn't "do it right," staff interrupts her efforts, corrects her re: positions, etc
Nonverbal Communication			
■ Staff (doctors as well as nurses) give reinforcement for breastfeeding (respect, smiles, affirmation) ■ Nurse (or any attendant) making mother feel comfortable and helping to arrange baby at breast for nursing ■ Mother sees others breastfeeding in hospital	■ Pictures of mothers breastfeeding ■ Literature on breastfeeding in understandable terms ■ Closed-circuit TV show in hospital on breastfeeding	■ Pictures of mothers bottle-feeding ■ Staff interrupts her breastfeeding session for lab tests, etc ■ Mother doesn't see others breastfeeding	■ Mother given infant formula kit and infant food literature ■ Mother sees official-looking nurses authoritatively caring for babies by bottle-feeding (leads to mother's own insecurities re: own capability of care)
Experiential			
■ If breastfeeding not immediately successful, staff continues to be supportive ■ Previous success with breastfeeding experience in hospital			■ Previous failure with breastfeeding experience in hospital

Source: US Department of Health and Human Services. Report of the Surgeon General's Workshop on Breastfeeding & Human Lactation. *Rockville, MD: US Department of Health and Human Services, Public Health Service, Health Resources and Services Administration; 1984. DHHS publication HRS-D-MC 84-2.*

B. **Initial Feeding.** While the mother may have read about proper positioning and latch-on, the real-life situation is different. Although many infants placed on the mother's chest or abdomen during their usually alert and active first hour after delivery will spontaneously find the nipple-areola and latch on to it, others may require assistance. While infant identification bands may be essential immediately after delivery, eye prophylaxis, vitamin K, weighing, and other routine procedures can be done after the first breastfeed has been successfully achieved. Ideally, the initial feed should not be interrupted and, as long as medically safe, the mother and infant should remain together. Skin-to-skin contact in the delivery room will maintain the newborn's body temperature in a normal range.

II. Breastfeeding Technique

A. **General.** Breastfeeding is natural, but it is also a learned skill. Teaching the mother the basics of correct breastfeeding technique reduces the chance of physical discomfort during feedings, improves infant attachment to the breast, and enhances milk transfer to the infant. Bedside teaching should be reinforced with written materials and/or videos.

B. **Positioning.** There are many different positions for the nursing mother to use, but regardless of position, she should be comfortable. Pillows and footstools may provide assistance. The baby should be positioned so that the head, shoulders, and hips are in alignment and the infant faces the mother's body. The football (or clutch) and side-lying positions may provide an advantage for mothers who have undergone cesarean delivery by avoiding contact with the surgical incision. The football (or clutch) position often is used for low birth weight or premature infants, or infants having trouble latching on, because it allows for good control of the infant's head and good visibility of the infant's mouth on the breast. (See Chapter 14.) No matter which position is used, it is important to avoid pushing on the back of the infant's head because doing so may cause the infant to arch away from the breast.

1. *Cradle Hold* (Figure 6-1). The mother's same-sided arm supports the infant at the breast on which he is nursing.

The infant's head is cradled near the mother's elbow while the arm supports the infant along the back, facing the mother, chest to chest.

2. ***Cross-cradle or transitional hold*** (Figure 6-2) uses the opposite arm to support the infant with the back of the head (below the occiput) and neck held in the mother's hand. This leaves the hand closest to the breast to support and position the breast as needed.

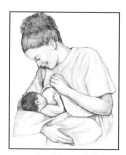

Figure 6-1. The cradle hold.

3. ***Football (or Clutch) Hold*** (Figure 6-3). The infant is positioned at the mother's side. The infant's feet and body are tucked under her arm and the infant's head is held in her hand facing the breast. If the infant pushes against the back of the chair with his feet, angle his legs and feet up the back of the chair.

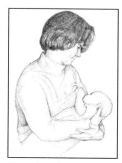

Figure 6-2. The cross-cradle hold.

4. ***Side-lying Position*** (Figure 6-4). The mother lies on her side facing the infant, who is also lying on his or her side. The infant faces the mother with the mouth at the level of the nipple.

C. **Latch-on.** To ensure proper latch-on, the infant should be held so that the mouth is opposite the mother's nipple and the neck is slightly extended, with the head, shoulders, and hips in alignment. While the infant is learning to nurse, proper latch-on is facilitated if the breast is supported with 4 fingers underneath and the thumb on top (C-hold, Figure 6-5A–C). Another way to present the nipple and areola is the scissors or V-hold, but only

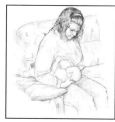

Figure 6-3. The clutch or football hold is an easy position to maintain and is particularly helpful after a cesarean delivery because it keeps the infant's weight off the incision.

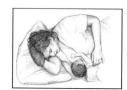

Figure 6-4. Side-lying position.

if the mother's fingers can open wide enough to keep the areola exposed to ensure adequate latch-on. The mother's fingers should be parallel to the infant's jaws and placed well behind the areola. An effective latch is crucial to breastfeeding success because it prevents sore nipples, ensures sufficient milk transfer, and adequately stimulates the breast to ensure plentiful continued milk production.

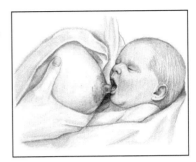

Figure 6-5A. The C-hold

1. **Rooting reflex** is elicited when the mother strokes the middle of the infant's lower lip with her nipple. The mother should wait patiently until the infant opens his mouth wide, and then quickly draw the baby to her breast, aiming the nipple toward the hard palate to facilitate the lower jaw taking in an adequate amount of the breast.

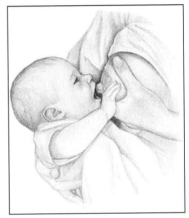

Figure 6-5B. Ensure the infant's mouth is wide open.

2. **Areola Grasp.** The infant should grasp the entire nipple and as much of the areola as comfortably possible (about 1 to 2 inches from the base of the nipple) and draw it into the mouth, perhaps as far as the circumareolar line. If the infant is well positioned, the nose and chin

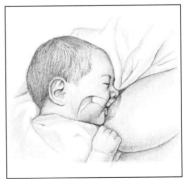

Figure 6-5C. This baby is properly latched on, with lips covering the areola and the nipple well inside the mouth.

will touch the breast, and the lips will be flanged outward around the breast tissue. The infant's tongue should be cupped beneath the nipple-areola complex and may be visible if the infant's lower lip is pulled down slightly. The infant's tongue compresses the lactiferous sinuses, located beneath the areola. The new father or other family members can be helpful in looking for these signs of good positioning and latch-on. When the infant is latched correctly, the mother will feel a gentle undulating motion but no pain with each suck.

3. **Sucking and Swallowing and Milk Transfer.** Once the infant is latched to the breast, suckling begins with rapid bursts and intermittent pauses. This will assist with stimulating the milk let-down reflex. Initially it may take a few minutes of suckling before a let-down occurs. As milk flow is established, the rhythm of suckling, swallowing, and pauses becomes slower and more rhythmic, approximately one suckle/swallow per second. Audible swallowing indicates milk transfer to the infant. A slight negative pressure exerted by the oropharynx and mouth holds the length of the breast in place and reduces the "work" to refill the lactiferous sinuses after they are drained. The milk is extracted, not by negative pressure, but by a peristaltic action from the tip of the tongue to the base. There is no stroking, friction, or in-and-out motion of the tongue; it is more of an undulating action. The buccal mucosa and tongue mold around the breast, leaving no space.

4. **Releasing the Latch** (Figure 6-6). At the end of nursing, the infant will often come off the breast spontaneously. If that does not occur, the mother can release the suction by inserting her finger gently into the corner of the infant's mouth.

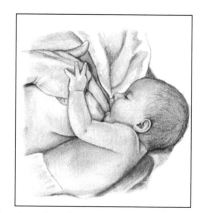

Figure 6-6. Releasing the latch.

This will minimize trauma to the nipple. The nipple should be observed; it should be elongated but otherwise have no creases or areas of trauma.

5. *Signs of incorrect latch* include indentation of the infant's cheeks during suckling, clicking noises, lips curled inward, frequent movement of the infant's head, lack of swallowing, and maternal complaint of pain. Swallowing may be difficult to hear when the newborn is taking small sips of colostrum, but as milk volume increases, swallowing should be heard easily. Later signs of incorrect latch-on include trauma to the nipples, pain, poor infant weight gain, and low milk supply.

III. Problem Solving

A. **Pain Management During and After Labor and Delivery.** To support the mother's desire to breastfeed, pain management should be balanced to ensure pain relief for the mother while avoiding excessive amounts of medication, particularly narcotics, that can have adverse effects on the infant's ability to nurse effectively.

1. *Intrapartum Narcotics.* The narcotic choice and dosing interval should be managed with the goal of minimizing adverse effects on the infant's ability to nurse effectively (Table 6-2). Meperidine is metabolized by mother and

TABLE 6-2. POSTPARTUM PAIN MANAGEMENT*			
Drug	*Onset IV*	*Onset IM*	*Neonatal Half-Life*
Meperidine	5 minutes	30–45 minutes	13–22 hours (63 hours for active metabolites)
Morphine	5 minutes	30–40 minutes	7 hours
Nalbuphine	2–3 minutes	15 minutes	4 hours
Butorphanol	1–2 minutes	10–30 minutes	Unknown (similar to nalbuphine in adults)
IV, intravenous; IM, intramuscular.			

infant via N-demethylation to form normeperidine, an active metabolite. Normeperidine is lipophilic, has a long half-life in the newborn, and may accumulate with regular breastfeeding. If possible, meperidine should be avoided intrapartum and postpartum in breastfeeding mothers. Morphine also is metabolized by mother and infant via N-demethylation, but forms inactive morphine-3-glucuronide and active morphine-6-glucuronide in a 9:1 ratio. Therefore, it has primarily inactive metabolites. Morphine is hydrophilic so there is less transfer into human milk. Nalbuphine is a synthetic narcotic with agonist-antagonist properties. It is excreted in the milk in clinically insignificant amounts and has a short half-life. Butorphanol has similar properties to nalbuphine.

2. *Epidural anesthesia* provides excellent and safe pain relief during labor. While the effect of epidural or intrathecal narcotics on sucking behavior and/or lactation success has not been adequately studied, there is ample evidence that regional administration of narcotics results in lower maternal levels than with parenteral administration, and does not inhibit the breastfeeding process.

3. *Trained labor support personnel,* or a companion, other than family, a doula, or other trained health professional providing one-to-one support, seems to be an effective method to support some women's desire to decrease the need for labor analgesia. While not necessarily trained breastfeeding experts, doulas have been shown to enhance the success of breastfeeding by providing consistent advice, encouragement, and reassurance.

4. *Postpartum pain relief* is usually well managed by non-narcotic medications such as nonsteroidal anti-inflammatory drugs (NSAIDs) or acetaminophen. When stronger medication is needed, oral narcotics are safely used and have minimal transfer to the breastfeeding infant. When possible, aspirin-containing products should be avoided.

    a. *Acetaminophen* is excreted into the breast milk in extremely low concentrations and is not highly protein bound. It is considered compatible with breastfeeding.

    b. *NSAIDs* generally have short half-lives and primarily inert metabolites. They are excreted into human milk in low or undetectable amounts and are considered compatible with breastfeeding. (See Chapter 12.)

    c. *Oral narcotics (fentanyl, codeine, propoxyphene, methadone, morphine)* are excreted in milk, but at low concentrations with short half-lives. They are compatible with breastfeeding.

    d. *Meperidine* may accumulate with regular use and should be avoided in breastfeeding mothers.

    e. *Aspirin* is metabolized into salicylate. Although transport into milk is limited, neonates eliminate salicylate very slowly. Therefore, caution must be exercised with more than occasional use.

   5. ***Postsurgical pain relief*** may be managed by the same medications mentioned previously. Severe pain may be managed by intrathecal narcotic, continuous epidural, use of a patient-controlled analgesia pump, or parenteral narcotics. Pain relief that requires parenteral administration of medication is best achieved with narcotics other than meperidine.

B. Cesarean Delivery. The incidence of breastfeeding may be 10% to 20% lower following cesarean compared with vaginal delivery. Causative factors have not been measured. After cesarean deliveries, clinicians concerned about maternal rest and recovery may be less likely to help the mother put the infant to the breast immediately or to encourage frequent feeding in the first 24 hours. Women undergoing planned cesarean delivery are more likely to breastfeed than those for whom the cesarean was not anticipated. Sometimes the unanticipated cesarean follows a long and difficult labor. In addition, some mothers view unplanned cesarean delivery as a distressing turn of events, a loss of control, or even a failure, factors that may inhibit let-down.

With active interventions to support breastfeeding in these high-risk situations, the initiation and duration of breastfeeding can be preserved. With assistance, the infant can be placed adjacent to the breast while avoiding the incision area. A side-by-side lying down position usually works best initially. Later, use of pillows and other position adaptations allows breastfeeding in the sitting or semireclining position. After cesarean delivery, the mother usually needs more help from the nursing staff and family members in lifting and positioning the infant. Compared with general anesthesia, regional anesthesia for cesarean delivery is preferable for maternal health and also has been associated with improved breastfeeding rates.

C. **Exhaustion** may affect breastfeeding outcome. Long and difficult labor may make it more difficult for the new mother to initiate breastfeeding and learn proper technique. Adequate support by educated personnel after delivery will help to overcome these obstacles to establishing successful breastfeeding. Additionally, when the new mother leaves the hospital, the many tasks facing her may be overwhelming. The new mother will be able to focus her energies on bonding with and breastfeeding her infant, as well as resting and recuperating from delivery, if she requests visitors and family members to help by changing diapers, cooking, and assisting with other children and household tasks. Postpartum depression is not uncommon, and new parents should be informed regarding the need for rest and how to identify more severe symptoms that would warrant contacting their physician. (See Chapter 9.)

IV. Hospitals Can Affect Breastfeeding Success

In 1984 the *Report of the Surgeon General's Workshop on Breastfeeding & Human Lactation* commented on hospital practices that influence breastfeeding. A hospital or birth center can facilitate breastfeeding success by implementing criteria set forth in the *Ten Steps to Successful Breastfeeding*. Hospitals have used a variety of strategies to encourage breastfeeding (Table 6-3).

Policies drive hospital systems. A written breastfeeding policy is an important tool for changing outdated routines. The single most difficult management issue is the control of routines and hospital

---

TABLE 6-3. TEN STEPS TO SUCCESSFUL BREASTFEEDING

Step 1—Have a written breastfeeding policy that is routinely communicated to all health care staff.

Step 2—Train all health care staff in skills necessary to implement this policy.

Step 3—Inform all pregnant women about the benefits and management of breastfeeding.

Step 4—Help mothers initiate breastfeeding within 1 hour of birth.

Step 5—Show mothers how to breastfeed and how to maintain lactation even if they should be separated from their infants.

Step 6—Give breastfeeding newborns no food or drink other than human milk, unless medically indicated.

Step 7—Practice rooming-in—allow mothers and infants to remain together 24 hours a day.

Step 8—Encourage breastfeeding on demand.

Step 9—Give no artificial teats or pacifiers to breastfeeding infants.

Step 10—Foster the establishment of breastfeeding support groups and refer mothers to them on discharge from the hospital or clinic.

The 1994 report of the Healthy Mothers, Healthy Babies National Coalition Expert Work Group recommended that the UNICEF-WHO Baby Friendly Hospital Initiative be adapted for use in the United States as the United States Breastfeeding Health Initiative, using the adapted 10 steps above.

Randolph L, Cooper L, Fonseca-Becker F, York M, McIntosh M. Baby Friendly Hospital Initiative feasibility study: final report. Healthy Mothers, Healthy Babies National Coalition Expert Work Group. Alexandria, Virginia: HMHB, 1994.

---

attitudes detrimental to maternal self-esteem and successful breast-feeding. Some policies may work against the physiology of lactation: taking the newborn away from the mother for routine procedures, supplementation of the breastfeeding infant without a medical indication, requiring pediatric clearance prior to the first feeding, and limiting maternal access to the infant. The following should be included in written hospital breastfeeding policy.

A. **Staff training** at all levels is critical to the successful support and promotion of breastfeeding. Without adequate staff education, families receive conflicting advice. Evidence-based lactation policies implemented by trained staff who offer accurate, consistent advice can make the difference between success and failure for breastfeeding women. Most caregivers indicate that their professional preparation did not result in adequate knowledge about the benefits of human milk and about the clinical management of breastfeeding. All staff should receive formal training in breastfeeding theory and management.

B. **Rooming-in and Feeding on Cue**

1. *Infant cues* can be used to determine when they should be fed: when they show signs of hunger (hand-to-mouth activity, smacking lips, rooting, eye movement in light sleep, movement of extremities) and not on a rigid schedule. Putting the baby to breast frequently, and whenever they demonstrate these cues, stimulates milk production and allows the full milk supply to develop as soon as possible, usually in 2 to 5 days.

2. *Rooming-in* where mother and infant are in close proximity so that the mother can recognize and respond to the feeding cues allows a better chance for successful initiation and establishment of breastfeeding.

3. *Time at breast.* Breastfeeding should continue at each breast without a time limit until the infant falls asleep or unlatches. Complete draining of the breast is essential for establishing a full milk supply.

C. **Latch-on,** as described above, is one of the most important factors in breastfeeding. The latch describes the way the infant takes the breast and transfers milk from the breast into the mouth.

D. **Supplementation**

1. *No supplements* (water, glucose water, formula) are needed for breastfeeding newborns unless a medical indication exists. Giving such supplements is likely to interfere with the process of successful initiation of breastfeeding by the mother and newborn.

2. *Hospital Incentives.* The hospital that pays fair market price for all formula and infant feeding supplies will strengthen corporate incentives to increase the scope and quality of its breastfeeding programs.

3. *Patient Incentives.* The routine distribution of products supplied free of charge by commercial interests, such as commercial baby bags containing samples of formula or formula samples alone, has been shown to be associated with less successful breastfeeding outcomes.

E. **Separation.** To support mothers in their desire to breastfeed, they should be taught how to express milk by hand or pump. (See Chapter 11.) If the infant is admitted to the neonatal intensive care unit, the need for this teaching will be immediate, but it should, in any case, take place before discharge and be reinforced in early visits along with other breastfeeding skills. When mothers and infants need to be separated, expression of milk is important, not only for infant feeding, but also to initiate and maintain the woman's milk supply during the separation. (See Chapter 10.)

F. **Pacifiers.** The most common reason women stop breastfeeding in the hospital setting is because of perceived inadequacy of their milk supply. Offering anticipatory guidance about normal milk production and normal weight loss for the newborn in the first few days can reassure the mother. The time a newborn spends sucking on a pacifier is time not spent suckling on the mother's breast, and the lack of stimulation can delay the arrival of the full milk supply, misleading the mother to think she is not making enough milk. The use of pacifiers in the early breastfeeding period has been shown to be associated with shorter breastfeeding duration and should be avoided until after breastfeeding is well established. Furthermore, the use of a pacifier may be a sign of impaired milk production.

G. **Support Following Discharge.** Discharge planning includes referrals and contact information for ongoing assistance with breastfeeding. (See Chapter 7.)

Selected References

Berens PD. Prenatal, intrapartum, and postpartum support of the lactating mother. *Pediatr Clin North Am.* 2001;48:365–375

Kramer MS, Chalmers B, Hodnett ED, et al. Promotion of Breastfeeding Intervention Trial (PROBIT): a randomized trial in the Republic of Belarus. *JAMA.* 2001;285:413–420

Kramer MS, Barr RG, Dagenais S, et al. Pacifier use, early weaning, and cry/fuss behavior. *JAMA.* 2001;286:322–326

Langer A, Campero L, Garcia C, Reynoso S. Effects of psychosocial support during labour and childbirth on breastfeeding, medical interventions, and mothers' well-being in a Mexican public hospital: a randomized clinical trial. *Br J Obstet Gynaecol.* 1998;105:1056–1063

Naylor AJ. Baby-Friendly Hospital Initiative. Protecting, promoting, and supporting breastfeeding in the twenty-first century. *Pediatr Clin North Am.* 2001; 48:475–483

Powers NG, Naylor AJ, Wester RA. Hospital policies: crucial to breastfeeding success. *Semin Perinatol.* 1994;18:517–524

US Department of Health and Human Services. *Report of the Surgeon General's Workshop on Breastfeeding & Human Lactation.* Rockville, MD: US Department of Health and Human Services, Public Health Service, Health Resources and Services Administration; 1984. DHHS publication HRS-D-MC 84-2

World Health Organization Division of Child Health and Development. *Evidence for the Ten Steps to Successful Breastfeeding.* Geneva, Switzerland: World Health Organization; 1998

Breastfeeding in the Hospital: The Postpartum Period

Adequate communication between obstetric and pediatric care professionals in the immediate postdelivery period will greatly facilitate helping the breastfeeding woman. It is equally important that all health care personnel involved in caring for mothers and infants possess basic breastfeeding knowledge so that they can provide accurate and consistent information. This chapter discusses issues relating to infants and mothers after delivery and before hospital discharge. Before discharge, anticipatory guidance regarding the breastfeeding process should be provided to the patient, her partner, and other supporting family members. Follow-up visits should be arranged. The patient should be given information on how to easily access further breastfeeding support if it is needed.

I. Breastfeeding Risk Factor History

A. **General.** Although most mothers can produce an adequate quantity of milk and most infants can nurse effectively and consume an adequate volume, specific maternal and infant factors can place an infant at risk for inadequate breastfeeding (Tables 7-1 and 7-2). It is assumed that risk factors for breastfeeding problems are assessed as part of routine prenatal care, although some mothers may present with limited or no prenatal care. Findings of the prenatal maternal breast examination that may adversely affect adequacy of milk production (such as inverted nipples, severely asymmetrical or tubular breasts, and prior breast surgeries) should be forwarded to the pediatric care professional. This information also should be discussed with the patient in a supportive and realistic fashion. In

TABLE 7-1. MATERNAL RISK FACTORS FOR LACTATION PROBLEMS

History/Social Factors

Early intention to breastfeed and bottle-feed

History of previous breastfeeding problems or breastfed infant with slow weight gain

History of hormone-related infertility

Significant medical problems (eg, untreated hypothyroidism, diabetes, cystic fibrosis)

Maternal age (eg, adolescent mother or advanced age)

Psychosocial problems, especially depression

Perinatal complications (eg, hemorrhage, hypertension, infection)

Intended use of combined oral contraceptives before breastfeeding is well established

Anatomic/Physiologic Factors

Lack of noticeable breast enlargement during pregnancy

Flat or inverted nipples

Variation in breast appearance (marked asymmetry, hypoplastic, tubular)

Previous breast surgery that severed milk ducts or nipple afferent nerves

Previous breast surgery to correct abnormal appearance or developmental variants

Previous breast abscess

Extremely or persistently sore nipples

Failure of lactogenesis stage 2 (milk did not noticeably come in)

Environmental Factors

Mother-baby separation or mother needing to pump

Adapted with permission from Pediatr Clin North Am. *2001;48:285.*

TABLE 7-2. INFANT RISK FACTORS FOR LACTATION PROBLEMS

Medical/Anatomic/Physiologic Factors

Low birth weight or premature (<37 weeks)

Multiples

Difficulty latching on to one or both breasts

Ineffective or unsustained suckling

Oral anatomic abnormalities (cleft lip/palate, micrognathia, macroglossia)

Medical problems (jaundice, hypoglycemia, respiratory distress, infection)

Neurologic problems (genetic syndromes, hypotonia, or hypertonia)

Persistently sleepy infant

Excessive infant weight loss

Environmental Factors

Formula supplementation

Effective breastfeeding not established by hospital discharge

Early discharge from hospital

Early pacifier use

Adapted with permission from Pediatr Clin North Am. *2001;48:285.*

---

particular, lack of breast growth during pregnancy is a red flag
and should be communicated from the obstetric to the pediatric care professional, as well as any other pertinent information about maternal perinatal conditions and delivery events.

B. **Maternal History.** Appropriate maternal history includes
amount and timing of prenatal care and education, medical
complications, obstetric complications, medical history (especially breast surgeries, infertility, endocrine problems, and past
breastfeeding difficulties), family history (atopy, breastfeeding
problems), and psychosocial history (substance abuse, mental
illness, sexual abuse, family support of breastfeeding).

C. **Infant History.** Appropriate history includes medical complications, postnatal feeding and elimination patterns, and infant temperament and sleep patterns.

II. Feeding Patterns

New mothers should be encouraged to nurse at each breast at each feed starting with the breast offered last at the prior feeding. This will help her achieve an optimal milk supply (Table 7-3). However, it is perfectly normal for a newborn to fall asleep after the first breast and refuse the second. It is preferable to allow an infant to drain the first breast well before switching him to the other breast. The mother should not interrupt a feeding just to switch to the second side. Typically, the infant will spontaneously release the first breast after sufficient draining. Timing each side is not necessary or desirable. Limiting the time at the breast has no effect on nipple soreness, but correct latch and positioning are crucial.

A. **Hunger Cues.** Many new parents expect their baby to cry when he is hungry and need to be informed that crying is a late sign of hunger and can result in an infant who is difficult to calm and latch to the breast. Anticipatory guidance and rooming-in 24 hours a day allow the parents to notice early infant hunger cues such as increased alertness, flexion of the extremities, mouth and tongue movements, cooing sounds, rooting, bringing the fist toward the mouth, or sucking on fin-

---

TABLE 7-3. MILK SUPPLY FOR BREASTFED NEONATES: THE FIRST WEEK

First 24 hours	Some milk may be expressed
Day 2	Milk should come in (lactogenesis stage 2)
Day 3	Milk should come in (lactogenesis stage 2)
Day 4	Milk should come in (lactogenesis stage 2)
Day 5	Milk should be present; breasts may be firm or leaking
Day 6+	Breasts should feel softer after nursing

Adapted with permission from Clin Perinatol. *1999;26:281–306.*

gers or the hand. Signs of satiety also need to be taught, such as nonnutritive sucking with longer pauses between sucking bursts, infant taking himself off the breast, disappearance of hunger cues, relaxed posture, and sleep.

B. **Feeding Frequency.** In addition to information regarding latch-on and positioning of the infant (Chapter 6), the mother should be instructed on expected breastfeeding routines, which can vary widely (Table 7-4). Typically, newborns will nurse 8 to 12 times or more in 24 hours for 10 to 15 minutes per breast. The interval between feedings is figured from the beginning of one nursing to the beginning of the next. Frequent breastfeeding in the first few days minimizes postnatal weight loss, decreases bilirubin levels, and helps establish a good milk supply. Although every 2 to 3 hours is the average, there is a great deal of variation from infant to infant and during a 24-hour period. Human milk empties from the stomach faster than formula. Without anticipatory guidance, new mothers often compare their infants to bottle-fed infants and misinterpret the

---

TABLE 7-4. FEEDING ROUTINE FOR BREASTFED NEONATES: THE FIRST WEEK

First hour	Infant put skin-to-skin in delivery room
2–4 hours	Infant/mother sleep
4–24 hours	Breastfeeding every 1.5 to 3 hours (8–12 × in 24 hours)
Day 2	Breastfeeding every 1.5 to 3 hours (8–12 × in 24 hours)
Day 3	Breastfeeding every 1.5 to 3 hours (8–12 × in 24 hours)
Day 4	Breastfeeding every 1.5 to 3 hours (8–12 × in 24 hours)
Day 5	Should hear baby swallow milk; start 1 longer interval (up to 5 hours)*
Day 6+	Continue frequent breastfeeding with 1 longer interval; baby appears satisfied

As long as the milk supply is established; may not be the norm for a term breastfed infant before 2 to 3 months.

Adapted with permission from Clin Perinatol. *1999;26:281–306.*

normal frequency of breastfeeding to mean they have insufficient milk. As infants get older, they nurse more efficiently, and the frequency and duration of feedings decrease.

C. **Nursing Styles.** Infants have been classified by their feeding behaviors. The key to appropriate counseling is recognizing the difference in infants and responding to them (Table 7-5).

D. **Infant Behaviors**

1. *Sleepy Infant.* After the usual 1 to 2 hours of quiet alertness immediately after birth (the ideal time to initiate breastfeeding), many infants fall into deep sleep, with only brief, partial arousals for several hours. This is a normal pattern and does not indicate a need for supplementation. Sometimes unwrapping, gentle massage, holding upright, motion, changing a diaper, talking, or holding the infant skin-to-skin against the mother's chest may arouse the sleepy infant. Infants have short wakeful periods throughout the first couple of days that can be missed.

TABLE 7-5. INFANT BREASTFEEDING STYLES

Attention to infant cues for feeding and the acceptance of a range of styles is helpful in optimizing breastfeeding.

Type	Description
Barracuda (or "Excited, effective")	Grabs the nipple and sucks energetically for 10 to 20 minutes
Excited Ineffective	Very eager and active at the breast, frustrated and crying when no milk results
Procrastinator ("Slow to start")	Waits until the milk appears before sucking, does well once started
Gourmet ("Slow feeder")	Licks and tastes little drops of milk before latch-on; attempts to hurry are met with vigorous infant protest
Rester ("Protracted feeder")	Prefers to breastfeed for a few minutes, then rest a few minutes, resulting in a longer than usual nursing time

Rooming-in, where the infant sleeps in close proximity to the mother, allows the mother to recognize subtle hunger cues. The newborn whose mother received a large quantity of narcotics or sedatives may have longer periods of sleep and may need to be awakened after 4 hours to feed.

2. *Fussy/unsettled infants* may be fretful after a feed, especially before lactogenesis stage 2 is complete. An extra minute or 2 at the breast, a diaper change, or a cuddle will usually satisfy the infant. If the infant is consistently fussy after every feeding, even after the milk supply is established, the breastfeeding mother and infant should be carefully assessed with regard to milk supply, milk transfer, and infant weight gain. Breastfeeding should commence when the infant is in the quiet alert state. If the infant is at an active alert or crying state, he may need to be consoled before he can be successfully breastfed.

3. *Crying* has been interpreted through the years as a sign of vigor, "good lungs," and general health. Crying results in increased work, energy expenditure, and swallowing of air, which may precipitate vomiting. In addition, crying depletes metabolic reserves, which may precipitate hypoglycemia, and disrupts early breastfeeding behavior. Crying is a very late sign of hunger. Babies who cry for a long time may become exhausted and go to sleep without nursing, or before they have finished the entire feeding. Frequent feeding will diminish crying episodes. Efforts should be made to minimize crying.

III. Hospital Assessment of the Breastfeeding Infant
(Table 7-6)

A. **Physical examination** of the infant should include a general examination, vital signs, growth percentiles and percentage weight change from birth, and a more detailed oral-motor examination (mandible size, frenulum, rooting, sucking). Presence of congenital anomalies and overall tone should be noted.

B. **Breastfeeding Observation.** It is helpful for the physician to observe a feeding and evaluate positioning, latch, milk letdown, and milk transfer. Also note maternal responses to the

TABLE 7-6. OVERVIEW: IN-HOSPITAL NEWBORN BREASTFEEDING HEALTH SUPERVISION

Breastfeeding Assessment

- Review maternal prenatal record, intrapartum record, and newborn recovery and transition records.
- Discuss timing and events of first feeding.
- Has mother previously breastfed?
- How is mother doing and how is she feeling about breastfeeding?
- Does newborn need to be awakened to feed?
- Does newborn easily latch on to breast and nurse eagerly?
- How many times has the newborn been to the breast within the first 24 to 48 hours?
- Is newborn receiving any supplements?
- What is the number of wet diapers in last 24 hours?
- What is the number of stools in last 24 hours?
- Are mother's breasts comfortable (no tenderness or pain)?
- Is mother taking any medications?
- How do family members feel about breastfeeding?

Examining Newborn and Mother

- Obtain birth weight and gestational age.
- Evaluate neurobehavioral condition of the newborn.
- Calculate newborn's weight gain or loss since birth.
- Observe breastfeeding.
- Examine mother's breasts or refer for examination, if needed.
- Perform newborn examination with attention to oral-motor examination.
- Assess state of hydration.
- Observe for jaundice.

Anticipatory Guidance

- Encourage breastfeeding on demand, approximately 8 to 12 times per 24 hours.
- During the first 24 to 48 hours, newborn may show little interest in breastfeeding.
- Newborns who do not awaken to feed should be aroused to feed at least every 4 hours.

TABLE 7-6. OVERVIEW: IN-HOSPITAL NEWBORN BREASTFEEDING HEALTH SUPERVISION (CONTINUED)

- Discourage use of pacifiers and discuss potential risks.
- Review normal breastfeeding patterns.
- Review normal elimination patterns.

Breastfeeding Interventions

- Supportive, nondisruptive care is important during first 24 to 48 hours.
- Attempt to identify signs of inadequate milk supply or intake and address potential contributing factors.
- Maintain lactation if mother and newborn are separated.
- Consider referral to lactation specialist if problems are ongoing.

Discharge Visit

- Congratulate parents on decision to breastfeed their baby.
- Review some of the benefits of breastfeeding.
- Remind mother to eat when hungry and drink when thirsty.
- Arrange for follow-up in office at 3 to 5 days of age or sooner if indicated.

Adapted from Checklists for Breastfeeding Health Supervision. *Elk Grove Village, IL: American Academy of Pediatrics; 1999.*

---

feeding (eg, painful, pleasurable, anxious, relaxed, etc). The hospital staff should observe and document these breastfeeding observations at least twice daily.

C. **Latch.** The infant's mouth should be wide open with lips flanged outward ("fish lips") encompassing the nipple and a significant part of the areola. (See Chapter 6.) Some of the factors that are important in assessing latch include the ability of the infant to latch, quality of the latch, presence of audible swallowing, characteristics of the anatomy and physiology of the nipple, maternal sensation, and whether the caregiver provides assistance with feeding.

D. **Weight Changes.** The most accurate appraisal of the adequacy of breastfeeding is the serial measurement of the infant's naked weight. Nearly all infants lose weight for the first 2 to 4 days after birth. Infants who are feeding well should not continue to lose weight after lactogenesis stage 2. (See Chapter 4.) A weight loss greater than 7% of birth weight may be excessive even if lactogenesis and milk transfer seem to be proceeding normally. In such a situation, milk production and transfer should be assessed. Once lactogenesis stage 2 is completed, an infant who did not lose excessive weight and who is nursing effectively should obtain enough milk to begin gaining weight by day 4 or 5 at a rate of approximately 15 to 30 g per day (1/2–1 oz per day). At this rate, most breastfed infants will exceed their birth weight by 10 to 14 days, and gain 150 to 210 g per week (5–7 oz per week) for the first 2 months. A breastfed infant who weighs less than birth weight at 2 weeks requires careful evaluation and intervention. Refer to Table 8-2 for overall mean weight gains for breastfed boys and girls.

E. **Elimination Patterns.** Urine output usually exceeds fluid intake for the first 3 to 4 days after birth, a physiologic response to contract the extracellular fluid space. Stooling and voiding patterns after the first few days are good indicators of adequate milk intake (Table 7-7). A journal kept by the mother recording feeding and elimination by the infant in the first few weeks can

---

TABLE 7-7. ELIMINATION PATTERNS IN BREASTFED NEONATES: THE FIRST WEEK

First 24 hours	1 wet diaper in 24 hours	1 meconium stool in 24 hours
Day 2	2–3 wet diapers in 24 hours	1 meconium stool in 24 hours
Day 3	4–6 wet diapers in 24 hours	Stool color changes
Day 4	Urine light yellow, 4–6 × in 24 hours	Transition stools
Day 5	Urine colorless, 6–8 × in 24 hours	3–4 yellow stools
Day 6+	Urine colorless, 6–8 × in 24 hours	≥4 stools; once established, stool frequency may diminish

Adapted with permission from Clin Perinatol. *1999;26:281–306.*

be helpful, but the benefits must be weighed against the potential for added stress.

1. ***Urine Output.*** By 5 to 7 days (usually a day or 2 after lactogenesis stage 2 is completed) the breastfed newborn should be voiding colorless, dilute urine 6 or more times per day.

2. ***Stool output and character*** also are particularly useful indicators of adequate milk intake. The normal green-black meconium stool should change to transitional green, then to soft, seedy, yellow stool by day 4 or 5 after birth. By 5 to 7 days of age, well-nourished breastfed infants usually pass a medium-sized yellow stool at least 3 to 4 times a day. Some infants stool after most feedings. After the first month the volume of each stool increases and the frequency decreases. Anticipatory guidance is essential because normal human milk stools are quite loose and may be confused with diarrhea if parents are accustomed to seeing the firm brown stools typical of formula-fed infants. Insufficient milk intake in an infant older than 5 days may be signaled by the presence of meconium stools, green-brown transitional stools, infrequent (<3 per day) stools, or scant stools.

F. **Hypoglycemia** is one of physicians' most commonly cited concerns regarding breastfed infants. The risk of hypoglycemia may be reduced by immediate and sustained mother-infant skin-to-skin contact and early initiation of breastfeeding. Blood glucose concentrations reach a nadir 1 to 2 hours after birth. An adaptive response to low blood glucose concentrations in breastfed infants is an elevated concentration of ketone bodies and other substrates, which act as alternate fuels for the infant until breastfeeding is established.

1. ***Signs and Symptoms.*** The clinical signs of hypoglycemia may be nonexistent, nonspecific, or include changes in the level of behavior (irritability, lethargy, stupor, coma), apnea, cyanotic episodes, hypothermia, hypotonia, tremor, seizures, temperature instability, and change in feeding patterns/responses.

2. **Causes.** In general, healthy term breastfed neonates do not develop symptomatic hypoglycemia. If they develop symptomatic hypoglycemia, an underlying illness must be excluded. Infants of diabetic mothers, infants who are small for gestational age, and premature infants are among the common groups of infants at risk for hypoglycemia.

3. **Evaluation.** Routine monitoring of blood glucose in asymptomatic, not at-risk, term neonates is unnecessary. Blood glucose concentrations should be measured in at-risk infants and/or those with clinical signs suggestive of hypoglycemia. Bedside screening tests should be confirmed by laboratory blood glucose measurements. At-risk infants and those with abnormal blood glucose concentrations should be monitored every 2 to 4 hours, prior to a feeding. Continue to monitor until several normal pre-feeding blood glucose concentrations are obtained. Serial monitoring does not preclude routine breastfeeding.

4. **Management.** Hypoglycemia can be reduced by early initiation of breastfeeding, within the first hour after delivery. Early breastfeeding is *not* precluded, even though an infant meets the at-risk criteria for glucose monitoring. The intervention in an asymptomatic breastfed infant is to increase the frequency of breastfeeding to every 1 to 2 hours and to recheck the blood glucose before the next feeding. If breastfeeding alone cannot correct and maintain an appropriate blood glucose concentration, expressed human milk or formula should be offered. Symptomatic hypoglycemia requires treatment with intravenous glucose. As long as the infant is clinically stable, breastfeeding should continue, even if intravenous glucose is provided.

G. **Feeding at the Breast Versus the Bottle**

1. **General.** There is a distinct difference between tongue and jaw movements of breastfeeding and bottle-feeding infants. In breastfeeding, breathing is coordinated with sucking and swallowing, usually in a 1:1:1 pattern. The rapid flow from a bottle may result in respiratory pause and shortened expiration. It is often assumed that breastfed infants who have difficulty obtaining milk will be more likely to prefer bottle-feeding if given the opportunity. Some infants may simply

prefer the more rapid, gravity-induced flow from a bottle. Because the introduction of a bottle has the potential to disrupt the development of effective breastfeeding behavior, its use should be minimized until breastfeeding is well established.

2. *Pacifiers.* Infant pacifier use has been independently associated with significant declines in the duration of breastfeeding. It is not clear whether the association is causal or a marker for preexisting breastfeeding difficulties. (See Chapter 6.)

IV. Hospital Assessment of the Breastfeeding Mother

A. **Nipple Pain.** Nipple soreness is the most common complaint of breastfeeding mothers in the immediate postpartum period. Actual nipple pain should not be considered normal. Nipple pain beyond mere soreness or discomfort or even soreness that continues beyond the beginning of a nursing episode or after let-down should be investigated immediately. If ignored, it can lead to other problems, such as engorgement, mastitis, or early cessation of breastfeeding. (See also Chapter 9.)

1. *Signs and Symptoms.* Early mild nipple discomfort is common among breastfeeding women. Transient nipple pain attributed to suction injury of the skin usually begins on the second postpartum day, increases between days 3 to 5, then improves. Severe nipple pain, or even discomfort that continues throughout a feeding, or that does not improve at the end of the first week, should not be considered a normal part of breastfeeding.

2. *Causes* of Sore Nipples in the Immediate Postpartum Period

   a. *Improper breastfeeding technique,* specifically poor position and improper latch, is the most common cause of nipple pain in the immediate postpartum period. Limited milk transfer occurs when the infant is attached incorrectly, resulting in poor infant weight gain and impaired milk production. Mothers with abdominal incisions from a cesarean delivery or other surgery should find comfortable positions, such as the football (or clutch) hold, to feed the infant.

b. *Trauma.* Other potential causes of nipple pain include sources of trauma that produce cracking, such as overzealous breast cleansing, failing to release suction before removing the infant from the breast, climate variables, and unique skin sensitivity. There is no need for nipple cleansing other than routine bathing. Counsel the mother to avoid using soap on the nipples because it can be irritating.

3. *Evaluation.* A feeding history, examination of the mother's breasts and nipples, and an oral-motor examination of the infant should accompany the observation of a feeding. The latch-on technique and infant positioning should be evaluated carefully. Infant suck also should be assessed. The mother should be asked about use of cleansers, abrasives, or any creams or ointments used on the breast. Rarely are bacterial or fungal cultures indicated. (See Chapter 9.)

4. *Management.* Limiting the time at the breast, even with the intention of gradually increasing nursing time, will not prevent nipple pain. Treatment for nipple pain depends on the underlying etiology. Skilled help with position and latch-on are primary interventions. Specific infections and dermatoses require directed therapy. (See Chapter 9.) Some creams and lotions can be irritating and result in allergic manifestations. Wound care specialists now suggest moisture-retaining occlusive dressings instead of dry heat for optimum healing. Pain may be helped by taking a pain reliever such as ibuprofen or acetaminophen a half hour before nursing. If severe trauma exists, it may be necessary either to manually or mechanically express milk until the tissue has healed well enough to resume breastfeeding. Nipple healing might be hastened if a small amount of milk is applied to the area after a feeding. Different breastfeeding positions also may be helpful in avoiding more sensitive or traumatized areas. If only one breast is affected, nursing should begin on the unaffected breast to achieve the let-down reflex and the infant moved to the affected breast when suckling may be less vigorous. Nipple pain also may be lessened by the use of a silicone nipple shield. (See Chapter 11.)

B. **Engorgement.** Normal breast fullness occurs due to vascular congestion during lactogenesis stage 2. Engorgement is the firm, diffuse, and painful overfilling and edema of breasts usually due to infrequent or ineffective milk removal. The woman may notice a low-grade fever. Therefore, the best treatment of engorgement is prevention by frequent breastfeeding. If left untreated, engorgement may lead to difficulties in latch and to mastitis. Engorgement should not be confused with a plugged milk duct, which can result in a localized lump in one area of the breast (Table 9-1). Engorgement also may occur later in the course of breastfeeding related to a missed feeding or an abrupt change in feeding frequency. (See Chapter 9.)

1. *Signs and Symptoms.* Engorgement usually occurs around the time of increased milk production on days 3 to 7, and can be most severe in primiparous women. The breasts become swollen, warm, and tender. In severe cases, the nipples can become flattened to the point the baby cannot grasp them. Engorgement is sometimes confused with mastitis, but with engorgement the temperature will rarely be higher than 38°C, systemic symptoms are absent, and the white blood cell count is normal. The swelling and tenderness of engorged breasts are bilateral, generalized, and not unilateral or localized as in an infection (See Table 9-1).

2. *Causes.* Engorgement may be the result of infrequent or ineffective nursing from such causes as sore nipples, a sleepy baby, or mother-baby separation. Engorgement is potentiated by vascular congestion, either due to hormonal responses or obstructed lymphatic drainage.

3. *Evaluation.* Examination of the breasts should be undertaken visually and by palpation of all aspects of both breasts, particularly noting redness, induration, tenderness, and asymmetry.

4. *Management.* The treatment is frequent and effective milk removal (Table 7-8). Once the engorgement is relieved, the mother needs to take steps to prevent its recurrence. Mothers should have ready access to an efficient pump or be trained in manual expression if separated from their infants.

TABLE 7-8. MANAGEMENT OF BREAST ENGORGEMENT

Moist warm packs for 20 minutes or a warm shower before feeding to encourage milk flow

Gentle massage of the breast with hand expression to ease attachment of the infant to the breast

Frequent and effective feedings every 1 to 3 hours

Frequent and effective draining of the breast by hand or pump if mother and baby are separated, or if the breast is so tense that latch is not possible

Cold packs for 20 minutes after feeding

Supportive bra to provide comfort to the heavy breasts

Analgesics (ibuprofen or acetaminophen) (See Chapter 6.)

V. Discharge Planning

A. **Education/Anticipatory Guidance.** The success of breastfeeding is measured in the duration of breastfeeding and of exclusive breastfeeding, not in the initiation of breastfeeding alone. Anticipatory attention to the needs of the mother and baby at the time of discharge from the hospital facilitates successful, long-term breastfeeding. It is assumed that the family had adequate preparation for breastfeeding during prenatal education sessions. Building on this, the patient should again receive basic education regarding breastfeeding. The education should be simple, targeted, and culturally sensitive, and recognize that hormonal factors and maternal fatigue may precipitate information overload.

1. *General Education.* This should include information about infant positioning, latch-on, expected feeding and elimination patterns, jaundice, and signs that warrant physician notification, which can be communicated in infant care classes given prior to discharge and individual instruction, and with the use of noncommercial literature or video presentations. Mothers should be given information on reputable local breastfeeding support groups. Short hospitalizations and limited extended family assistance

heighten the need for adequate support after hospital discharge. Support groups increase women's confidence in their breastfeeding abilities. Strategies that provide face-to-face contact seem to be most effective, but providing a 24-hour telephone source for assistance is also valuable. Breastfeeding mothers should receive instruction on manual and mechanical milk expression methods so that they can maintain their milk supply and obtain milk for feeding if the mother and infant are separated. Discharge packs containing infant formula, pacifiers, and/or commercial advertising materials should not be given to a breastfeeding mother. The spouse and other family members should also be encouraged to provide assistance for the new mother in a way that is supportive of breastfeeding. They may assist with the evaluation of breastfeeding, burping, cuddling, carrying, and bathing the infant, as well as helping the mother with other household chores.

2. ***Basic Breast Care.*** Information regarding basic breast care should also be given to the mother. She should be instructed that little special care is required outside of avoiding the use of harsh soaps and detergents directly on the nipple and areola. The use of a comfortable, non-constraining nursing bra during lactation is advised. If an underwire-type bra is used, care should be taken to ensure that it fits properly and does not compress any tissue, which could lead to poor drainage and the potential for plugged ducts. The woman should also be counseled regarding the use of breast pads to absorb leakage. These can either be reusable pads made of cloth or disposable pads. If disposable pads are chosen, those backed with plastic liners should be avoided to reduce the possibility of inducing sore nipples from constantly being moist. Reusable pads should be changed frequently (when moist) and laundered.

B. **Maternal Nutrition.** Recommendations for healthy eating should also be given to the new mother. Care should be taken to avoid implying that her milk will not be adequate if her diet is not perfectly balanced. (See Chapter 9.)

C. **Contraception.** The new mother should be asked about plans for contraception prior to hospital discharge. This should be addressed again at the postpartum visit. The patient should be counseled that she might require the use of a vaginal lubricant to treat vaginal dryness during lactation. Various contraceptive options affect lactation in different ways. (See Chapter 13.)

D. **Follow-up**

   1. *General Support.* Every breastfeeding mother should be provided with names and phone numbers of individuals who can provide advice on a 24-hour-a-day basis, as well as on a less intensive basis. Although the primary physicians' offices provide general support to the breastfeeding mother, other community-based resources exist, such as peer support groups (eg, La Leche League). Contact information should be shared and mothers encouraged to participate.

   2. *Pediatric Follow-up.* Before discharge, an appointment should be made for an office visit when the infant is 3 to 5 days old. (See Chapter 8.) If the mother is ready for discharge but the infant is not, every effort should be made to allow the mother to remain in the hospital either as a continuing patient or as a "mother-in-residence" with access to the infant for continued exclusive breastfeeding.

   3. *Maternal Follow-up.* Assessment of breastfeeding should be an integral part of the postpartum obstetric evaluation. If the woman has undergone cesarean delivery, she may be seen at 1 to 2 weeks after delivery. (See Chapter 9) At the routine 4- to 6-week postpartum visit the obstetric care professional should assess breastfeeding and provide support for the patient's decision to breastfeed. (See Chapter 9.)

E. **Return to Work.** The physician can discuss plans with the new mother who intends soon after delivery to return to work outside the home or to attend school. The timing of the return to work and a plan to adjust the infant's feedings and the milk supply should be discussed well before the anticipated date of return. (See Chapters 8 and 10.)

F. **Continued Communication Among Caregivers.** Any issues
that are brought up regarding breastfeeding that could affect
the breastfed child should be communicated from the obstetric
care professional to the pediatric care professional (and reverse,
as appropriate).

Selected References

Dewey KG, Nommsen-Rivers LA, Heinig MJ, Cohen RJ. Risk factors for suboptimal infant breastfeeding behavior, delayed onset of lactation, and excess
neonatal weight loss. *Pediatrics.* 2003;112:607–619

Eidelman AI. Hypoglycemia and the breastfed neonate. *Pediatr Clin North Am.*
2001;48:377–387

Howard CR, Howard FM, Lanphear B, deBliecki EA, Eberly S, Lawrence RA. The
effects of early pacifier use on breastfeeding duration. *Pediatrics.* 1999;
103:e33

Merewood A, Philipp BL. Implementing change: becoming baby-friendly in an
inner city hospital. *Birth.* 2001;28:36–40

Neifert MR. Early assessment of the breastfeeding infant. *Contemp Pediatr.*
1996;13:142–166

Neifert MR. Clinical aspects of lactation. *Clin Perinatol.* 1999;26:281–306

Neifert MR. Prevention of breastfeeding tragedies. *Pediatr Clin North Am.*
2001;48:273–297

Wight NE. Management of common breastfeeding issues. *Pediatr Clin North Am.*
2001;48:321–344

Chapter 8

Maintenance of Breastfeeding—The Infant

Skilled anticipatory guidance and positive support are critical to the maintenance of lactation. A good understanding by the physician of common breastfeeding issues can help to foster a growing, healthy infant and a mother with a good milk supply who is comfortable and confident with breastfeeding. Issues common to breastfeeding maintenance in the infant are addressed in this chapter.

I. **Insufficient Milk Syndrome**

The lack of milk, either real or perceived, is a common reason for discontinuing breastfeeding. Insufficient milk syndrome is an imprecise term because it refers to failure of mother's milk production, either primary or secondary, or failure of the infant to extract milk. Because most infants leave the hospital between 24 and 72 hours of age, insufficient intake and dehydration are problems that may be seen in follow-up. However, problems that arise from insufficient intake can be prevented with appropriate interventions.

A. **Signs and symptoms** in the infant of insufficient intake include delayed bowel movements, decreased urinary output, early jaundice, an inconsolably hungry baby, lethargy, and/or a loss of more than 7% of birth weight. Generally, there are noticeable abnormalities in milk supply (Table 7-3), feeding (Table 7-4), and elimination patterns (Table 7-7).

B. **Causes** of insufficient milk intake either may be related to failure of the mother to produce milk or failure of the infant to extract milk. (See Tables 7-1, 7-2, 8-1.) Although primary lactation failure is rare (and often heralded by a lack of breast growth during pregnancy), delayed lactogenesis stage 2 may occur with retained placental fragments, primary pituitary insufficiency, diabetes, or certain maternal medications. Mothers who have had breast surgery are also at risk of insufficient milk production and/or inability to transfer the milk, especially if nerves and ducts have been severed. (See Chapter 3.) Insufficient milk supply more commonly is caused by inappropriate early feeding routines, including the use of supplements. Occasionally an infant may not be able to extract milk effectively, leading to a gradual decrease in milk supply. Such is the case with orally fed premature infants, especially borderline premature infants (34–37 weeks) and infants with neurologic problems or oral anomalies. Any factor that limits milk removal may result in diminished milk synthesis because local factors in the breast govern milk production. (See Local Regulation of Milk Production in Chapter 4 [page 51] to read about feedback inhibitor of lactation.)

C. **Evaluation.** A review of the perinatal history (Tables 7-1 and 7-2) will often identify maternal and/or infant factors to be addressed. A mother whose breasts did not enlarge during pregnancy, or do not become full by 5 days postpartum, may

---

TABLE 8-1. POTENTIAL CAUSES OF PRIMARY INSUFFICIENT MILK SYNDROME

Anatomic variants of the breast

    Breast hypoplasia

    Tubular breasts

    Marked breast asymmetry

Breast surgery

    Reduction

    Augmentation

    Breast abscess

    Breast cancer

    Radiation therapy

Endocrine abnormalities

    Pituitary insufficiency

---

have structural or hormonal problems resulting in inadequate milk supply. Direct observation of a breastfeeding may reveal improper latch, positioning, or inadequate infant effort. Objective measures of infant growth should be performed before beginning any intervention. Although significant weight loss usually indicates a problem with milk supply and/or transfer of milk to the infant, weight loss also may occur in infants with increased insensible water loss from hospital radiant warmers or from prolonged crying episodes. It also should be noted that weight loss may be an artifact of the scale. Electronic infant scales are available that can accurately measure pre- and post-feeding weights to estimate the volume of milk ingested (Chapter 11). One report that evaluated infants in the first few weeks found a high predictability of maternal lactation insufficiency if the weight change from before to after the feeding was less than 45 g. Manual milk expression or mechanical milk expression techniques may be needed to ascertain total milk volume before feeding or residual milk volume in the breast after a feeding. If the residual milk volume is high (>30 mL), this may be a reason for concern. It should be understood that these extra measures may contribute to the mother's feeling of inadequacy as opposed to less invasive procedures such as observing a feeding or performing a physical examination.

D. **Management.** The major goal in management is to increase milk production and milk transfer.

1. *Primary management* depends on the cause but usually involves increasing the frequency and effectiveness of breastfeeding. Mothers also may need to mechanically express milk after each breastfeeding to increase stimulation and breast drainage.

2. *Supplementation* adversely affects establishing a full milk supply by decreasing the frequency and completeness of breast draining, leading to milk stasis and reduced milk supply. However, supplementation is necessary if milk production does not increase with increased frequency of breastfeeding with the infant properly latched on, milk supply is markedly inadequate, or signs of dehydration and/or malnutrition already are present.

3. **Supplements** are given when there is inadequate milk intake. Fluids preferred for supplementation are expressed mother's own milk, pasteurized donor human milk (if available), or infant formula. Glucose water is not a preferred fluid. Glucose water provides significantly fewer calories and no alternate substrates and does not stimulate intestinal motility as does milk. Depending on the circumstances, if dehydration and/or malnutrition are present, the infant should be given enough supplemental milk to produce improved weight gain. Breastfeeding should continue with the addition of the supplemental milk after nursing. Sometimes only 1 to 2 oz of supplemental milk are needed per feeding. At the same time, the mother should continue milk expression techniques to increase milk production. As milk production increases, the need for supplemental fluids will diminish.

4. **Perceived Inadequate Milk Supply.** If the objective evaluation reveals that milk supply is adequate, it is important to reassure the mother that her milk supply is adequate and provide her with the knowledge to assess its adequacy. Even with appropriate prenatal education, many women and many cultures do not appreciate that colostrum is milk, and that the volumes produced in the first 2 to 5 days (2–20 mL per feeding) are adequate for the infant.

II. Jaundice

The association between breastfeeding and jaundice is observed in 2 distinct entities: *breastfeeding jaundice* and *breastmilk jaundice*.

A. **Breastfeeding Jaundice.** Severe jaundice is the most frequent reason for readmission of term and near-term infants. Many of these infants are breastfed. Poor breastfeeding management is often a contributing factor. Severe jaundice may be part of the clinical picture of the dehydrated, malnourished breastfed infant in the first week after birth. (See Insufficient Milk Syndrome on page 101.) Markedly elevated levels of unconjugated serum bilirubin, usually greater than approximately 25 mg/dL, may cause *acute bilirubin encephalopathy* manifest as lethargy, hypotonia, and poor feeding that progresses to chronic encephalopathy, known as *kernicterus*, with permanent brain injury manifest by athetoid cerebral palsy, auditory dysfunction, and paralysis of upward gaze. In recent years approximately 75% of infants who had kernicterus were breastfed. This almost always is a preventable outcome.

1. **Signs and Symptoms.** In their first week these infants have rising serum unconjugated bilirubin levels and poor milk intake. Usually a history is obtained of decreased maternal milk production and/or poor milk intake by the infant. Dehydration, weight loss, failure to gain weight, and/or hypernatremia also may be observed. (See Insufficient Milk Syndrome on page 101 and Tables 7-1 and 7-2.) Borderline premature infants of 35 to 37 weeks' gestation have been noted to be at particularly high risk for developing kernicterus, especially if breastfeeding. Clinicians cannot assume that these infants feed like term infants. In the hospital, these infants seem to feed adequately because milk production has not maximized. Once home, as milk production increases, these premature infants may not be capable of ingesting larger volumes. Thus they often have more breastfeeding problems and also have less well-developed hepatic mechanisms for disposal of bilirubin. Closer observation of borderline premature infants is indicated.

2. **Causes.** Breastfed infants who have an insufficient milk intake during the early days may have an increase in serum unconjugated bilirubin due to an exaggerated enterohepatic circulation of bilirubin. This entity also is known as *breast non-feeding jaundice* because it is similar to *starvation jaundice* in adults.

3. **Evaluation** is similar to that for insufficient milk syndrome. Serum total, unconjugated, and conjugated bilirubin should be monitored initially, then total serum bilirubin should be followed serially. Other causes of jaundice (hemolytic, infection, metabolic) should be considered to ensure optimal overall management.

4. **Management**

    a. Establishment of good breastfeeding practices that ensure adequate milk production and adequate intake of milk by the infant will prevent *breastfeeding jaundice.* (See Management on page 103.)

b. A plot of serum bilirubin on a bilirubin nomogram prior to discharge is helpful to predict future risk.

c. Follow up all breastfed infants on the third to fifth day after birth to assess general health and breastfeeding competency, as well as for the presence of jaundice. Early detection of jaundice will permit correction of any breastfeeding problems and initiation of diagnostic procedures.

d. Close monitoring of serum bilirubin is necessary to determine when to initiate phototherapy and/or perform an exchange transfusion. Breastfed infants should follow the same criteria for intervention as formula-fed infants. AAP recommendations have been published.

e. Breastfed infants usually may continue to receive human milk if phototherapy is initiated.

B. **Breastmilk Jaundice.** In many breastfed infants, serum unconjugated bilirubin concentrations will remain elevated, and in a few infants this may last for as long as 6 to 12 weeks. In formula-fed infants serum bilirubin levels decline, reaching values of less than 1.5 mg/dL by the 11th or 12th day after birth. In contrast, by week 3, 65% of normal, thriving breastfed infants have serum bilirubin concentrations above 1.5 mg/dL, and 30% will be clinically jaundiced. It has been suggested that the elevation in serum bilirubin may be protective against oxidative injury because bilirubin has been shown to be an effective antioxidant in vitro.

1. *Signs and Symptoms.* Because this is a normal response to breastfeeding, other than jaundice, the infants appear healthy and are thriving. The infants are growing normally and manifest no abnormal clinical signs, suggesting hemolysis, infection, or metabolic disease.

2. *Causes.* Mature human milk contains an unidentified factor that enhances the intestinal absorption of bilirubin resulting in *breastmilk jaundice.* As the production of the factor diminishes over time and the infant's liver matures, serum bilirubin concentrations eventually return to normal.

3. *Evaluation*

   a. Evaluate severity of jaundice based on cephalocaudal progression of jaundice.

   b. Check total serum bilirubin if clinical examination indicates elevated level.

   c. Check unconjugated and conjugated bilirubin if jaundice persists (eg, >3 weeks).

   d. Ensure no other etiologies of prolonged unconjugated hyperbilirubinemia.

       i.   Galactosemia

       ii. Hypothyroidism

       iii. Urinary tract infection

       iv. Pyloric stenosis

       v.   Low-grade hemolysis

4. *Management*

   a. Breastfeeding should be continued.

   b. Parents should be reassured.

   c. Persistent rise in serum bilirubin may necessitate a diagnostic challenge by interrupting breastfeeding for 24 to 48 hours. Following interruption of breastfeeding, the serum bilirubin will decline markedly and not rise to prior levels with resumption of breastfeeding.

   d. If breastfeeding is interrupted, the mother should be encouraged and helped to maintain her milk supply.

   e. The mother may be reluctant to resume breastfeeding because of the association between breastfeeding and jaundice. A positive attitude on the part of the health care professionals and assurance that this will not occur later may avoid termination of breastfeeding.

III. **Appetite and/or growth spurts** are considered "transient lactational crises."

   A. **Signs and Symptoms.** The infant acts hungrier than usual and may not be satisfied, leading the mother to believe her milk supply is insufficient and that she should start supplemental fluids or introduce complementary foods to satisfy her baby's appetite.

B. **Causes.** Approximately one third of breastfeeding mothers experience these "spurts" one or more times during lactation; most occur during the first 3 months of lactation (typically around 2–3 weeks, 6 weeks, and 3 months) and are of short duration.

C. **Evaluation.** History and physical examination are unchanged. Verify that no new medications have been introduced.

D. **Management.** Extra breastfeeding over a few days will stimulate an increased milk supply to enable the infant to resume a more normal feeding pattern. Anticipatory guidance regarding infant feeding patterns often eliminates supplementation and premature weaning. If the problem persists more than 3 or 4 days, the nursing dyad should be evaluated to determine the adequacy of the mother's milk supply and the infant's weight gain.

IV. Nursing Refusal

A. **Signs and Symptoms.** An infant's sudden refusal to nurse, often called a nursing strike, can occur at any time and is often perceived by the mother as a personal rejection or as evidence that her milk is bad or inadequate. The mother frequently responds by weaning.

B. **Causes.** Nursing strikes are patterns of infant behavior that are associated either with the onset of the mother's menses; change in maternal diet; a change in maternal soap, perfume, or deodorant; or maternal stress. Infant nasal obstruction, gastroesophageal reflux disease, and teething also can cause nursing strikes. The older breastfeeding infant might suddenly refuse to nurse when the mother goes back to work, the infant is offered a bottle, or there is separation of the dyad. Occasionally infants will refuse to feed from one breast. Sometimes this occurs after an episode of mastitis when the milk tastes slightly saltier. If the reason can be identified and changed, nursing will usually resume quickly.

C. **Evaluation.** History and physical examination are unchanged.

D. **Management.** When a baby refuses the breast, efforts to restore breastfeeding may take several days or longer. Infants may nurse more willingly when they are sleepy or just awakening. Other methods to reestablish the nursing relationship include making feeding special and quiet with no distractions; increasing the amount of cuddling and stroking, including skin-to-skin care; and using cobathing as a relaxation, reattachment strategy. Avoiding the bottle and using other methods of feeding, such as cup feeding, are often successful in overcoming breast refusal. Mothers should be advised to maintain their milk supply by manual or mechanical expression techniques so breast refusal is not compounded by insufficient maternal milk supply.

V. **Ankyloglossia,** commonly known as tongue-tie, is a congenital oral anomaly that may result in difficulty with suckling and could lead to sore nipples, low milk supply, poor weight gain, maternal fatigue, and frustration. It may affect breastfeeding more than bottle-feeding because of the differences in tongue movements.

A. **Signs and Symptoms.** The infant is unable to extend the tongue forward over the gum line, preventing peristaltic compression of the nipple and areola, reducing the effectiveness of the suckling effort. Milk intake may be low and the infant may become frustrated. Frantic suckling may traumatize the nipple. Maternal pain may lead to withdrawal of the breast and/or inhibition of milk let-down.

B. **Cause.** Abnormally short and/or thick lingual frenulum.

C. **Evaluation.** Careful oral evaluation of the infant is needed, assessing the ability to extend the tongue beyond the lower gum border and observing for restriction of tongue mobility. The mother should be evaluated for nipple pain or evidence of nipple trauma. Impending lactation failure is an indication for the surgical procedure.

D. **Management.** The anterior portion of a tight or thick frenulum may be divided with a scissors in a procedure called frenotomy. Anesthesia is not usually required and suturing is not necessary. The infant should be observed for bleeding from the site of division, although this is usually minimal or absent because the ligament binding the tongue is relatively avascular. The infant can be put to the breast a few minutes after the procedure.

VI. Growth Patterns of Breastfed Infants

The conclusions drawn from plotting the growth of a breastfed infant on some growth charts may be erroneous if the growth chart does not adequately reflect the normal growth of the breast-feeding infant.

A. **Growth Charts.** The Centers for Disease Control and Prevention (CDC) May 2000 growth charts include a more heterogenous group of infants than earlier charts, but still include relatively few infants who were breastfed for more than a few months. The CDC growth charts show that healthy breastfed infants maintain their length-for-age percentiles but may show slight reductions in weight-for-age percentiles beginning at 8 months. Studies attempting to provide additional food to breastfed infants in later infancy failed to change this pattern of weight gain. Most authorities assume this is normal growth of the breastfed infant. The World Health Organization (WHO) currently is developing a new international reference based on growth of healthy infants optimally breastfed throughout the first year.

B. **Growth faltering** is a concern when the weight-for-age (or weight-for-length) is more than 2 standard deviations below the mean or over a period of time weight-for-age crosses more than 2 percentile channels downward on the growth chart. Nutritional assessment of the infant with slow weight gain or faltering linear growth includes an evaluation of milk supply and infant intake, appropriateness of complementary foods, intake of micronutrients (eg, zinc, vitamin D), and the feeding environment. The principles in the assessment of insufficient milk syndrome also should be considered for these infants. Published data on the growth of exclusively breastfed girls and boys during the first year may assist in evaluating an infant whose growth is questionable (Table 8-2).

TABLE 8-2. AVERAGE OF MEAN VALUES FOR PUBLISHED GAINS IN WEIGHT FOR HEALTHY EXCLUSIVELY BREASTFED INFANTS

Interval (months)	Girls (g/d)	Boys (g/d)
0–1	30	33
1–2	28	34
2–3	22	23
3–4	19	20
4–5	15	16
5–6	13	14
6–7	12	11
7–8	10	12
8–9	8	9
9–10	11	10
10–11	8	6
11–12	7	9

Adapted with permission from J Pediatr. 1994;124:32–39 and Pediatrics. 1992;89:1035.

VII. Vitamin and Mineral Supplementation

A. Fat-Soluble Vitamins

1. *Vitamin K* deficiency results in hypoprothrombinemia and hemorrhage. Vitamin K sufficiency depends on production by the intestinal flora. The gut of the newborn is essentially sterile and the intestinal flora of the breastfed infant produce relatively less vitamin K. The content of vitamin K in human milk is low. Therefore, to ensure vitamin sufficiency, a single dose of vitamin K (0.5–1.0 mg IM) is given to all newborns at delivery (Chapter 2).

2. *Vitamin D* requirements can be met by sunlight exposure, but it is not possible to define what is adequate sunlight exposure for a given infant. Furthermore, in recent

years concern about the risk of later skin cancer has led to
the recommendation against sunlight exposure even in
young infants, and for the use of sunscreen ointments,
which also reduce cutaneous vitamin D production. An
adequate intake of vitamin D for infants (200 IU/day) is
not met with human milk alone. Cases of rickets in
infants caused by inadequate vitamin D intake and limited exposure to sunlight have been reported. Thus
infants who are breastfed, without supplements of vitamin D, are at increased risk of rickets. A dose of 200
IU/day started by 2 months is recommended. Maternal
dietary supplementation does not preclude the need for
infant vitamin D supplementation.

3. ***Vitamin A*** supplementation is not needed in the breastfed infant in most areas of the world. In some developing
countries, vitamin A deficiency has been found in breastfed infants and children.

B. **Water-soluble vitamin** concentrations in human milk may
be affected by maternal diet. This only becomes a problem if
the mother's diet lacks adequate intakes of water-soluble vitamins. Maternal malnutrition and alcoholism are situations
where nutritional rehabilitation should include a multivitamin
supplement for the mother. Mothers who are strict vegetarians (vegans) may not receive adequate vitamin B_{12} from their
diet alone, and this may result in low B_{12} concentrations in
their milk. Their infants may present with vitamin B_{12} deficiency without obvious symptoms in the mother. Therefore,
vegan mothers should receive a multivitamin supplement to
ensure adequate availability of micronutrients. In these circumstances, water-soluble vitamin supplements do not need
to be given to the infant.

C. **Multivitamins** should be given to human milk–fed premature infants.

D. **Iron** reserves present at birth are a critical factor determining
the risk of anemia during infancy. In normal full-term infants,
who generally have adequate iron reserves, there is little risk
of anemia with exclusive breastfeeding prior to 9 months of
age, although biochemical indices of low iron status may

occur in some between 6 and 9 months. At about 6 months, iron should be given in the form of iron-containing or iron-fortified complementary foods, or iron drops can be given (1 mg/kg/day). Iron-fortified infant cereal and/or meats are good sources of iron. The risk of iron deficiency anemia is much greater in premature or low birth weight infants because the iron stores at birth are smaller. Iron needs for such infants are likely to be best met by an iron supplement (2 mg/kg/day) beginning by 2 months. The dose of iron provided by multivitamin preparations containing iron is not likely to meet the needs of the breastfed premature infant.

E. **Fluoride** supplementation of breastfed infants is not recommended during the first 6 months. Thereafter, if the local water supply is less than 0.3 ppm, a supplement of 0.25 mg/day is recommended. Maternal fluoride intake does not affect the fluoride content of human milk.

VIII.   Complementary Feeding (Duration of Exclusive Breastfeeding)

The timing of introduction of complementary foods into the diet of the breastfed infant is difficult to define with precision, and indeed there may not be a single optimal age for all infants. The recommendations by the WHO and others for exclusive breastfeeding for approximately 6 months are intended for populations, and do not dictate the management for individual infants. The AAP and ACOG recommend exclusive breastfeeding for the first 6 months.* Most authorities recognize that many infants are developmentally ready to accept complementary foods prior to this time. There are some data demonstrating additional benefits to exclusive breastfeeding for 6 months compared with 4 months, especially in developed countries. Decisions about the introduction of complementary foods for individual infants need to be based on a number of

---

* There is a difference of opinion among AAP experts on this matter. The Committee on Nutrition supports introduction of complementary foods between 4 and 6 months of age where safe and nutritious complementary foods are available, while the Section on Breastfeeding recommends exclusive breastfeeding for the first 6 months of life.

considerations, including birth weight, postnatal growth rate, and developmental readiness. Infants who were born prematurely or small for gestational age may need micronutrients provided by complementary foods earlier, especially iron and zinc. To delay the introduction of complementary foods beyond 6 months is not recommended due to increasing risk of micronutrient deficiencies.

IX. Sleep Patterns

Lack of sleep, in mother and infant, is a frequent parental concern. Parent and physician expectations regarding sleep are shaped by cultural norms, which may not be based on normal physiology.

A. **Mother.** In early stages of establishing breastfeeding, it is important that the infant nurse at least 8 to 12 times per 24 hours, which implies feedings at least every 1.5 to 3 hours, including during the night. Mothers with continuous rooming-in during hospitalization sleep for the same duration as mothers whose infants are taken to the nursery. Once a mother's milk supply is well established, a single, longer sleep interval of about 5 hours may be possible for some term infants, but is not the norm for exclusively breastfed infants in the first 2 to 3 months.

B. **Cosleeping.** The concern of nighttime feedings can be lessened by allowing the infant to sleep in close proximity to the mother, enabling intermittent nursing throughout the night while leaving the mother's sleep relatively undisturbed. Some families may prefer a cosleeper attachment to the bed or a bedside bassinet. Bedsharing, or cosleeping, is the most common sleeping arrangement for most of the world, including developed countries, and has beneficial effects on the success of breastfeeding. Families who choose this type of sleeping arrangement need guidelines for safe cosleeping because bed sharing may be hazardous under certain conditions. If a mother chooses to have her infant sleep in her bed to breastfeed, care should be taken to use a supine sleep position, avoid soft surfaces or loose covers, avoid waterbeds, and ensure that no entrapment possibilities exist. Adults (other than parents), children, or other siblings should avoid sharing a bed with an infant. Obese parents should not sleep with an infant. Parents who choose to share a bed with their infant should not smoke or use substances, such as alcohol or drugs, which may impair arousal.

X. Dental Health

The risk of dental decay exists for the breastfed child as it does for the bottle-fed child. Early childhood dental caries results from a complicated combination of factors including genetics, general nutrition, preventive dental care, and the presence or absence of *Streptococcus mutans,* which usually is acquired from the mother or another adult through close oral contact. Breastfeeding has been implicated in the disease, but population-based studies do not support a definitive link between prolonged breastfeeding and dental caries. Children should see a dentist as early as 6 months and no later than 6 months after the first tooth erupts or 12 months of age (whichever comes first).

XI. Infant illness, such as fever, upper respiratory infection, colds, or diarrhea, is reduced overall if breastfeeding is maintained.

Because of its low solute load, human milk enables the ill infant to maintain hydration despite fever, diarrhea, or other increased fluid losses. Continued breastfeeding helps lessen the severity and duration of the diarrhea and helps preserve gut mucosal integrity (Chapter 2). With significant respiratory symptoms, an infant may feed better at the breast than with a bottle because the infant has more control over the milk flow and breastfeeding requires less energy expenditure. Human milk can be expressed mechanically and fed via tube if the infant is unable to suckle. In addition to the appropriateness of human milk for a sick infant, there is the added comfort of nursing because of the closeness with the mother.

XII. Readmission to the Hospital

As breastfeeding rates have increased, so have readmissions for excessive weight loss, dehydration, hyperbilirubinemia, and hypernatremia that result from inappropriate breastfeeding routines and inadequate follow-up. During any hospitalizations, efforts should be made to continue breastfeeding while supplying appropriate supplemental nutrition to the infant and providing lactation evaluation and interventions to recover successful breastfeeding. The milk supply should be increased through appropriate feeding routines and, if indicated, mechanical breast pumping. Every effort should be made to keep the mother and infant together. When the breastfeeding mother requires hospitalization, efforts should also be made to continue the breastfeeding relationship either by having the infant stay with the mother through the hospitalization or by bringing the baby to the mother one or more times per day to complement mechanical milk expression. (See Chapter 10.)

XIII. **Breastfeeding Guidance During Preventive Pediatric Health Care Visits**

Lactation is a dynamic process, as is growth and development, so the practitioner should be mindful of the changing agenda at each follow-up visit. Incorporation of breastfeeding assessments, encouragement, and anticipatory guidance may enhance successful breastfeeding outcomes. A summary of key points for each follow-up visit from 3 to 5 days to 12 months of age is found in Tables 8-3 through 8-9.

XIV. **Breastfeeding in the Second Year and Beyond**

Breastfeeding should be continued, with appropriate complementary foods, for as long as the mother and infant mutually desire. In societies where children are allowed to nurse as long as they wish, they usually self-wean, with no arguments or emotional trauma, between 3 and 4 years of age. Physicians may be surprised to discover that their patients are actually nursing much longer than they believe. Mothers may fail to disclose that they are continuing to nurse an older infant or child because they perceive that their physician may not approve of or support their continued breastfeeding.

The studies demonstrating advantages of breastfeeding for infants and mothers suggest that many of the benefits are directly related to the duration of breastfeeding. The composition of human milk does not change markedly from

12 to 24 months, including most nutrients and bioactive factors. Because the human immune system may not mature completely for several years, the constituents of human milk continue to support host defense of the infant. Breastfeeding also promotes comfort and caring. A strong attachment to the mother during the early years may have a positive neurobehavioral effect. Long-term breastfeeding seems to be a mutually positive experience for mother and child.

XV. **Weaning** can mean either the beginning of a process of gradual introduction of complementary feedings and decreased breastfeeding or the complete cessation of breastfeeding. Weaning is a complex process involving nutritional, microbiological, immunologic, biochemical, and psychological adjustments.

A. **Infant-led weaning** can be confused with a nursing strike. Reasons commonly cited when infants attempt to wean from the breast include inadequate milk supply (eg, due to illness, return to work) and infant illness.

B. **Mother-led weaning** should be done gradually by replacing one feeding at a time with solids, a bottle, or a cup, depending on the infant's age and stage of development. The bedtime breastfeeding is often the last to be eliminated. Occasionally sudden weaning is necessary because of severe illness in the mother or prolonged separation of the mother and infant. Mothers should use manual or mechanical methods of milk expression to relieve breast fullness; wear a supportive, comfortable bra; and be alert to signs of a plugged duct or breast infection. Other measures such as cold compresses may help in reducing engorgement. Rapid weaning may increase the mother's risk of developing mastitis. The infant should receive extra cuddling and holding, as should the mother.

TABLE 8-3. FIRST NEWBORN OFFICE VISIT: 3 TO 5 DAYS OF AGE (48 TO 72 HOURS AFTER DISCHARGE)

Breastfeeding Assessment

- What is the number of feedings in last 24 hours?
- What is the number of wet diapers in last 24 hours?
- What is the number of stools in last 24 hours?
- Does newborn need to be awakened to feed?
- Does newborn easily latch on to breast and nurse eagerly?
- Is newborn receiving any vitamin, mineral, or dietary supplements or non-milk liquids?
- How is mother doing and how is she feeling about breastfeeding?
- Are mother's breasts comfortable (not tender or painful)?
- Has mother previously breastfed?
- Is mother taking any medications or dietary supplements?
- How is mother's nutrition?
- Does mother have weight reduction diet or other dietary restrictions?
- How do family members feel about breastfeeding?

Examining Newborn and Mother

- Calculate newborn's weight gain or loss since birth.
- Perform routine newborn examination with attention to oral-motor examination.
- Assess state of hydration.
- Observe for jaundice.
- Observe breastfeeding.
- Examine mother's breasts or refer for examination, if needed.
- Consider using test weight to estimate volume of milk consumed by newborn if there is concern regarding adequacy of intake.

Anticipatory Guidance

- Encourage breastfeeding on demand.
- Review normal breastfeeding patterns.
- Discourage use of pacifiers and discuss potential risks.
- Avoid long nighttime intervals without feeding.
- Review normal elimination patterns.
- Reinforce the importance of the care of the mother.

Breastfeeding Interventions

- Attempt to determine and treat the cause of inadequate milk supply before supplementing.
- Consider referral to lactation specialist if problems are ongoing.
- Identify an appropriate peer support group.

Closing the Visit

- Congratulate parents on decision to breastfeed their newborn.
- Review some of the benefits of breastfeeding.
- Remind mother to take the time to establish regular food and fluid intakes to meet her needs.
- Arrange for appropriate follow-up until weight gain is adequate and breastfeeding is going well.

Adapted from Checklists for Breastfeeding Health Supervision. *Elk Grove Village, IL: American Academy of Pediatrics; 1999.*

TABLE 8-4. 1-MONTH OFFICE VISIT

Breastfeeding Assessment

■ What is infant's feeding pattern?

■ What is the number of feedings per 24 hours?

■ Is infant breastfeeding on demand?

■ What is the number of wet diapers and stools per 24 hours?

■ Is infant receiving any vitamin, mineral, or dietary supplements or non-milk liquids?

■ How is mother feeling?

■ How does mother perceive her milk supply?

■ Evaluate mother's nutrition.

■ Does mother have weight reduction diet or other dietary restrictions?

■ How do family members feel about breastfeeding?

Examining Newborn and Mother

■ Calculate newborn's weight change since birth and since previous visit. (Table 8-2)

■ Complete examination.

■ Observe breastfeeding if weight gain is inadequate or feeding ineffective.

■ Consider using test weight to estimate volume of milk consumed by infant if there is concern regarding adequacy of intake.

Anticipatory Guidance

- Usually breastfeeding 8 to 12 times per 24 hours.
- Encourage unrestricted breastfeeding.
- Discuss and encourage exclusive human milk feedings.
- Review importance of continuing nighttime feedings.
- Discourage use of pacifiers and discuss potential risks.
- Discuss vitamin D supplement by 2 months.
- Discuss mother's plans to return to school or work.
- Review maternal nutrition.
- Explain techniques for expressing and storing milk.
- Discuss common over-the-counter medications.
- Remind mother to have postpartum visit with breast examination and family planning discussion.

Breastfeeding Interventions

- Attempt to determine and treat the cause of inadequate milk supply before supplementing.
- Consider referral to lactation specialist if problems are ongoing.

Closing the Visit

- Commend mother on ongoing breastfeeding success.
- Review some of the benefits of breastfeeding.
- Encourage continued breastfeeding if baby is to be enrolled in a child care program (See Chapter 10).

Adapted from Checklists for Breastfeeding Health Supervision. *Elk Grove Village, IL: American Academy of Pediatrics; 1999.*

TABLE 8-5. 2-MONTH OFFICE VISIT

Breastfeeding Assessment

- What is infant's feeding pattern?
- Is infant content with feedings?
- Is infant breastfeeding on demand?
- Has infant had any feedings other than human milk?
- How does mother feel?
- How does mother perceive her milk supply?
- Is mother taking any medications or dietary supplements?
- How is mother's nutrition?
- Is mother restricting any foods?
- How do family members feel about breastfeeding?

Examining Infant and Mother

- Calculate infant's weight change since birth and since previous visit. (Table 8-2)
- Routine examination.
- Observe breastfeeding if weight gain is inadequate or feeding ineffective.

Anticipatory Guidance

- Usually breastfeeding 8 to 12 times per 24 hours.

- Encourage unrestricted breastfeeding.

- Review importance of nighttime feedings.

- Discuss exclusive human milk feedings.

- Stools may become less frequent in normally breastfeeding infant.

- Discuss the breastfeeding infant who is teething.

- Begin vitamin D supplement if not already started.

- Review maternal nutrition.

- Discuss mother's plans to return to school or work.

- Explain techniques for expressing and storing milk.

- Discuss common over-the-counter medications.

- Ascertain that the mother had her postpartum visit.

Breastfeeding Interventions

- Attempt to determine and treat the cause of inadequate milk supply before supplementing.

- Consider referral to lactation specialist if problems are ongoing.

Closing the Visit

- Commend mother on ongoing breastfeeding success.

- Review some of the benefits of breastfeeding.

- Encourage continued breastfeeding if baby is to be enrolled in a child care program. (See Chapter 10.)

Adapted from Checklists for Breastfeeding Health Supervision. *Elk Grove Village, IL: American Academy of Pediatrics; 1999.*

TABLE 8-6. 4-MONTH OFFICE VISIT

Breastfeeding Assessment

- What is baby's feeding pattern?
- Is baby content with feedings?
- Is baby breastfeeding on demand?
- Is the baby's longest sleep pattern at night? If not, when?
- Has baby had any feedings (liquids or solids) other than human milk? If so, what?
- How does mother perceive her milk supply?
- Is mother taking any medications?
- How is mother's nutrition?
- How do family members feel about breastfeeding?
- Has mother returned to work/school or planned to return?

Examining Baby and Mother

- Calculate baby's weight change since birth and since previous visit. (Table 8-2)
- Observe breastfeeding if weight gain is inadequate, feeding is ineffective, or mother has concerns.
- Routine examination.

Anticipatory Guidance

- Usually breastfeeding 6 to 12 times per 24 hours.
- Discuss exclusive human milk feedings until about 6 months of age.
- Encourage unrestricted breastfeeding.
- Review importance of nighttime feedings.
- Stools may become less frequent in normally breastfeeding baby.
- Discuss breastfeeding the baby during teething.
- Discuss the increasing distractibility of the baby during feedings.
- Continue vitamin D supplement.
- Review maternal nutrition.
- Discuss mother's plans to return to school or work.
- Explain techniques for expressing and storing milk.
- Discuss common over-the-counter medications.

Breastfeeding Interventions

- Attempt to determine and treat the cause of inadequate milk supply before supplementing.

Closing the Visit

- Commend mother on ongoing breastfeeding success.
- Review some of the benefits of breastfeeding.

Adapted from Checklists for Breastfeeding Health Supervision. *Elk Grove Village, IL: American Academy of Pediatrics; 1999.*

TABLE 8-7. 6-MONTH OFFICE VISIT

Breastfeeding Assessment

- What is baby's feeding pattern?
- Is baby content with feedings?
- Is the baby's longest sleep period at night? If not, when?
- Has baby had any feedings other than human milk? If so, what?
- How does mother perceive her milk supply?
- Is mother taking any medications?
- How is mother's nutrition?
- How do family members feel about breastfeeding?
- Has mother returned to work/school or planned to return?

Examining Baby and Mother

- Calculate baby's weight change since birth and previous visit. (Table 8-2)
- Observe breastfeeding if weight gain is inadequate.
- Complete examination.

Anticipatory Guidance

- Usually breastfeeding 6 to 12 times per 24 hours.
- Review importance of continued breastfeeding.
- Discuss readiness for introduction of complementary foods. Offer solid foods 1 to 2 times per day.
- Discuss importance of iron-containing foods.
- Discuss offering supplemental fluids in a cup (limit juice to 4 oz per day).
- Discuss the increasing distractibility of the baby during feedings.
- Discuss breastfeeding the baby during teething.
- Introduce fluoride supplement if indicated. Continue vitamin D.

Breastfeeding Interventions

- Discuss plan for breastfeeding and return to work.
- Discuss plan for introducing solid foods.

Closing the Visit

- Commend mother on ongoing breastfeeding success, especially if baby was exclusively breastfed for 6 months.
- Review some of the benefits of continued breastfeeding.

Adapted from Checklists for Breastfeeding Health Supervision. *Elk Grove Village, IL: American Academy of Pediatrics; 1999.*

TABLE 8-8. 9-MONTH OFFICE VISIT

Breastfeeding Assessment

- What is baby's feeding pattern?
- Is the baby's longest sleep period at night? If not, when?
- What other foods does baby take? Is baby receiving iron-containing foods?
- Is baby receiving vitamin D, other supplements?
- Is mother taking any medications?
- How is mother's nutrition?
- How do family members feel about breastfeeding?

Examining Baby and Mother

- Calculate weight change since birth and since previous visit. (Table 8-2)
- Observe breastfeeding if weight gain is inadequate, feeding is ineffective, or mother has concerns.
- Complete examination.
- Obtain hematocrit or hemoglobin measurement.

Anticipatory Guidance

- Usually breastfeeding frequency is decreasing.
- Review importance of continued breastfeeding.
- Continue vitamin D supplement.
- Discuss importance of iron-containing foods and foods rich in protein (meats/poultry).
- Discuss offering supplemental fluids in a cup (limit juices to 4 oz per day).
- Discuss breastfeeding the baby during teething.
- Discuss behavior of the older breastfeeding baby.
- Discuss new communication skills that relate to breastfeeding behaviors.
- Discuss pressure to wean by family or friends.
- Remind mother to have her annual breast examination.
- In the next few months, infant should transition to regularly scheduled feedings.

Breastfeeding Interventions

- If baby is gaining weight and mother is satisfied with feeding behavior, interventions usually are not indicated.

Closing the Visit

- Commend mother on ongoing breastfeeding success.
- Review some of the benefits of breastfeeding.

Adapted from Checklists for Breastfeeding Health Supervision. *Elk Grove Village, IL: American Academy of Pediatrics; 1999.*

TABLE 8-9. 12-MONTH OFFICE VISIT

Breastfeeding Assessment

- What is baby's feeding pattern?
- Is the baby's longest sleep period at night? If not, when?
- What other foods does baby take?
- Is mother taking any medications?
- How is mother's nutrition?
- How do family members feel about breastfeeding?

Examining Baby and Mother

- Calculate weight change since birth and since previous visit.
- Complete examination.
- Consider obtaining hematocrit or hemoglobin measurement, if indicated.

Anticipatory Guidance

- Usually breastfeeding frequency is decreasing.
- Review importance of continued breastfeeding.
- Discuss importance of iron-containing foods.
- Discuss offering supplemental fluids in a cup.
- Discuss breastfeeding the baby during teething.
- Discuss infant eating pattern to include 3 meals and 2–3 snacks per day.
- Discuss behavior of older breastfeeding baby.
- Discuss new communication skills that relate to breastfeeding behaviors.
- Discuss pressure to wean by family or friends.
- Discuss appropriate weaning techniques.
- Review maternal nutrition.
- Recommend that mother obtain routine breast examination from her physician.

Breastfeeding Interventions

- Provide indicated support or intervention.

Closing the Visit

- Commend mother on successfully breastfeeding for 12 months.
- Review some of the benefits of breastfeeding a toddler.

Adapted from Checklists for Breastfeeding Health Supervision. *Elk Grove Village, IL: American Academy of Pediatrics; 1999.*

Selected References

American Academy of Pediatrics Committee on Fetus and Newborn. Controversies concerning vitamin K and the newborn. *Pediatrics.* 2003:112:191–192

American Academy of Pediatrics Work Group on Breastfeeding. *Checklists for Breastfeeding Health Supervision: Breastfeeding Promotion in Pediatric Office Practices.* Elk Grove Village, IL: American Academy of Pediatrics; 1999

American Academy of Pediatrics Section on Dentistry. Oral health risk assessment timing and establishment of the dental home. *Pediatrics.* 2003;111:1113–1116

American Academy of Pediatrics Committee on Nutrition. Complementary feeding. In: Kleinman RE, ed. *Pediatric Nutrition Handbook.* 5th ed. Elk Grove Village, IL: American Academy of Pediatrics; 2004:103–115

American Academy of Pediatrics Task Force on Infant Sleep Position and Sudden Infant Death Syndrome. Changing concepts of sudden infant death syndrome: implications for infant sleeping environment and sleep position. *Pediatrics.* 2000;105:650–656

American Academy of Pediatrics Subcommittee on Hyperbilirubinemia. Management of hyperbilirubinemia in the newborn infant 35 or more weeks of gestation. *Pediatrics.* 2004;114:297–316

Black LS. Incorporating breastfeeding care into daily newborn rounds and pediatric office practice. *Pediatr Clin North Am.* 2001;48:299–319

Dewey KG. Nutrition, growth, and complementary feeding of the breasfed infant. *Pediatr Clin North Am.* 2001;48:87–104

Dewey KG, Heinig MJ, Nommsen LA, Peerson JM, Lonnerdal B. Growth of breast-fed and formula-fed infants from 0 to 18 months: the DARLING study. *Pediatrics.* 1992;89:1035–1041

Gartner LM, Greer FR; American Academy of Pediatrics Section on Breastfeeding, Committee on Nutrition. Prevention of rickets and vitamin D deficiency: new guidelines for vitamin D intake. *Pediatrics.* 2003;111:908–910

Gartner LM, Herschel M. Jaundice and breastfeeding. *Pediatr Clin North Am.* 2001;48:389–399

Griffin IJ, Abrams SA. Iron and breastfeeding. *Pediatr Clin North Am.* 2001;48:401–413

Krebs NF, Reidinger CJ, Robertson AD, Hambidge KM. Growth and intakes of energy and zinc in infants fed human milk. *Pediatrics.* 1994;124:32–39

Kramer MS, Guo T, Platt RW, et al. Infant growth and health outcomes associated with 3 compared with 6 mo of exclusive breastfeeding. *Am J Clin Nutr.* 2003;78:291–295

Kramer MS, Kakuma R. The optimal duration of exclusive breastfeeding: a systematic review. *Adv Exp Med Biol.* 2004;554:63–77

Kreiter SR, Schwartz RP, Kirkman HN Jr, Charlton PA, Calikoglu AS, Davenport ML. Nutritional rickets in African American breast-fed infants. *J Pediatr.* 2000;137:153–157

Neifert MR. Prevention of breastfeeding tragedies. *Pediatr Clin North Am.* 2001;48:273–297

Powers NG. How to assess slow growth in the breastfed infant. Birth to 3 months. *Pediatr Clin North Am.* 2001;48:345–363

■ Chapter 9 ■

Maintenance of Breastfeeding—
The Mother

Support for the breastfeeding mother continues beyond the immediate postpartum period. The obstetric care professional should assess the breast at various postpartum visits and be aware of the evaluation and management of various maternal problems and complications related to lactation.

I. Postpartum Follow-up Visits

A. Routine Obstetric Visit. The mother's routine follow-up visit to her obstetric care professional is scheduled for 4 to 6 weeks postpartum. Obstetric care professionals should encourage the mother to bring the baby to this visit.

1. *Assess Breastfeeding.* This visit is an ideal time to observe the infant breastfeeding, specifically assessing position, latch, and milk transfer. Information about perceived breastfeeding problems or concerns of the mother can be elicited.

2. *Provide Support.* Obstetric support for the patient's decision to breastfeed has been shown to improve breastfeeding continuation. This is an ideal time to praise the success of her breastfeeding experience and allow the patient to explore any of her concerns.

3. *Breast Examination.* The physician should perform a breast examination to evaluate any signs of trauma, infection, or breast masses. It may be helpful to have the mother nurse her infant prior to the examination to decrease engorgement of tissue that could obscure physical

examination findings. The obstetric care professional can also encourage continuation of breastfeeding and point out the recommendations for exclusive breastfeeding. The patient also should be advised to continue her regular breast self-examinations and report any unusual findings to her health care professional.

4. *Plans for Return to Work.* The physician should discuss plans for the new mother to return to work outside the home at this visit, including options for feeding and milk expression. Milk expression should begin prior to return to work so that there is an adequate supply of stored milk to allow for daily variations in the amount of milk consumed by the infant. (See Chapter 10.)

5. *Resources.* Mothers should have names and phone numbers of individuals who can provide lactation advice on a 24-hour-a-day basis. Mothers also should know of peer support groups with contact information and be encouraged to participate. (See the Appendix.)

B. **Post-Cesarean Delivery.** If the mother has undergone a cesarean delivery, she may have an earlier visit than the typical 4- to 6-week postpartum interval. Although this visit is primarily focused on detecting surgical complications, it is well timed to assist with any early breastfeeding complaints, especially because mothers with cesarean deliveries may have more difficulty establishing and sustaining lactation.

II. Maternal Breastfeeding Issues—Short Term

Nipple pain and engorgement are the most frequent complaints of lactating women and may present early in the immediate postpartum period, but also may arise at any time in lactation.

A. **Nipple Pain** is a concern at any time. (See Chapter 7.) Infection is one cause of nipple pain beyond the immediate postpartum period.

B. **Nipple *Candida* infections** are not uncommon. A usual source is thrush in the infant.

1. *Symptoms.* Breast infections due to *Candida* may present with nipple pain, itching, or burning sensation or "shooting" breast pains that radiate back toward the chest wall

and persist or worsen after feeding is complete and the breast is drained. The nipple and areola may appear erythematous or shiny or have white patches. However, in some cases there may be no external signs.

2. *Causes.* Predisposing factors for *Candida* infections of the breast include diabetes, steroid use, immune deficiency, antibiotic use, nipple trauma, and the use of plastic-lined breast pads, which keep the nipples moist continuously.

3. *Evaluation.* *Candida* breast infection can be treated based on clinical symptomatology alone if no other diagnosis is apparent. It is difficult to prove that *Candida* is the causative organism in all situations. Because yeast is ubiquitous, cultures of skin surfaces may represent skin flora and be positive even in asymptomatic mothers. Milk or skin surface cultures for *Candida*, therefore, are not helpful and not performed routinely.

4. *Management.* Treatment of breast infections due to *Candida* should be undertaken by treating the *mother and infant simultaneously* when either of them is symptomatic. The mother's partner also may need treatment.

    a. *Antifungal Therapy.* A variety of antifungal agents is available and effective. Typically, mothers are treated with a topical antifungal agent, such as ketoconazole, nystatin, or miconazole. The antifungal cream is applied to the mother's breast after feeding and an antifungal solution is swabbed on the inside of the infant's cheeks after feeding. The infant's diaper area also may need treatment. Nystatin has poor oral absorption so side effects are rare, though resistance may be a clinical concern. This therapy is usually continued for 14 days, or at least several days after symptoms have resolved.

    b. *Gentian Violet.* Other topical treatment options include the use of 0.25% to 1% gentian violet swabbed on the affected areas for up to 3 days. Gentian violet may cause permanent staining of clothing and temporary violet discoloration of the infant's mouth and the maternal breast.

c. *Oral fluconazole* may be prescribed if the nipples are not significantly better after several days of topical treatment, or in cases of recurrent candidiasis.

d. *Additional Management.* Any objects in contact with the infant's mouth (pacifiers, nipples) or the mother's breast (breast pump equipment) should be washed in hot soapy water and boiled on a daily basis. Clothing, such as bras and blouses, should be laundered using a dilute bleach solution or dried in sunlight daily. If used, disposable nursing pads are preferred. Leaving the breasts exposed to air and applying good wound care principles may assist with rapid healing. Other sites of yeast infection also should be checked, such as yeast vaginitis or "jock itch" in her partner and diaper rash in the infant. Regardless of the treatment regimen employed, the mother should be instructed on appropriate hygiene to prevent reinfection.

C. **Engorgement** (Chapter 7) refers to the swelling and distention that results from inefficient draining of the breast. Engorgement usually occurs around the time milk production increases, approximately days 3 to 7 postpartum. Engorgement also may occur later in the course of breastfeeding related to a missed feeding or an abrupt change in feeding frequency. Engorgement should not be confused with a plugged duct, which can result in a localized lump or cord in one area of the breast, nor with mastitis, which can result in fever, systemic flu-like symptoms, and an elevated white blood cell count (Table 9-1). Engorgement may be the result of infrequent or ineffective nursing from causes such as sore nipples, a sleepy infant, or mother-infant separation.

The breast must be examined to rule out related problems such as plugged ducts or mastitis. If left untreated, engorgement can lead to difficulties in properly latching the infant to the breast and to mastitis. The best treatment of engorgement is prevention. Frequent breastfeeding or pumping of the breasts (8 to 12 times per day from both breasts) is the best way to prevent engorgement.

TABLE 9-1. COMPARISON OF FINDINGS OF ENGORGEMENT, PLUGGED DUCT, AND MASTITIS

Characteristics	Engorgement	Plugged Duct	Mastitis
Onset	Gradual, immediately postpartum	Gradual, after feedings	Sudden, after 10 days
Site	Bilateral	Unilateral	Usually unilateral
Swelling and heat	Generalized	May shift; little or no heat	Localized, red, hot, swollen
Pain	Generalized	Mild, but localized	Intense, but localized
Body temperature	<38.4°C (101°F)	<38.4°C	>38.4°C
Systemic symptoms	Feels well	Feels well	Flu-like symptoms

Adapted with permission from Breastfeeding: A Guide for the Medical Professional. *5th ed. St Louis, MO: Mosby; 1999:276.*

D. Plugged Ducts (Milk Stasis)

1. *Symptoms.* A plugged duct is a localized blockage of milk, frequently presenting as a painful knot in the breast. This lump may decrease in size with nursing.

2. *Causes.* This condition may be caused by an abrupt change in the feeding schedule, inadequate draining of the breast, failure to vary nursing positions, or wearing tight and constricting clothing (such as a poorly fitting underwire bra). Especially when the condition recurs in the same breast segment, the cause may be anatomic variations leading to plugged ducts. Rarely, what is considered a plugged duct may be a tumor, benign or malignant, that is blocking the duct.

3. *Evaluation.* Plugged ducts are easily differentiated from engorgement and mastitis and are not associated with fever or other signs of systemic illness (Table 9-1). If the plugged

duct does not resolve within 48 to 72 hours or if fever develops, the patient should be seen and evaluated by a health care professional.

4. *Management.* The treatment for plugged ducts is to apply moist heat prior to feeding and massage the affected area before and during nursing. If possible, start feedings with the affected breast first. Attempt different positions to allow better drainage of the particular part of the breast that is affected. Ensure that the patient is not compressing the breast tissue, such as indenting the breast with the finger(s) to provide a breathing space for the infant. Changing the infant's position during the feed also may help to empty the plugged area.

E. **Mastitis** is defined typically as a unilateral bacterial infection of the breast, occurring in 2% to 3% of lactating women.

1. *Symptoms.* Mastitis most commonly presents as a single area of localized warmth, tenderness, edema, and erythema in *one* breast more than 10 days after delivery. The highest incidence occurs in the second and third weeks postpartum. Depending on the severity of the infection, the area of inflammation can range from a few centimeters to almost the entire breast. Mastitis may present with a sudden onset of breast pain, myalgia, and fever that can be dramatic. Sometimes mastitis presents with flu-like symptoms such as fatigue, nausea, vomiting, and headache.

2. *Causes.* The infection commonly enters through a break in the skin, usually a cracked nipple. However, milk stasis and congestion resulting from engorgement, or plugged ducts, also can lead to mastitis. Fifty percent of causative organisms are penicillin-resistant *Staphylococcus aureus.* Other organisms seen are *Escherichia coli,* Group A *streptococcus, Peptostreptococcus, Haemophilus influenzae, Klebsiella pneumoniae,* and *Bacteroides.*

3. *Evaluation.* Perform a careful examination of the breast to verify the diagnosis and to rule out abscess formation. A bacterial culture of the milk usually is not indicated, because skin flora will contaminate a culture and may mask the true organism.

4. *Management.* Mastitis needs to be treated as soon as it is discovered. The following steps should be taken:

   a. *Prescribe an antibiotic* that is effective against penicillin-resistant *Staphylococcus,* and administer a 10- to 14-day course. Safe antibiotics for therapy include first-generation cephalosporins or oxacillin. If the patient is allergic to penicillin, erythromycin and its derivatives are also effective.

   b. *Instruct the mother to continue nursing* because the milk is not harmful to the infant. Frequent feeding is recommended. If the mother can tolerate feeding on the affected breast first, this is preferable. However, if this is too painful, the mother may begin on the unaffected breast until symptoms subside. The affected breast should be drained at each feeding by nursing and/or pumping. In an occasional circumstance, manual expression or a breast pump may be needed to remove the milk from the breast due to more severe pain prohibiting breastfeeding. Weaning should not be recommended during mastitis and may predispose the mother to developing a breast abscess.

   c. *Encourage fluid intake* to ensure hydration.

   d. *Recommend bed rest* until the mother's fever has subsided for at least 24 hours. She can have the baby with her and should seek help from family members.

   e. *Analgesics.* Symptomatic relief can be achieved with mild analgesics (acetaminophen or ibuprofen), warm or cold packs (whatever works best), and a supportive bra.

   f. *Severe cases* of mastitis that do not respond rapidly to outpatient therapy will require admission to the hospital and parenteral therapy.

F. **Recurrent and/or Chronic Mastitis**

   1. *Symptoms* are the same as with acute mastitis but persist beyond treatment.

   2. *Causes.* Recurrent or chronic mastitis usually results from incomplete treatment of mastitis or the use of an

ineffective antibiotic. Patients with mastitis typically feel improved after only a short course of antibiotics and should be counseled to comply with the entire duration of therapy. Another cause of recurrent mastitis is a failure to treat underlying predisposing factors such as persistent nipple trauma and fissuring, or an obstructive lesion.

3. *Evaluation.* In cases of recurrent infection, a thorough breast examination should be performed after resolution of infection to rule out any underlying solid or cystic masses. An ultrasound examination also may be useful.

4. *Management.* A midstream culture of expressed milk may prove helpful. Generally, midstream milk cultures do not grow pathogens. The patient should be counseled on compliance with a full 2-week course of therapy and any potential predisposing factors should be addressed. In some circumstances, a longer course of antibiotics may be needed.

G. **Breast abscess** is a walled-off area of the breast that contains purulent material and occurs in 5% to 11% of women with mastitis.

1. *Symptoms.* The presenting signs and symptoms are similar to mastitis with the added finding of a defined tense or fluctuant mass in the breast. Persistent symptoms of mastitis after 48 to 72 hours of therapy should prompt investigation for a possible underlying abscess.

2. *Causes.* If mastitis is not promptly treated or treatment is not adequate, abscess formation is possible.

3. *Evaluation.* The breast should be carefully evaluated to rule out other causes of a breast mass.

4. *Management.* Prompt treatment with incision and drainage, antibiotics, and complete draining of the breast every few hours is required. In these cases the abscess fluid should be cultured so that the appropriate antibiotic can be prescribed. In some cases hospitalization and parenteral antibiotics will be necessary. Feeding from the contralateral breast can be continued with the term healthy infant. Feeding from the affected breast will depend on practical con-

siderations. If the incision can be made far enough from the areola to allow successful latch, then breastfeeding on the affected breast can be undertaken. If there is no breastfeeding, then milk must be emptied via mechanical or manual methods. Sometimes applying pressure over the incision with sterile dressing during feeding or pumping helps avoid a fistula.

H. Milk Leakage

1. *Symptoms.* Milk leakage refers to the involuntary loss of milk from the breast. Milk may leak from the opposite breast as the baby suckles and the milk lets down. It is a common event for breastfeeding women. This is usually more pronounced early in the course of lactation and subsides to some degree as milk volume and frequency of feeding adapts to the needs of the infant.

2. *Causes.* Milk leakage is a physiologic event and may occur when the milk ejection, or let-down reflex, occurs. Simply thinking about the infant may make the milk let down and cause leaking. The absence of leaking does not imply a reduction in the volume of milk or inadequacy of supply.

3. *Evaluation.* No specific evaluation is required.

4. *Management.* The mother should be reassured about this physiologic event and instructed on the use of appropriate, preferably disposable, nursing pads. Pressing firmly against the nipples with the palms of the hands at the time of the let-down reflex can minimize leaking.

III. Postpartum Mood Changes—Postpartum Blues and Depression

Postpartum blues or mild depression is a common condition following childbirth, estimated to occur in up to 80% of new mothers. Moderate to severe postpartum depression or postpartum psychosis is less common, occurring in 8% to 10 % of women. Because these conditions may affect not only the health of the woman, but also the care of her child(ren), including breastfeeding, their acknowledgment and treatment are important.

A. **Symptoms** of postpartum blues are transient and are characterized by mild sadness or weepiness. Symptoms of postpartum depression mimic other types of depression and may include changes in sleep patterns, appetite changes, fatigue, sadness, hopelessness, apathy, or persistent crying. In rare cases, symptoms may be severe and involve thoughts of harming self or infant, or an inability to care for self or infant, signaling postpartum psychosis.

B. **Causes.** Postpartum mood changes may be caused by sudden hormonal changes, fatigue, stress, sleep deprivation, or a combination of these. Risk factors for developing depression include prior history of depression, prior postpartum depression, positive family history, and adjustment difficulties related to childbirth. Medical problems, such as hypothyroidism, should be considered.

C. **Evaluation.** Symptoms and coping mechanisms should be discussed with the patient.

D. **Management.** Transient or mild mood changes require support. If the new mother's symptoms do not resolve rapidly, she should be referred to her mental health care professional for further assistance. Depending on the severity of the condition, pharmacologic therapy may be required. If pharmacologic therapy is needed, tricyclic antidepressants and selective serotonin reuptake inhibitors can be used during lactation. (See Chapter 12.)

IV. Maternal Breastfeeding Issues—Long Term

A. **Maternal Illness.** A breastfeeding mother with an illness, whether it is acute or chronic, often finds that advice regarding breastfeeding during illness is inconsistent among medical professionals. Factors to consider include whether lactation worsens the mother's illness, milk composition or supply will be affected, and will the infant be affected by the mother's illness or medication usage. The answer to all of these questions is usually no, and breastfeeding may proceed. The physicians involved in the mother's care should communicate fully to ensure the best and most consistent advice and management.

1. ***Acute Illness.*** During an immediate postpartum illness the
   infant should be allowed to room in with the mother, or
   at least be brought to her for breastfeeding at frequent
   intervals. The mother's milk supply should be established
   and maintained through continued breastfeeding, or breast
   pumping. Most acute illnesses (ie, maternal respiratory
   infections, gastroenteritis) are compatible with breastfeeding, and breastfeeding can provide the infant with
   protective antibodies. Interruption of breastfeeding at the
   time of onset of maternal symptoms may increase the risk
   of the child developing the infection.

2. ***Chronic Illness.*** A chronic illness may have a greater
   effect on a mother's ability to breastfeed because of
   changes in her own functioning, changes in milk supply,
   and the possible side effects of her medications on the
   infant. Mothers should be given information regarding
   the risks and benefits of breastfeeding to herself and her
   infant. Most chronic illnesses are compatible with breastfeeding, and breastfeeding can be one activity that helps
   to normalize the mother's experience with her infant.
   Cancer chemotherapy and radiation treatment may
   require temporary interruption of breastfeeding. (See
   Chapters 3 and 11.)

3. ***Diagnostic studies,*** especially those requiring radioisotopes,
   may require temporary "pump and dump" strategies to
   protect the infant. (See Chapters 3 and 11.)

4. ***Surgery and Anesthesia.*** When a nursing mother is
   required to have surgery, either urgently or electively, the
   patient and her health care professional should consider
   options for anesthesia and postoperative analgesia that
   meet the mother's health and comfort needs and have
   little effect on the breastfeeding infant. (See Chapter 6.)
   Hospital policies and support should encourage and be
   compatible with lactation maintenance, particularly if the
   procedure dictates a prolonged hospital stay. Whenever
   possible, arrangements should be made for pumping and
   storage of milk before and after the procedure in the case

of a prolonged separation. Postoperatively, the mother should pump or feed at least every 3 hours to maintain her milk supply and avoid engorgement.

B. **Maternal Nutrition During Lactation.** The assessment of maternal nutritional status is important to ensure the adequacy of the diet. In adequately nourished women, additional caloric intake and fluid intake do not enhance milk volume. Unless there is malnutrition, the mother's diet generally does not affect milk composition.

1. *Fluid intake* during lactation does not affect milk volume. Breastfeeding women should drink to satisfy their thirst. Mothers are encouraged to drink fluids and to note whether their urine is pale yellow, indicative of adequate fluid intake. Inadequate fluid intake also may be associated with constipation.

2. *Energy Intake.* The Dietary Reference Intake for energy during the first 6 months of lactation is an additional 500 kcal per day above the usual diet appropriate for the woman's height, normal weight, and level of activity. From 7 to 9 months of lactation, the energy intake declines to an additional 400 kcal per day. When sufficient calories are not consumed, the mother's own nutrient reserves are affected. Intakes less than 1,500 kcal per day may cause maternal fatigue and lower milk volume.

3. *Nutrient Intake.* Specific nutrient needs generally are higher in lactation than in pregnancy (Table 9-2). The milk contents for most nutrients are unrelated to maternal intake. Milk concentrations of water-soluble vitamins, however, reflect maternal intake, and a normal diet provides adequate vitamin levels. Strict vegetarians (vegans) who avoid all animal products are at risk for vitamin B_{12} deficiency and should be advised to take a vitamin B_{12} supplement. If the mother's vitamin B_{12} stores are depleted, her milk will also be low in this nutrient, and vitamin B_{12} deficiency may develop in the infant. Unusually high intakes of some nutrients (vitamin B_6, vitamin D, iodine, selenium) will increase their concentration in milk. The contents of some nutrients in milk may be maintained at a satisfactory

	Dietary Reference Intakes[†]			Percentage Increase During Lactation Over Non-reproducing Adult Women
Nutrient	**Adult Women[‡]**	**Pregnancy**	**Lactation**	**Lactation %**
Energy, [§] kcal	19–50 years	↑340 kcal/d 2nd Trimester ↑452 kcal/d 3rd Trimester	↑500 kcal/d 0–6 mo ↑400 kcal/d 7–9 mo	↑
Protein,[∥] g	46	71	71	54
Vitamin C,[∥] mg	75	85	120	60
Thiamin,[∥] mg	1.1	1.4	1.4	27
Riboflavin,[∥] mg	1.1	1.4	1.6	45
Niacin,[∥] ng NE	14	18	17	21
Vitamin B_6,[∥] mg	1.3	1.9	2	54
Folate,[∥] μg DFE	400	600	500	25
Vitamin B_{12},[∥] μg	2.4	2.6	2.8	17
Pantothenic acid,[¶] mg	5	6	7	40
Biotin,[¶] μg	30	30	35	17
Choline,[¶] mg	425	450	550	29
Vitamin A,[∥] μg RE	700	770	1300	86
Vitamin D,[¶] μg	5	5	5	0
Vitamin E,[∥] mg μ-TE	15	15	19	27
Vitamin K,[¶] μg	90	90	90	0
Calcium,[¶] mg	1,000	1,000	1,000	0
Phosphorus,[¶] mg	700	700	700	0
Magnesium,[∥] mg	310	350	310	0
Iron,[∥] mg	18	27	9	-50
Zinc,[∥] mg	8	11	12	50
Iodine,[∥] μg	150	220	290	93
Selenium,[∥] μg	55	60	70	27
Fluoride,[¶] mg	3	3	3	0

TABLE 9-2. DIETARY REFERENCE INTAKES FOR LACTATING WOMEN*

Adapted with permission from J Nutr. 2003;133:1997S–2002S.
* NE, niacin equivalents; DFE, dietary folate equivalents; RE, retinal equivalents; TE, tocopherol equivalents.
[†] Values are from the Institute of Medicine.
[‡] Assumes age >19 years. Women <19 years have greater nutrient needs for calcium (1,300 mg), phosphorus (1,240 mg), and zinc (13 mg).
[§] Calculations are based on recommended intakes per day, assuming 9 months is equivalent to 270 days.
[∥] Recommended Dietary Allowance (RDA), the average daily dietary intake level that is sufficient to meet the nutrient requirements of nearly all (97% and 98%) individuals in a life stage and gender group and based on the Estimated Average Requirement (EAR).
[¶] Adequate Intake (AI), the value used instead of an RDA if sufficient scientific evidence is not available to calculate an EAR.

level at the expense of maternal stores, especially folate and calcium. For this reason, folic acid supplementation (400 μg per day) should continue. There are no recommendations for calcium supplementation if Dietary Reference Intakes are met, although calcium losses occur from maternal skeleton. These losses are restored after weaning. The variation in total milk fat content is not affected by diet. Some studies suggest that maternal body fat stores are correlated with milk fat content. The pattern of fatty acids, however, is affected by maternal diet. A maternal diet high in polyunsaturated fatty acids may increase the proportion of these fatty acids in the milk. Most practitioners encourage the continued intake of prenatal vitamins during lactation.

4. *Weight Loss.* Lactating women eating self-selected diets generally lose weight at the rate of 0.5 to 1 kg (approximately 1–2 lb) per month in the first 4 to 6 months of lactation. Approximately 20% of women, however, do not lose weight during this time. Women can lose as much as 1 lb per week without compromising milk volume. For the lactating woman who had an elevated body mass index before pregnancy or who desires to lose weight more quickly, moderate increase in physical activity is more desirable than significant restriction in caloric intake. Rapid weight loss should be discouraged because it can decrease milk volume. Weight loss drugs and liquid diets are not recommended during lactation, and a weight-reduction diet in general is discouraged during the first 4 to 6 weeks postpartum. The average time to return to prepregnancy weight is 5 months. Mothers should be given sound nutritional advice to ensure adequate nutrient intake.

V. Breast Evaluation While Nursing

A. **Screening for Breast Masses.** The incidence of breast malignancy during pregnancy and lactation is estimated at 1:3,000 to 1:10,000 women. Approximately 3% of women diagnosed with breast cancer will be either pregnant or lactating. With increased childbearing in more advanced years, this number is expected to increase. Delay in diagnosis has been reported in pregnant and breastfeeding women. If a breastfeeding mother notices a lump in her breast that doesn't decrease with breastfeeding or one that increases in size, prompt evaluation should be pursued. If the mass persists, diagnostic tests should be performed. (See Chapter 3.)

1. *Diagnostic mammography* is safe during lactation, but normal findings should not be completely reassuring in the presence of a palpable mass. If a mammogram is performed, the woman should either nurse her infant or express milk from her breasts immediately prior to the mammogram to allow optimal visualization.

2. *Ultrasound* can provide further assistance in evaluating palpable breast masses (solid or fluid-filled) during lactation.

B. **Diagnostic studies,** including needle biopsy or fine needle aspiration, can also be performed without significant interruption of lactation. Most breast masses identified and biopsied during pregnancy and lactation are benign (80%) and can be biopsied without harm to mother, fetus, or infant. About 30% have pathology specific to the lactating breast. Benign pathology specific to the lactating breast includes lactating adenoma, infarcted fibroadenoma, hypertrophied breast tissue, galactoceles, mastitis/inflammatory lesions, and papillomas.

C. **Bloody nipple discharge** is a relatively frequent finding associated with nipple trauma and engorgement in early lactation, typically occurring around day 3 to 7. Evaluation of the nipple for trauma and adjustment of problems associated with latching the infant may resolve the problem. Occasionally women will complain of reddish-brown milk as ducts become distended and capillaries leak (ductal ectasia or rusty pipe syndrome). This usually resolves within the first week. If the milk is blood-tinged it is usually well tolerated by the infant, though occasionally it may be associated with vomiting and blood-tinged stools in the infant. If the bloody nipple discharge is persistent and from only a single milk duct, further evaluation is required. Most commonly, this will be caused by an intraductal papilloma. Intraductal carcinoma is rare and may also be associated with a mass in the affected breast.

D. Recommendations for Breast Evaluation During Lactation

1. *Regular Breast Self-Examinations.* Although technically difficult, some women choose to continue to do regular breast self-examinations during lactation.

2. *Clinical breast examinations* should be performed by a physician at the onset of pregnancy, in the postpartum period, and annually thereafter even while lactating.

3. *Mammograms.* Routine screening mammograms in contrast with diagnostic mammograms as outlined above should be delayed until several months after weaning.

4. *Biopsy,* if indicated, is safe during pregnancy and lactation.

5. *Breast cancer* diagnosed during pregnancy and lactation generally has the same prognosis, stage for stage, as premenopausal breast cancer diagnosed outside of pregnancy and lactation. Early diagnosis is important and treatment should not be delayed. Early referral to a breast surgeon for further evaluation of a breast abnormality is indicated if there is any cause for concern.

6. *Lactation* is possible (even if unilateral) after most breast surgeries and breast cancer treatments.

Selected References

Berens PD. Prenatal, intrapartum, and postpartum support of the lactating mother. *Pediatr Clin North Am.* 2001;48:365–375

Committee on Nutritional Status During Pregnancy and Lactation. *Nutrition During Lactation.* Washington, DC: National Academies Press; 1991

Kalkwarf HJ. Hormonal and dietary regulation of changes in bone density during lactation and after weaning in women. *J Mammary Gland Biol Neoplasia.* 1999;4:319–329

Krebs NF, Reidinger CJ, Robertson AD, Brenner M. Bone mineral density changes during lactation: maternal, dietary, and biochemical correlates. *Am J Clin Nutr.* 1997;65:1738–1746

Labbok MH. Effects of breastfeeding on the mother. *Pediatr Clin North Am.* 2001;48:143–158

Picciano MF. Pregnancy and lactation: physiological adjustments, nutritional requirements and the role of dietary supplements. *J Nutr.* 2003;133: 1997S–2002S

Chapter 10

Supporting Breastfeeding During Separation

There are circumstances, such as maternal hospitalization, return to work, or school attendance, in which an interruption in continuity of breastfeeding may occur by necessity. The physician can help the mother by providing guidance on specific strategies and appropriate plans for continued breastfeeding.

I. **Maternal employment and school attendance** are the most frequent reasons for mother-infant separation during lactation. Anticipatory guidance should be practiced so that health care professionals can discuss options for continued breastfeeding. Counseling and discussion of strategies should begin prenatally, continue during visits to the physician, and be included in the instruction provided in breastfeeding classes.

A. **Support for Breastfeeding in the Workplace**

1. *On-site Child Care.* Some employers have lactation programs to encourage continued breastfeeding for mothers who return to work. These may include on-site lactation specialists or a contract with community or hospital lactation specialists and on-site child care facilities in which a mother can breastfeed during breaks.

2. *Off-site Child Care.* In the absence of a corporate program, at minimum the breastfeeding mother should have access to appropriate facilities at work (Table 10-1). Although there is no legal mandate for employers to support breastfeeding, the creative use of scheduled breaks and lunchtime combined with strategies such as a double pump kit that allows milk to be expressed from both breasts

---

**TABLE 10-1. FACILITIES NECESSARY TO
SUPPORT BREASTFEEDING IN THE WORKPLACE**

1. Private place for milk expression (office, break room, lounge), preferably with a lock on the door

2. Breast pump either supplied by workplace or brought by mother

3. Sink for washing hands before handling pump equipment or milk and for rinsing equipment

4. Storage refrigerator or cooler with ice packs for milk (separate from general employee lunch or break refrigerator to avoid milk tampering)

5. Comfortable seating for milk expression or breastfeeding

---

simultaneously may facilitate maintenance of a milk supply. Milk expression should occur at least once for every 4-hour period of separation. The off-site child care selected should be compatible with the parents' beliefs and the mother's desire to continue breastfeeding. Areas to be addressed when interviewing a prospective caregiver are shown in Table 10-2.

B. **Advocacy for breastfeeding** in the workplace is needed when employers are not supportive.

　1. *Providing literature* that discusses the benefits of breastfeeding and demonstrates the cost savings of breastfeeding

---

**TABLE 10-2. QUESTIONS FOR PARENTS TO ASK A PROSPECTIVE
CHILD CARE PROFESSIONAL**

1. What has been your previous experience with breastfeeding and the use of expressed human milk?

2. Do you agree with our/my general philosophy and style of parenting?

3. Will you follow specific instructions in terms of feeding expressed human milk?

4. Will you be willing to attempt to soothe the baby or wait a brief period for the feeding if I am delayed at work?

5. Will you follow our/my plan for introducing cereal, solids, and juices?

---

to the employer may be helpful. Health care professionals may need to write letters or contact employers or school administrators in support of the health care interests of the infant and mother and the need for continued breast-feeding.

2. *Professionals' Role.* Health care professionals should advocate for insurance or managed care coverage for the cost of a pump to allow the mother to continue milk expression at work. All health care professionals should advocate for supportive legislation and policies at the local, state, and national levels.

C. **Options for continued breastfeeding after return to work or school** should be considered before the beginning of mother-baby separation. The mother should ideally discuss her desire to continue breastfeeding with her supervisor or human resources director, or with a school guidance counselor or administrator prior to maternity leave or childbirth. The physician also may need to discuss breastfeeding with the employer or school official.

D. **Preparing for the Return to Work or School**

1. Strategies for the mother to prepare for separation are shown in Table 10-3.

2. Medical students and residents pose unique situations due to the schedule and workload demands. House staff who have had successful experiences with breastfeeding are likely to be more knowledgeable, strong advocates for breastfeeding, and role models for their peers and patients when they become practitioners. Medical school administrators and residency training program directors and faculty should support and encourage breastfeeding among their students and residency staff. Optimal support may involve flexibility in terms of work assignments or accommodation of part-time scheduling for a period.

II. **Separation Due to Newborn or Infant Illness**
Prematurity or neonatal illness may preclude continuous rooming-in or necessitate discharge of the mother before the infant's

---

TABLE 10-3. SUGGESTED STRATEGIES FOR THE MOTHER WHO IS RETURNING TO WORK OR SCHOOL

A. Preparation prior to the day of separation

1. Arrange as long a period of maternity leave as feasible.

2. Make arrangements with the employer/school before the day.

3. Practice using the breast pump at least 2 weeks before the planned separation.

4. Begin milk expression early to allow storage of a sufficient supply.

5. Introduce alternative methods of feeding in advance.

6. Experiment with different types of bottle nipples or cups to find one that the infant prefers.

7. Encourage the father, or other relatives or friends, to provide assistance with household chores or with the care of other children to ease the transition.

8. Leave the infant or child with the caregiver for brief periods prior to the first day.

9. Let the caregiver practice giving the baby a bottle or cup before the separation.

---

discharge. Strategies to promote continued bonding and stimulation of milk production include skin-to-skin contact and facilities or rooms that permit overnight stays of the mother to maximize the amount of time she can spend with the infant. These "mother-in-residence" programs also permit the infant to remain in the room with the mother either continuously or intermittently. If physical separation of mother and infant is required, the mother should be provided with a hospital-grade electric pump. Strategies to assist breastfeeding if the infant is ill are addressed in Chapters 11 and 14.

III. Separation Due to Maternal Illness or Surgery

A. **Acute minor maternal illness,** including fever, should not interrupt breastfeeding. By the time maternal symptoms develop, the infant has already been exposed to the infectious agent. Continued breastfeeding is protective to the infant. (See Chapters 8 and 9.)

TABLE 10-3. SUGGESTED STRATEGIES FOR THE MOTHER WHO IS RETURNING TO WORK OR SCHOOL (CONTINUED)

B. Preparations at the work/school site

1. Enlist the support of coworkers (or teachers, principals, or guidance counselors) who are breastfeeding or who have breastfed in the past.

2. Arrange gradual return to work schedule if possible, beginning with half days.

3. If returning to work full time, consider starting on a Thursday or Friday to avoid having to work a full 5-day stretch the first week back at work.

4. Breastfeed just before leaving the infant and as soon as mother and infant are reunited at the end of the day.

5. Allow the infant to breastfeed as often as desired in the evening and overnight to encourage continued milk supply. Having baby close by at night may facilitate frequent feedings.

6. Remember to pack the breast pump, kit, bottles, and other equipment ahead of time.

7. Take a cooler or bag with "blue ice" for transporting expressed milk home or for storage while away.

8. Take a picture of the infant (or consider having a blanket with the baby's smell or a tape recording of the baby's coos, squeals, or cries) to use when expressing to facilitate the milk ejection reflex (let-down).

9. Have a change of clothing available in case of milk leaks or spills.

10. Wear clothing with a pattern or wear a jacket over a blouse or dress to conceal accidental leaks or spills.

11. Wear 2-piece outfits or commercially available clothing designed for breastfeeding women that allow easy access to the breasts for feeding or expressing milk.

B. **Planned elective surgery,** if it cannot be postponed, should prompt a discussion with the surgeon and anesthesiologist to select the most appropriate medications for anesthesia, pain control, and other therapies. (See Chapters 6, 8, 9, and 12.) Continued nursing or having the infant visit at intervals to breastfeed should be considered whenever possible. Family and/or friends should be encouraged to assist in caring for the infant during such visits. In some hospitals, breastfeeding infants may be kept with mothers in postoperative units. Milk should be expressed and stored in advance of the procedure in case there is a longer than expected interruption in breastfeeding. In the event of a more serious maternal condition or emergency surgery, the mother should be provided an electric pump and assisted in the collection and storage of breast milk.

IV. **Milk expression** should continue on a regular basis throughout the period of separation to maintain supply and prevent engorgement.

    A. **Unanticipated Separation.** The frequency of milk expression should approximate the frequency at which the infant would be breastfeeding (every 2–3 hours for the newborn, every 4–5 hours for the older baby) to maintain an adequate milk supply.

    B. **Anticipated separation** occurs in situations where there is elective surgery or return to work or school. Milk should be expressed before the anticipated absence and stored for later use. Milk volume can be increased by increasing the frequency of milk expression 1 to 2 weeks before the anticipated date.

V. **Bottle-feeding**
If the mother desires that the baby learn to drink from a bottle, she should consider introduction of the bottle gradually, a few weeks before its anticipated need. Acceptance of a bottle is more likely if someone other than the mother offers it. The mother should be outside the range of sight or smell of the baby when the bottle is offered, and the bottle-feeding should not take place in the same location as the usual nursing location. The breastfed infant will typically accept expressed human milk from the bottle better than infant formula. If the bottle is not accepted on the first attempt, repeat introductions may be necessary, approximately once every day or two. Trying another style, size, or shape of nipple may be helpful. If the baby does use a pacifier, a nipple that is similar in size and shape to the pacifier may be helpful. Attempting the feeding when the infant is hungry, but not crying inconsolably, will enhance the chances for positive acceptance of the bottle. For

babies who continue to refuse bottles, a small cup can be used to offer the feeding using a technique that has been used in premature and term babies to provide supplemental feedings. (See Chapter 11.)

Selected References

Auerbach KG. Maternal employment and breastfeeding. In: Riordan J, Auerbach KG, eds. *Breastfeeding and Human Lactation.* 2nd ed. Sudbury, MA: Jones and Bartlett Publishers; 1999

Biagioli F. Returning to work while breastfeeding. *Am Fam Physician.* 2003;68: 2201–2208

Bocar DL. Combining breastfeeding and employment: increasing success. *J Perinat Neonatal Nurs.* 1997;11:23–43

Cohen R, Mrtek MB, Mrtek RG. Comparison of maternal absenteeism and infant illness rates among breast-feeding and formula-feeding women in two corporations. *Am J Health Promot.* 1995;10:148–153

Corbett-Dick P, Bezek SK. Breastfeeding promotion for the employed mother. *J Pediatr Health Care.* 1997;11:12–19

Duckett L. Maternal employment and breastfeeding. *NAACOGS Clin Issu Perinat Womens Health Nurs.* 1992;3:701–712

Gielen AC, Faden RR, O'Campo P, Brown CH, Paige DM. Maternal employment during the early postpartum period: effects on initiation and continuation of breast-feeding. *Pediatrics.* 1991;87:298–305

Greenberg CS, Smith K. Anticipatory guidance for the employed breast-feeding mother. *J Pediatr Health Care.* 1991;5:204–209

Healthy Child Care America Campaign. American Academy of Pediatrics; www.healthychildcare.org

Meek JY. Breastfeeding in the workplace. *Pediatr Clin North Am.* 2001;48: 461–474

Pantazi M, Jaeger MC, Lawson M. Staff support for mothers to provide breast milk in pediatric hospitals and neonatal units. *J Hum Lact.* 1998;14:291–296

US Department of Health and Human Services, Office of Women's Health, American Association of Health Plans. *Advancing Women's Health: Health Plans' Innovative Programs in Breastfeeding Promotion.* Washington, DC: US Government Printing Office; 2001

Chapter 11

Breastfeeding Technology

Breastfeeding technology refers to breast pumps, breast shells, nipple shields, feeding-tube devices, weighing scales, and milk storage methods, any or all of which can be very useful in supporting women to initiate and continue breastfeeding.

I. **Manual and mechanical milk expression** techniques are effective in helping to initiate and maintain milk production during infant-mother separation, maternal or infant illness, inability of the infant to latch to the breast, and poor maternal milk production.

   A. **Manual milk expression** works well during short-term separation and to alleviate engorgement or sore nipples (Figure 11-1). These simple steps can be mastered by the mother after some practice (Table 11-1).

   B. **Mechanical expression** of milk can be accomplished using a manual, small battery-operated or hospital-grade electric breast pump (Figure 11-2A and B). Mechanical expression works best for those planning to express their milk on a regular, ongoing basis, such as for a return to work or school or in case of maternal or infant illness. See Table 11-2 for a list of common questions used to evaluate breast pumps before purchase.

      1. *Manual breast pumps* are available in 3 styles.

         a. *Piston or Cylinder Pumps.* For intermittent pumping this is a simple and effective device. It is unlikely to be adequate to increase milk production or maintain supply if there is prolonged mother-infant separation. Mothers who choose to use a hand pump need to be instructed on how to use it properly because lateral epicondylitis (tennis elbow) has been associated with the use of trombone-action style hand pumps.

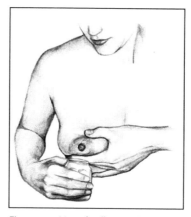

Figure 11-1. Manual milk expression.

TABLE 11-1. MANUAL MILK EXPRESSION TECHNIQUE

1. Wash hands thoroughly.

2. Gently massage the breast from the outside quadrants toward the areola; avoid applying deep pressure or friction.

3. A washcloth with warm water may be placed on the breast about 5 minutes before milk expression.

4. Place the hand with the fingers below and the thumb above about 3 cm away from the nipple base. Press toward the chest wall and then compress the thumb and fingers together, rolling them toward the nipple. Move the hand around the areola to reach all of the areas that cover the pooled milk in the lactiferous sinuses. Use the free hand to massage the breast from the outer quadrants toward the nipple. Do not squeeze the nipple.

5. The manual method can take 20 to 30 minutes for adequate draining of both breasts.

TABLE 11-2. QUESTIONS TO ANSWER BEFORE OBTAINING A BREAST PUMP

- Is the pump for short- or long-term use?
- What will the pump cost?
- How much does the pump weigh?
- How comfortable is the pump?
- Does it drain the breast efficiently?
- How easy are the pump and collection kits to clean?
- Are there clear written instructions on how to use the pump?
- Can a standard bottle be used to collect milk with the pump?
- How many suction cycles are there per minute?
- Does the pump cycle on its own?
- Are there variable collection cup sizes available?
- Are there mechanisms to prevent pump contamination?
- How quiet is the pump?
- How long are the electrical cords?
- Can it pump both breasts at the same time?
- Is the pump approved for use in the hospital, if applicable?
- What is the manufacturer's warranty?
- Is the pump meant for a single owner or for multiple users?
- Does the pump come with a case or a tote bag?
- Do you have to use 2 hands to operate the pump?
- Is the pump efficient and effective?

Adapted from **Pediatric Clinics of North America**, *Volume 48, Slusser W and Frantz K, Questions to ask before buying a breast pump. pages 506–507, copyright 2001, with permission from Elsevier.*

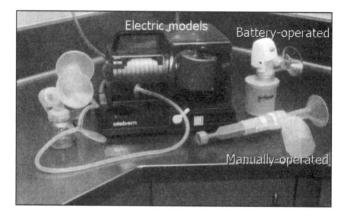

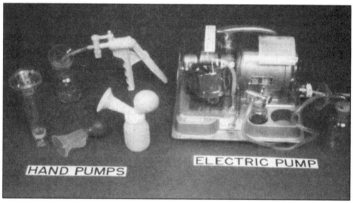

Figure 11-2A and B. Various styles of electric and manual breast pumps.

    b.   Squeeze-handle pumps are effective at removing milk, but some women develop fatigue in their hand after prolonged use.

    c.   Rubber bulb (bicycle horn) pumps are not recommended because of the potential for bacteria build-up inside the rubber bulb and contamination of the milk.

  *2. **Battery-operated and electric pumps*** generally are lightweight and have variable frequency (2–76 cycles per minute), suction pressures (8–360 mm Hg), and capabilities for double pumping. The electric breast pump with automatic cycling yields milk that has a higher calorie content (secondary to increased fat concentration from complete breast drainage) compared with the milk expressed by manual methods. Guidelines for mechanical milk expression are found in Table 11-3.

3. **Breast Pump Maintenance**

    a. *Assembly.* A knowledgeable person should demonstrate to the family how to assemble and disassemble a pump.

    b. *Cleaning.* Each mother should have her own collection kit and storage containers, which should be rinsed to remove milk residue; cleaned with hot, soapy water; and dried in the air after each use. Dishwasher cleaning also is adequate. Bottled or boiled water should be used for cleaning parts where the water supply is potentially contaminated. Manufacturer's instructions

---

TABLE 11-3. GENERAL GUIDELINES FOR MECHANICAL MILK EXPRESSION

- Wash hands before beginning to express milk.
- To initiate and maintain milk supply for a hospitalized infant, begin as soon as possible and continue at a frequency of 8 times in 24 hours. After a supply is established, the frequency can be reduced. For other situations, the frequency can be less.
- Ten minutes of pumping each breast is sufficient for maintenance of adequate milk production, preferably from both breasts simultaneously.
- Develop relaxation techniques, such as sitting in a comfortable environment. Think about the infant, look at a photograph of the infant, or sit at the bedside of the hospitalized infant. Gently massage the breast before and during milk expression.
- It is unnecessary to discard the first few milliliters of milk.
- A pump collection kit should be used only by one mother unless it is sterilized between use. Verify manufacturer's instructions prior to sterilizing.
- Pumps categorized for in-home single users should be used by only one mother.
- Routine microbiologic surveillance is costly and not supported by milk culture data.
- Review recommendations verbally and in written form for washing and cleaning of pump equipment. (Instructions usually accompany the pump.)

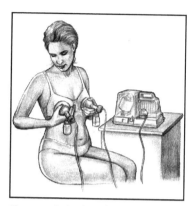

Figure 11-3A. An electric breast pump that allows collection of milk from both breasts simultaneously is best for mothers who express milk on a routine basis, especially if they have a hopsitalized infant.

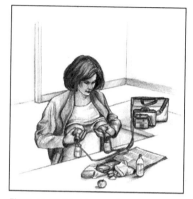

Figure 11-3B. Double pumping system.

should be followed. When more than one mother is using the same breast pump, as in a hospital lactation room, hospital staff should be responsible for cleaning the pump daily, examining for milk backup, and regularly checking the suction settings.

c. *Double Pumping System.* Long-term mother/baby separation warrants a breast pump that is capable of simultaneous double pumping because of the time saved, higher amount of prolactin released, and potential for greater milk production (Figure 11-3A and B).

d. *Fitting the Flange.* The opening where the breast meets the collection kit needs to be wide enough to allow the nipple to easily move in and out without pain, but not so large that milk removal is impaired. Some collection kits have breast shield inserts to accommodate for different nipple sizes.

4. *Economics of Pump Purchase/Rental.* If a physician prescribes a breast pump for a patient, some health insurance companies and the Special Supplemental Nutrition Program for Women, Infants, and Children (WIC) will cover the cost of a breast pump rental or purchase. In addition, many employee breastfeeding support programs support the cost of purchasing or renting the equipment.

II. Nipple Shields and Breast Cups and Shells

A. **Nipple shields** are made of latex or silicone and provide a thin protective barrier over the nipple and areola with holes at the tip to allow the transfer of milk (Figure 11–4A and B). Nipple shields are used to help an infant latch on to a flat or inverted nipple or an engorged breast, protect sore nipples, reduce an excessively rapid milk flow, and sometimes entice an infant to the breast who is accustomed to the nipple of a bottle. The shields have been used frequently to help premature infants transition from tube feeding to breastfeeding. Because of the potential to interfere with milk transfer and reduce stimulation of the areola, the health care professional should monitor infant weight gain to ensure adequate milk intake.

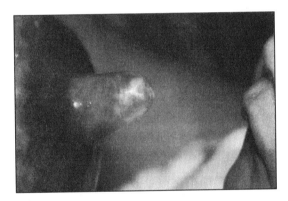

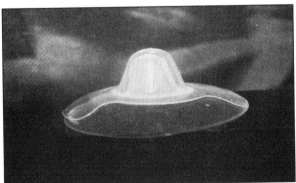

Figure 11-4A and B. Nipple shields.

B. **Breast cups and shells** are made of hard polypropylene, silicone, or other hard plastic and are designed in a cup shape with air holes on one side and one larger hole on the other side for the nipple to protrude through the opening into the cup or shell. They help in the relief of sore nipples, and in preventing milk from leaking onto clothes. The most important features of breast cups/shells are the air holes for ventilation, sufficient size to prevent overflow of milk onto the clothes, and a large enough nipple opening for comfort. They are worn inside the bra between breastfeedings. Although they are sometimes used for correcting inverted nipples during the prenatal and postpartum period, there is no evidence that they are effective.

III. Supplemental Feeding Methods

For the infant who is unable or unwilling to suckle at the breast, there are other methods of providing expressed human milk, such as with feeding-tube devices, cups, and bottles, and via the finger-feeding technique.

A. **Feeding-tube devices** are very thin, soft plastic feeding tubes that are attached to a milk container at one end with the other end placed adjacent to the mother's nipple and fixed to the breast with a small piece of tape (Figure 11-5). The device helps deliver milk to the infant while the infant is suckling at the breast and is used to supplement a breastfeeding if milk intake is inadequate, or the mother wishes to relactate or induce lactation. The use of such a device allows the infant to receive additional nutrition during breastfeeding while providing the stimulation for the mother to increase her milk supply. The use of feeding-tube devices requires supervision. Although the feeding-tube device improves stimulation at the breast so that a breast pump may not be needed, in some cases mothers will use the feeding-tube device and the breast pump.

B. **Cup feeding** is an alternative to bottle-feeding when breastfeeding is not an option (Figure 11-6). For term infants, duration of the feeding session, volume of milk ingested, and infant physiologic stability do not differ between cup feeding and bottle-feeding methods. Benefits of cup feeding for the premature infant also have been reported. For some infants bottle-feeding

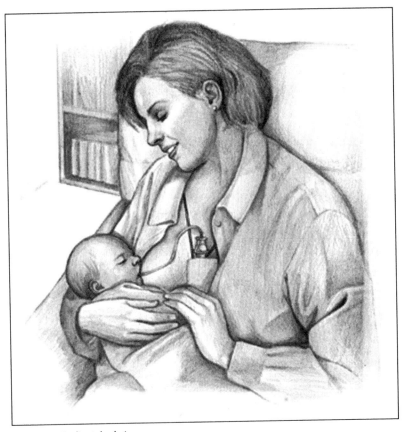

Figure 11-5. Feeding-tube device.

may interfere with the establishment of breastfeeding, so cup feeding is a reasonable alternative. It entails using a small plastic or glass medicine cup filled with milk. Infants are fed in a semi-upright position with head and upper back support. Infants can be stimulated to root by stroking the lower lip with the edge of the cup. The infant sips or laps the milk when the cup is placed against the infant's lower lip and tilted so that the milk is available,

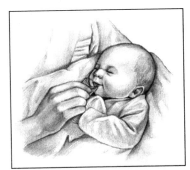

Figure 11-6. Cup feeding.

but not poured or dripped into the infant's mouth. Some infants may not be able to sustain the sipping or lapping effort to get an adequate volume, or may lose significant amounts due to dribbling of milk.

C. **Bottle-feeding.** Bottles are not recommended for the first few weeks until breastfeeding is well established. Because the tongue and oral-motor structures are used differently for bottle-feeding and breastfeeding, and because breastfed infants become accustomed to the soft, supple human nipple, bottle nipples or pacifiers may not be accepted readily. During a bottle-feeding, the infant should be held in a somewhat flexed position resting in the arms of the caregiver. The bottle should be introduced by touching the lower lip of the infant to elicit the rooting reflex, then slipping the bottle nipple in the mouth once the infant's mouth opens. In some infants, early introduction of bottles may lead to ineffective suckling at the breast or result in breast refusal. There may be a need to introduce bottles to infants whose mothers expect to be separated from them in the near future. (See Chapter 10.)

D. **Other temporary feeding methods** to deliver milk to the infant when breastfeeding is not possible include using a medicine dropper or syringe, or holding a feeding tube with a finger near the junction of the hard and soft palates. These methods avoid delivering milk by bottle and artificial nipple. When using a syringe or a medicine dropper, avoid squeezing or pushing the milk into the baby's mouth. Allow the infant to suck the milk out by enticing the infant with a few drops placed on the infant's lip. No long-term studies have examined the risks and benefits of such alternative methods.

E. **Intragastric (orogastric, nasogastric) tube feeding** usually is used when an infant is premature or too ill to suckle at the breast. There are 2 ways milk can be fed by this method: intermittent bolus and continuous infusion. For the bolus technique, milk flows by gravity into the tube. A continuous infusion requires that the syringe of milk be placed on a syringe infusion pump and then attached to the feeding tube. Because the fat will separate from the milk on standing, efforts should be made to ensure that the separated fat is not left behind

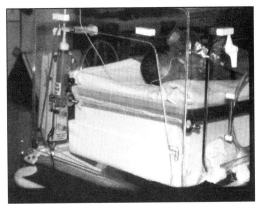

Figure 11-7. Orientation of syringe in continuous tube-feeding system. Schanler RJ. Special methods in feeding the preterm infant. In: Tsang R, Nichols BL, eds. Nutrition in Infancy. *Philadelphia, PA: Hanley & Belfus, Inc.; 1988:315–325.*

when the milk is fed. To ensure the best delivery of fat with the continuous tube-feeding method, a single syringe infusion pump with the shortest length of tubing is used. The syringe should be oriented with the tip upright and the syringe emptied completely after each use (Figure 11-7). With continuous feedings, syringe systems should be changed every 3 to 4 hours.

IV. **Test weighing** is a procedure to measure milk intake by weighing the infant before and after a feeding. The net intake in grams (closely approximating volume in milliliters) is obtained by subtracting the pre-feed weight from the post-feed weight. Test weighing is generally used as a research tool to assess the adequacy of milk intake and evaluate milk production after changes in lactation performance. Short-term use of an electronic baby scale can be useful for estimating milk intake in the premature infant during the transition from the hospital to the home. A sensitive scale (± 2 g sensitivity) with a digital readout and computerized integration to correct for infant movement is recommended. Test weighing on a non-electronic scale is not reliable and not recommended. Although it has been used to estimate milk intake from a single feeding, for best estimates of milk intake, test weighing should be performed at each feeding for at least 24 hours because there is variation from feed to feed. The infant must wear the same clothing and diaper before and after the feeding to obtain an accurate reflection of intake. Test weighing can interfere with successful breastfeeding when it is used without medical indication and supervision.

V. Milk Storage

Human milk should be stored in a cool, safe place to maximize its preservation and minimize contamination. Human milk has significant immunologic protection that also protects it from contamination. However, when expressed into collection containers, some skin bacteria mix with the milk. Nevertheless, when stored in the refrigerator (4°C [39°F]) bacterial counts decrease over 6 hours. See Table 11–4 for milk storage guidelines.

A. General Storage Guidelines

1. *Room Temperature* (25°C [77°F]). The consensus is that fresh human milk can be maintained or used at room temperature for up to 4 hours. Continuous intragastric tube-feeding syringes used in neonatal nurseries generally remain at room temperature for up to 4 hours.

2. *Refrigeration* (4°C [39°F]). Milk fed within 48 hours of collection can be refrigerated without significant bacterial proliferation.

TABLE 11-4. SUGGESTED GUIDELINES FOR MILK STORAGE AND USE FOR ALL INFANTS

Storage Method and Temperature	Maximum Amount of Time for Storage
Room (25°C [77°F])	4 hours*
Refrigerator (4°C [39°F])	48 hours
Previously thawed refrigerated milk	24 hours
Freezer (-20°C = 0°F)	3 months (approximately)

*Continuous milk infusions for tube-feeding neonates generally remain at room temperature for 3 to 4 hours.

3. *Freezing* (-20°C = 0°F) is the preferred method of storing milk that is not intended to be fed within 24 hours. Single milk expressions should be packaged separately for freezing. Unlike heat treatment, freezing preserves many of the nutritional and immunologic properties of human milk. When frozen appropriately, milk generally can be stored for as long as 3 months before levels of free fatty acids increase (evidence for rancidity). Milk should not be stored on the door of the freezer. Optimally, freezers should have a thermometer and an alarm and should be opened only infrequently, especially if used for long-term storage. Some clinicians permit long-term storage for up to 6 months.

4. *Thawing.* Milk should be thawed rapidly, usually by holding the container under running tepid (not hot) water. Milk should never be thawed in a microwave oven. After milk is fully thawed, it should not be refrozen but stored in a refrigerator until used. Thawed milk should be used within 24 hours or discarded. For hospitalized infants, expressed human milk remaining in a bottle after a feeding should be discarded.

B. **Milk storage containers** should have caps that provide an airtight seal. In the hospital setting, all containers for frozen expressed milk must carry a standardized label that includes the infant's name, medical record number, and date and time milk was expressed. Some hospitals request that mothers list medications and/or current illnesses on the label to ensure communication about the acceptability of the milk with hospital staff. Policies should be developed to avoid feeding one mother's milk to someone else's infant. In the child care setting milk also must be labeled clearly.

1. *Rigid plastic* storage containers made of polycarbonate (clear hard plastic), polypropylene (frosted hard plastic bottles), or other hard plastic are recommended for long-term storage of expressed human milk.

2. *Glass* containers also can be used for long-term storage, but care must be taken to ensure they don't get overfilled and/or crack.

3. *Soft plastic* (polyethylene) storage bags have potential for contamination from nicks in the bags, loss of nutrient properties (especially fat and fat-soluble vitamins), loss of milk because of spillage, and high cost. They are not recommended for hospitalized premature infants, and some experts discourage their use for all infants. Polyethylene bags specifically designed for storing human milk, however, may be convenient for the workplace/school if mothers bring their milk home at the end of the day. If they are used, the milk should be poured into rigid containers before freezer storage.

C. **Cleaning collection/storage containers** should begin with a rinse to remove adherent milk, then wash with hot soapy water, and dry in the air. Dishwasher cleaning also is adequate.

VI. **Donor human milk** is milk contributed by women other than the biological mother of the receiving infant. Donor milk generally is used as a replacement if mother's milk is not available. This milk is collected and stored through a milk bank. Because of the risk of disease transmission, banked donor milk must be pasteurized. Use of banked donor milk must be preceded by a discussion of the potential benefits of pasteurized human milk versus the potential risks of its use. The Human Milk Banking Association of North America (HMBANA) is the source for information, policies, and procedures related to donor milk. All member banks of the HMBANA are required to follow established guidelines, such as carefully selecting and monitoring donors, following strict procedures for heat treatment and storage of donated milk, and evaluating processed milk. Health care professionals interested in potential uses of donor human milk should consult HMBANA (www.HMBANA.com) or a member milk bank.

VII. **Bacteriologic Surveillance of Mother's Own Milk**
Human milk potentially can be a mode of transmission of infection. This particularly is a concern when breast pumps are used. For example, the rubber bulb portion of the bicycle horn type of breast pump cannot be cleaned or sterilized properly so its use is not recommended. Electric breast pumps that are disinfected

inadequately also may serve as a potential source of infection in neonatal nurseries. Expressed milk may contain bacterial flora of the skin.

A. **Bacteriologic cultures** of a mother's own milk may, under rare circumstances, be indicated to assess unexplained infections in infants. For example, some clinicians culture milk if an infant becomes infected with an unusual organism. Routine culture is costly and not done.

B. **Bacteriologic Screening Results.** Bacteria found on screening usually are identical to that found on the mother's skin and nipples. Generally, gram-positive organisms are found (usually $<10^5$ organisms/mL), but no gram-negative organisms.

C. **How to Deal With a Positive Culture.** If the organism is pathogenic and/or present in large quantities, the breast pump and the mother's equipment should be examined for contamination. The mother's milk expression technique also should be evaluated.

Selected References

Bier JB, Ferguson A, Anderson L, et al. Breast-feeding of very low birth weight infants. *J Pediatr.* 1993;123:773–778

Blaymore Bier JA, Ferguson AE, Morales Y, Liebling JA, Oh W, Vohr BR. Breast-feeding infants who were extremely low birth weight. *Pediatrics.* 1997;100:e3

Blenkharn JI. Infection risks from electrically operated breast pumps. *J Hosp Infect.* 1989;13:27–31

Feher SD, Berger LR, Johnson JD, Wilde JB. Increased breast milk production for premature infants with a relaxation/imagery audiotape. *Pediatrics.* 1989;83:57–60

Hill PD, Aldag JC, Chatterton RT. Effects of pumping style on milk production in mothers of non-nursing preterm infants. *J Hum Lact.* 1999;15:209–216

Howard CR, de Blieck EA, ten Hoopen CB, Howard FM, Lanphear BP, Lawrence RA. Physiologic stability of newborns during cup- and bottle-feeding. *Pediatrics.* 1999;104:1204–1207

Howard CR, Howard FM, Lanphear B, et al. Randomized clinical trial of pacifier use and bottle-feeding or cupfeeding and their effect on breastfeeding. *Pediatrics.* 2003;111:511–518

Human Milk Banking Association of North America. *Guidelines for the Establishment and Operation of a Donor Human Milk Bank.* West Hartford, CT: Human Milk Banking Association of North America; 1994

Human Milk Banking Association of North America. *Recommendations for Collection, Storage, and Handling of a Mother's Milk for Her Own Infant in the Hospital Setting.* West Hartford, CT: Human Milk Banking Association of North America; 1993

Lang S, Lawrence CJ, Orme RL. Cup feeding: an alternative method of infant feeding. *Arch Dis Child.* 1994;71:365–369

Meier PP. Breastfeeding in the special care nursery. Prematures and infants with medical problems. *Pediatr Clin North Am.* 2001;48:425–442

Meier PP, Engstrom JL, Fleming BA, Streeter PL, Lawrence PB. Estimating milk intake of hospitalized preterm infants who breastfeed. *J Hum Lact.* 1996;12: 21–26

Robbins ST. *Infant Feedings: Guidelines for Preparation of Formula and Breastmilk in Health Care Facilities.* Chicago, IL; American Dietetic Association; 2004

Slusser W, Frantz K. High-technology breastfeeding. *Pediatr Clin North Am.* 2001; 48:505–516

Sosa R, Barness L. Bacterial growth in refrigerated human milk. *Am J Dis Child.* 1987;141:111–112

Zinaman MJ, Hughes V, Queenan JT, Labbok MH, Albertson B. Acute prolactin and oxytocin responses and milk yield to infant suckling and artificial methods of expression in lactating women. *Pediatrics.* 1992;89:437–440

Chapter 12

Medications and Breastfeeding

The use of a medication by the breastfeeding mother continues to be a common reason for unnecessarily stopping breastfeeding. Usually this occurs because the mother gets incorrect advice as to what drugs are safe for the breastfed infant. The goal of successful maternal therapy during lactation is to provide the necessary therapeutic compounds to the breastfeeding mother while minimizing the amount of drug passed through the milk to the child, and those amounts that are transferred do not cause any significant changes in the child.

I. **Sources of information on medications and breastfeeding** include the AAP Committee on Drugs statement and references by Briggs et al and Hale (see Selected References and Appendix). *The Physician's Desk Reference* generally is not a source of information on the significance of medication exposure to the infant via human milk.

II. **Pharmacologic Principles**
    There are several factors that enhance drug transfer into human milk, including low molecular weight, high lipid solubility, long half-life, low protein binding, drug metabolites with long half-life, and acid-base characteristics that favor the transfer of weak bases. Intestinal drug absorption may be unpredictable in the neonate due to lower gastric pH. The neonate's intestinal tract has higher permeability, which may permit greater drug uptake. The action of intestinal glucuronidases favors the release of free drug and enhanced intestinal absorption. In addition, the neonate may have less protein binding of drugs, greater blood-brain barrier permeability, and less body fat to store drugs. Immature hepatic and renal

excretory metabolism and greater red blood cell sensitivity further compromise the newborn infant. The neonate, with delayed renal and hepatic clearance of drugs, is exposed to even greater effects when the mother uses medication with active metabolites. Lastly, drug effects through milk may be additive to the drug levels acquired transplacentally.

There are practices, however, to minimize drug exposure during breastfeeding. Because drugs disappear from maternal circulation with a known half-life, it is possible to minimize the amount transferred to the infant by recommending that drug dosing occur just at the conclusion of the feeding. In some cases, the drug can be substituted with a safer drug, or the therapy can be delayed. The avoidance of breastfeeding at peak plasma drug concentration is helpful.

III. Drug Categories

A. Social Drugs

1. *Cigarette smoking* exposes the infant to nicotine and other compounds, including cyanide and carbon monoxide, directly via milk and indirectly by secondhand smoke. Cigarette smoking may affect milk production, impair let-down, and result in behavioral changes in the infant. Despite these concerns, breastfeeding should be encouraged because of its protection against respiratory illnesses, which are more common in the infant living in a home with smokers. (See Chapter 3.) Pregnancy and lactation are opportune times to counsel the mother on smoking cessation to protect her health as well as her infant's.

    a. *Smoking cessation* may be achieved through counseling with or without the use of pharmacologic aids.

        i. Nicotine patches are designed to deliver a precise amount of nicotine transdermally over a definite period. Because nicotine appears in milk, there is a slight risk that the breastfed infant may exhibit signs of restlessness, jitteriness, poor feeding, and abnormal sleep patterns. Other forms of nicotine replacement (eg, gum, inhalers) may be less predictable in dosage/timing.

ii. Bupropion is a centrally acting drug also used in children with attention deficit disorder and related behavioral problems. The exposure of small infants to a drug with its major action in receptors and neurotransmitters in the central nervous system is discussed under Maternal Depression (page 176). It is not known whether there are any long-term effects of chronic exposure to bupropion in the breastfed infant.

2. *Alcohol* (ethanol) is one prototype of drug demonstrating rapid transport into milk. It is lipid-soluble, is not ionized, and has low molecular weight. Concentrations in milk are very close to maternal plasma concentrations. The Institute of Medicine recommends lactating women limit alcohol intake to 0.5 g or less of alcohol per kilogram of maternal body weight per day. For a 60-kg woman, this represents the equivalent of 2 cans of beer, 2 glasses of table wine, or 2 oz of liquor. (See Chapter 3.) There is evidence that the consumption of alcohol by the mother may decrease the amount of milk ingested by the infant. Perhaps this is related to taste. Chronic or binge drinking of alcoholic beverages may diminish milk production. Mothers should be counseled against excess ingestion of alcoholic drinks. Some clinicians recommend avoiding breastfeeding for 2 hours after ingesting alcohol; others suggest that the mother wait until she no longer feels the effects of the alcohol.

3. *Caffeine* is transferred but the amount in milk is usually less than 1% of the amount ingested by the mother. Because no caffeine is detected in the infant's urine with maternal consumption of up to 3 cups of coffee a day, it is unlikely that the infant has measurable exposure to caffeine. The amount of caffeine in carbonated beverages (soft drinks) is quite low, usually less than 50 mg/12 oz can, but there are some soft drinks with higher concentrations. The transport of other substances that may be in caffeinated beverages has not been measured.

4. *Drugs of abuse* are contraindicated for breastfeeding mothers.

B. **Anticoagulation.** Unfractionated and low molecular weight heparin given to the mother are safe for the breastfed infant because they do not cross into milk. Warfarin is also safe because of its very low concentration in milk due to very high binding of the drug to maternal plasma protein. There are no alterations in the breastfed infant's prothrombin time in mothers who are taking warfarin.

C. **Asthma** therapy emphasizes prophylaxis through the use of corticosteroids, usually by inhalation. For treatment of acute asthma attacks, beta-agonists and leukotriene-blocking agents are used.

   1. *Steroids* are transferred into milk in extremely small quantities, and transfer from oral inhalers is even smaller. The use of steroids to treat asthma in the breastfeeding mother is safe for the infant.

   2. *Beta-agonists* such as albuterol are associated with very small transfer to the breastfed infant and seem to be safe.

   3. *Theophylline* is rarely used now for either prophylaxis or treatment of acute asthma and ordinarily will not be an issue for the breastfeeding mother. Irritability in the infant, however, has been reported.

   4. *Newer agents* such as zileuton inhibit leukotriene formation, and zafirlukast and montelukast block leukotriene action. No information on their concentration in milk is available and there are no reports of effects on the breastfed infant.

D. **Maternal depression,** often accompanied by anxiety, carries significant risk for child development (Chapter 9). If the mother has been successfully treated for depression before delivery, there are strong arguments for her to continue her medication in the postpartum period. Antidepressants are thought to alter the concentration of neurotransmitters in the central nervous system, particularly in the interneuronal space. Some of the drugs are effective in inhibiting uptake of a neurotransmitter, thus prolonging pharmacologic action. Older antidepressants, such as the tricyclics nortriptyline and amitriptyline, have a good safety profile in breastfeeding, including long-term infant developmental follow-up. However, the tricyclics are used infrequently because of bothersome side effects. Newer antidepressants, such as the serotonin selective reuptake inhibitors (SSRIs), are better tolerated and are widely prescribed during pregnancy and lactation. The SSRIs generally exhibit low concentrations in human milk—usually less than 50% of maternal plasma level. A sensitive measure of SSRI intake is the depletion of platelet serotonin levels. Some investigations find that breastfed infants exposed to SSRIs via milk demonstrate no effect on platelet serotonin levels. Many infants, especially older than 4 months, may have no detectable serum levels of the drug after passage through milk. Infants younger than 4 months may have detectable levels and, in the case of some drugs (fluoxetine), the infant plasma level may be close to the accepted therapeutic range for adults. There have been a few reports of infants who exhibited restlessness, irritability, colic, poor weight gain, and sleep disorders when their mothers took fluoxetine. For the other SSRIs, no adverse effects have been described. Two often-used SSRIs, fluoxetine and sertraline, have active metabolites and half-lives that are on the order of days, and accumulation may occur in the very young infant. The concern about exposure of the breastfed infant to these compounds is that there are no long-term studies indicating either safety or adverse effects.

Long-acting benzodiazepines (diazepam), especially if associated with chronic use, may accumulate in milk and produce symptoms in the infant, such as lethargy, sedation, and poor suck. Sporadic use of long-acting drugs and the use of short-acting drugs (lorazepam, midazolam, oxazepam) pose less of a risk.

E. **Diabetes** therapy generally does not present any concerns for breastfeeding. In some cases, breastfeeding may reduce maternal insulin needs.

1. *Insulin* does not cross into human milk.

2. *Oral Hypoglycemics.* There are little data concerning the use of the oral hypoglycemics and virtually none on newer agents. Tolbutamide is usually compatible with breastfeeding. Other drugs should be used with caution by mothers who breastfeed. This is based on the experience

with their use in pregnancy, which can result in severe and prolonged hypoglycemia in the newborn. The best advice for using these agents during lactation is to avoid them until lactation is well established, the infant is gaining weight satisfactorily, and the parents discuss with the pediatric care professional the need to monitor the infant's blood glucose. Newer data on glyburide are encouraging. There is poor transplacental transfer of this drug likely due to high protein binding and a short elimination half-life. For the same reason, there may be limited transfer into milk. Until safety during lactation is established, however, these agents also should be used with caution.

F. **Gastrointestinal Disorders**

1. *H_2 receptor blocking agents* (famotidine, ranitidine, and cimetidine) seem to be safe during lactation. All of these compounds have been given directly to young infants to treat reflux and in hospitalized children to decrease production of gastric acid and minimize the occurrence of peptic ulcers. Likewise, the use of the protein pump inhibitor omeprazole also seems to be quite safe during lactation, although concentrations in milk have not been documented.

2. *Inflammatory Bowel Disease.* The treatment of inflammatory bowel disease (Crohn disease, ulcerative colitis) may require the use of multiple medications, either sequentially or simultaneously. These include corticosteroids (by enema and orally) and anti-inflammatory drugs such as sulfasalazine, mesalamine, and olsalazine. The anti-inflammatory drugs have as their active moiety 5-aminosalicylic acid. This substance is rapidly cleared from the plasma of adults and if it does appear in milk, it is in very low concentrations.

3. *Antimetabolites.* Inflammatory bowel disease occasionally may be treated with an antimetabolite drug, such as 6-mercaptopurine or methotrexate. Previous editions of the AAP policy statement reported that these drugs were contraindicated during breastfeeding because of potential cytotoxicity. However, there exist no data to support this, and the amount transferred may be inconsequential to the

baby. These drugs should not be given to lactating mothers without fully informing the parents about the possible immune suppression and effects on growth, even in small amounts, to the breastfed infant. If used, the infants should be monitored for neutropenia.

G. **Hypertension.** The treatment of adult hypertension often involves combinations of drugs. Currently there are 4 classes of antihypertensive drugs that are used: 1) diuretics, 2) beta blocking agents, 3) angiotensin converting enzyme inhibitors/ angiotensin receptor blockers (ACE inhibitors), and 4) calcium channel blocking agents.

1. *Diuretics* Seem to be safe during lactation. Hydrochlorothiazide and chlorothiazide have been used for decades and no problems have been described in the breastfed infant.

2. *Beta-Blocking Agents.* The drugs within this class that seem to be safest for use during pregnancy are propranolol, sotalol, and metoprolol. Atenolol and acebutolol may present problems to the breastfed infant. One case report describes cyanosis and bradycardia in a 5-day-old infant whose mother was receiving atenolol. The milk concentration was 2 to 3 times the simultaneous maternal plasma concentration. It is prudent to avoid atenolol and acebutolol in the breastfeeding mother. The infant of any mother who needs to take a beta-blocking agent should be monitored, especially for heart rate, feeding problems, respiratory pattern, and activity.

3. *ACE inhibitors* are excreted in limited quantities into milk. There are no reports of problems using these drugs.

4. *Calcium channel blocking agents* are the newest of the antihypertensive agents. Little is known about their excretion in milk, but it does seem that nifedipine is excreted in small amounts and is safe during breastfeeding. The same is also true of verapamil, the calcium channel blocking agent with the longest clinical use. Diltiazem is one of the newer agents, and one study shows that the average dose presented to the infant was less than 1% of the maternal dose. This drug also is probably safe during breastfeeding.

H. **Infectious disease** treatment is probably the most frequent cause for the use of drugs in the lactating woman. Generally, all antibiotics are transferred to milk. Many of them are also used for the treatment of infectious diseases in pediatrics. The doses received by the breastfed infant always are less than what would be given directly to the infant for therapy. There exist some specific concerns for certain antibiotics.

1. *Sulfonamides* should not be given to a breastfeeding mother whose infant is jaundiced or in the age group where jaundice may develop. This is because of the possible displacement of bilirubin from albumin in the infant's plasma by sulfonamides, which may increase the risk of kernicterus. In addition, there are concerns that these drugs may increase the risk of hemolysis in infants with a deficiency of glucose-6-phosphate dehydrogenase. Because sulfonamides are rarely used in today's management of infectious disease, they should not present a problem because other drugs are available.

2. *Tetracycline.* There are numerous statements in reviews of drugs in milk cautioning against the use of tetracycline during breastfeeding. There is no published evidence to support this. The amount of tetracycline that might appear in milk is extremely low, and there are no reports of adverse effects on the infant's gastrointestinal tract or on calcified tissues, such as bone and teeth. Tetracyclines are not commonly used because they have been replaced by more effective and safer antibiotics.

3. *Metronidazole.* The caution against metronidazole seems related to its in vitro ability to cause chromosomal damage. This has not been described in humans receiving the drug or in infants breastfeeding from mothers who receive the drug. Metronidazole is an antibiotic that is occasionally used in infants for the treatment of *Giardia* and some anaerobic infections, and is used in pregnancy. Metronidazole seems to be safe for the breastfed infant.

4. *Quinolone* (nalidixic acid) and **fluoroquinolone** (ciprofloxacin, ofloxacin) antibiotics have reasonably long half-lives, which allow once- or twice-a-day dosing. They

are well absorbed from the gastrointestinal tract, permitting the early switch from intravenous to oral therapy and hence discharge from the hospital and increased compliance. Some of these drugs may interfere with cartilage formation in juvenile mammals. This has resulted in a warning label that they are not to be used in anyone younger than 18 years. However, some pediatric studies involving long-term use in patients with cystic fibrosis have not shown any cartilage damage as measured by serial magnetic resonance imaging of joints. Furthermore, ciprofloxacin is approved for limited use in children and the oldest quinolone, nalidixic acid, has been labeled for pediatric use for more than 30 years, although it is now rarely used in the pediatric population. There have been no reported adverse effects of this drug on growth. The amount that would be transferred into human milk is extremely low and if there is no other choice for maternal therapy, a short (1- to 2-week) exposure to quinolones may be acceptable for the breastfed infant.

   5. *Antifungal agents* currently given orally, including fluconazole, are safe for the infant and have been used for direct infant therapy.

I. **Migraine** headache treatment in adults is divided into prophylaxis of attacks and treatment of the acute episode. Drugs that are used for prophylaxis of migraine are verapamil, amitriptyline, propanolol, sertraline, cyproheptadine, valproic acid, and gabapentin. Sertraline and amitriptyline are antidepressants. (See Maternal Depression on page 176.) No milk concentration data have been found for cyproheptadine and gabapentin. All of the other drugs seem safe for the breastfed infant.

   1. *The initial therapy for acute migraine headache* may range from nonpharmacologic measures, such as rest, darkened room, and a wet cloth to the forehead, to some of the newest drugs. The use of acetaminophen and nonsteroidal anti-inflammatory drugs (NSAIDs) is acceptable during lactation because most are weak acids and highly protein bound. The NSAIDs include ibuprofen, naproxen, and ketoprofen. There are products that contain

a combination of acetaminophen with caffeine. All of these compounds are safe during lactation. The amount of acetaminophen and/or ibuprofen that might be transferred during lactation is only a small fraction of the dose given to infants for fever and pain. (See Chapter 6.)

2. *The Triptan* family contains the following compounds: sumatriptan, naratriptan, rizatriptan, and zolmitriptan. The only one for which data exist is sumatriptan, and the excretion in milk is extremely low and has not caused adverse effects in the breastfed infant.

3. *The Ergot* family contains a number of compounds including methylergonovine, which is used to contract the uterus and decrease bleeding immediately after birth. Methylergonovine has a very short half-life of 0.5 to 2 hours and, after a single dose, probably would not interfere with lactation. The intravenous form of ergotamine is dihydroergotamine, which has a very long half-life. An oral ergot is methysergide. Ergotamines may inhibit prolactin release and thus interfere with lactation. Because alternatives exist with the triptan family, it is prudent not to use drugs in the ergotamine family during lactation.

J. **Pain management** in the breastfeeding mother can be achieved by appropriate doses of either acetaminophen or NSAIDs such as ibuprofen and naproxen. More severe pain, such as that occurring immediately after birth or after surgery, is best managed with the use of appropriate doses of morphine because morphine has primarily inactive metabolites. See Chapter 6 for a discussion of pain management during lactation.

K. **Seizure Management.** A significant number of antiepileptic drugs is available. Many of the drugs that were once used as standard management for seizure disorders have been replaced. For example, phenytoin and phenobarbital are rarely used in adults. Phenobarbital has low protein binding, and sedation has been reported in breastfed infants exposed to the drug through milk. Most adults receive carbamazepine or valproic acid as single drug agents with the addition of lamotrigine or tiagabine for complex seizure disorders. There are single case reports that indicate infant problems. Cholestasis with carbamazepine has been reported, and thrombocytopenia and anemia with valproic acid. An older publication has described methemoglobinemia in the infant of a mother taking phenytoin. Lamotrigine taken by the breastfeeding mother may be associated with therapeutic levels in the infant. Given the widespread use of these agents over a period of many years, it is uncertain that these few case reports were indeed connected with exposure from secretion into milk. Regardless of which drug or drugs the mother needs for the control of her epilepsy, it would be prudent not only to clinically observe the baby, but also to measure drug concentrations in the infant's plasma on a regular basis, especially in very young infants in the first 2 months of life.

L. **Thyroid hormone** (levothyroxine) is transmitted into milk in extremely small quantities and will not change the thyroid function of the infant. Women with hyperthyroidism have a choice of 2 drugs for therapy: propylthiouracil and methimazole. Propylthiouracil is the preferred drug because about 75% of it is bound to maternal plasma protein in contrast to methimazole, which has almost no protein binding. Thus the amount of propylthiouracil secreted is quite small; usually less than 1% of the therapeutic dose goes to the infant. Thyroid function of the infant is not altered by maternal use of propylthiouracil. With chronic ingestion, iodides, being of low molecular weight, may be transferred to milk and in the infant may interfere with thyroid function. Occasional doses, however, used to protect the thyroid may not be a problem. Chronic use of iodine-containing cough and cold medications should be avoided.

M. **Radioactive Isotopes.** If a diagnostic radioisotope is to be administered to a breastfeeding mother, she should be told how long she likely is to be unable to breastfeed, based on the half-life of the radioisotope chosen. This will allow her to express and freeze milk in advance for her infant's use while she is unable to breastfeed. When she stops breastfeeding temporarily (for example 24–48 hours for some thyroid scans), she should be counseled to express and discard her milk during the time required for treatment. Mothers who receive therapeutic radioactive isotopes will probably not be able to breastfeed because the dose of radiation remains high for a sustained period. A nuclear medicine physician should be consulted.

N. **Galactagogues** are drugs that stimulate the production of milk. Galactagogues should be used in conjunction with usual efforts to increase milk production (frequent breastfeeding and milk expression). Metoclopramide commonly is used to increase milk production early in lactation or at any time when milk production seems to be falling. Short-term use of metoclopramide (usually not exceeding 14 days) seems safe. Studies differ as to the success in sustained increase in milk production with this drug. The drug may have multiple effects on the mother's central nervous system, including sleepiness, depression, or extrapyramidal signs. Short-term use of metoclopramide seems safe because it seldom is used for more than 14 days.

Other galactagogues, such as thyrotropin-releasing hormone and human growth hormone, may increase milk production through increasing prolactin secretion or working additively with prolactin to sustain normal lactation. There has been insufficient study of these hormones, and they are too expensive to be recommended for routine use to stimulate lactation. Oxytocin spray (40 IU/mL) was commercially available in the past to improve milk ejection, but it is no longer manufactured. Some practitioners have used the available dilute intravenous oxytocin (10 IU/mL) as nasal drops or spray (4 drops instead of 1).

O. **Herbal Remedies.** Many cultures have relied on herbs and other substances to improve milk production. There have been no scientific studies of these preparations to prove or disprove their value as galactagogues. The use of herbal remedies in the United States is extremely prevalent. Federal legislation in 1994 removed them from the rigorous safety and effectiveness provisions that the US Food and Drug Administration applies to prescription drugs. Herbal preparations are considered to be dietary supplements. Lactating women who ask about using herbal preparations should be informed that the composition, purity, and efficacy, as well as effect on either lactation or infant physiology, are unknown.

P. Environmental agents may affect breastfeeding. Table 7 of the AAP policy statement "The Transfer of Drugs and Other Chemicals Into Human Milk" (page 236) describes food and environmental agents that have been reported to have some relationship to breastfeeding. There is a lack of evidence that silicone breast implants pose a problem for the breastfeeding mother.

Selected References

American Academy of Pediatrics Committee on Drugs. The transfer of drugs and other chemicals into human milk. *Pediatrics.* 2001;108:776–789

Benowitz NL, Dempsey DA. Pharmacotherapy for smoking cessation during pregnancy. *Nicotine Tob Res.* 2004;6(suppl 2):S189–S202

Neal B, MacMahon S, Chapman N. Blood Pressure Lowering Treatment Trialists' Collaboration. Effects of ACE inhibitors, calcium antagonists, and other blood-pressure-lowering drugs: results of prospectively designed overviews of randomised trials. *Lancet.* 2000;356:1955–1964

Briggs GG, Freeman RK, Yaffee SJ. *Drugs in Pregnancy and Lactation.* 6th ed. Baltimore, MD: Williams & Wilkins; 2001

Hale TW. *Medications and Mothers' Milk: A Manual of Lactational Pharmacology.* 11th ed. Amarillo, TX: Pharmasoft Medical Publishing; 2004

Howard CR, Lawrence RA. Xenobiotics and breastfeeding. *Pediatr Clin North Am.* 2001;48:485–504

Ito S. Drug therapy for breast-feeding women. *N Engl J Med.* 2000;343: 118–126

Pahor M, Psaty BM, Alderman MH, et al. Health outcomes associated with calcium antagonists compared with other first-line antihypertensive therapies: a meta-analysis of randomised controlled trials. *Lancet.* 2000;356:1949–1954

US Pharmacopeia Convention, Inc. *USP DI Volume I: Drug Information for the Health Care Professional.* Taunton, MA: Micromedix; 2001

Chapter 13

Contraception and the Breastfeeding Mother

A woman should be encouraged to consider her future plans for child-bearing and desired birth spacing during prenatal care, and be given information and services that will help her meet her goals so she can devote her time and energy to her new infant.

I. Contraceptive Counseling

A. **Rationale.** An unplanned pregnancy within a year after birth not only may cause nutritional and emotional stress but also may negatively affect a mother's commitment to ongoing breastfeeding.

B. **Opportunities for Counseling.** Frequent visits with a health care professional in the antepartum and postpartum periods provide many opportunities to discuss contraceptive plans.

1. *Antepartum.* An antepartum visit presents an opportunity to explore a mother's attitudes about contraception; her experience with different contraceptive methods; her preferred method(s); and her thoughts on birth spacing or, alternatively, sterilization. The advantages and disadvantages of different methods can be reviewed in relation to her health profile and her decision to breastfeed.

2. *Immediate Postpartum.* At the time of discharge counseling after birth, the mother's contraceptive plan can be reviewed and reinforced or revised. Consideration may be given to the potential risk of unintended pregnancy before a return visit if breastfeeding may not meet lactation amenorrhea criteria to ensure resulting anovulation.

3. *Postpartum Office Visit.* The postpartum visit, typically 4 to 6 weeks after delivery, is an ideal time to assess the adequacy of breastfeeding frequency and duration in providing natural contraception. If the mother needs or wants more protection from unintended pregnancy, options can be discussed and initiated.

II. Contraceptive Options

A. Methods Not Using Exogenous Hormones

1. *Lactational Amenorrhea Method (LAM).* The LAM has been shown to be highly effective in a variety of cultural, health care, and socioeconomic settings. The LAM is most appropriate for women who plan to exclusively breastfeed 6 months or longer. If the infant is breastfed exclusively (or is very rarely given supplemental formula feedings), and if the mother has not experienced her first postpartum menses, breastfeeding provides more than 98% protection from pregnancy in the first 6 months following delivery. For optimal effectiveness, intervals between feedings should not exceed 4 hours during the day or 6 hours at night. Feeding practices other than direct breastfeeding, such as pumping, may reduce the vigor and frequency of suckling. This in turn may alter the maternal neuroendocrine response and hence increase the probability that ovulation will resume. An alternative method of contraception should be used if the mother's description of the extent of her breastfeeding suggests it may not be adequate to suppress ovulation. In addition, mothers using LAM should be provided standard counseling about strategies to prevent sexually transmitted diseases.

2. *Barrier Methods.* The advantage of barrier methods of contraception, including pre-lubricated latex condoms, the diaphragm, and spermicides, is the absence of any effect on breastfeeding. Condoms have additional, non-contraceptive advantages including effective protection against sexually transmitted diseases. The disadvantage of barrier methods is suboptimal effectiveness in typical use, with failure rates of approximately 10% to 20% across different barrier

methods. These data are based on normally menstruating women and thus are likely applicable to the breastfeeding woman once menses resume.

3. *Intrauterine devices (IUDs)* offer safe, effective long-term contraception and may be considered for all women who seek a reversible, effective, and coitally independent birth control method. They offer long-term pregnancy protection (5–10 years depending on the product chosen). They may be conveniently inserted at the time of the postpartum visit. Some evidence suggests that breastfeeding women have easier IUD insertions, fewer post-insertion complaints, and a lower rate of removal for adverse side effects compared with women who are not breastfeeding. Uterine perforation at IUD insertion does not seem to be more common in breastfeeding women. The advantage of IUDs, in addition to contraceptive effectiveness of 99% or greater, is the fact that they have no affect on breastfeeding. It should be noted that some IUDs contain a progestin; advantageous characteristics of progestins in relation to breastfeeding are described below.

B. **Methods Using Exogenous Hormones.** These are a readily accepted and highly effective means of preventing pregnancy. There are, however, potential disadvantages that relate to the postpartum state in general and to breastfeeding mothers in particular, and these disadvantages vary by hormonal method.

1. *Progestin-Only Contraceptives*

    a. *Advantages.* Progestin-only contraceptives, including progestin-only tablets ("minipills"), depot medroxyprogesterone acetate (DMPA), and levonorgestrel implants, do not affect the quality of human milk and may slightly increase the volume of milk and duration of breastfeeding compared with nonhormonal methods. Progestin-only methods are the hormonal contraceptives of choice for breastfeeding mothers.

    b. *Timing.* There is no scientific evidence that proscribes the initiation of progestin-only contraception in the early postpartum period. However, the typical 2- to

3-day postdelivery decrease of progesterone is part of the physiologic process that initiates lactation. Thus there is theoretical concern that giving progestins in the first few days before lactation is established could interfere with optimal lactation. Contraception is not needed in the first 3 weeks postpartum because of a delay in return of ovulation in all women, and this delay is extended for women who breastfeed exclusively. Health care professionals should consider initiating progestin-only contraception at 6 weeks in those women who are breastfeeding exclusively and at 3 weeks in others. There may, however, be practical reasons for initiating contraception in the immediate postpartum period, such as uncertainty about the opportunities for follow-up visits.

2. *Combination Oral Contraceptives*

   a. *Disadvantages.* The disadvantages of combination oral contraceptives (COCs) include the potential contribution of the estrogen component to the known hypercoagulable state of the postpartum period and the recognized negative effect of COCs on milk production. Estrogen also may be transferred into the milk.

   b. *Timing.* The most conservative recommendation, that of delaying combined oral contraceptive use until at least 6 months after birth, largely emanates from earlier studies of COCs that used higher doses of estrogen. Most contemporary formulations have 35 μg or less of estrogen, which likely has a lesser effect on the quality and quantity of milk. While progestin-only preparations remain the oral contraception of choice for breastfeeding women, COCs can be considered after 6 weeks postpartum if breastfeeding is well established and the infant's nutritional status is monitored.

Selected References

Abdulla KA, Elwan SI, Salem HS, Shaaban MM. Effect of early postpartum use of the contraceptive implants, NORPLANT, on the serum levels of immunoglobulins of the mothers and their breastfed infants. *Contraception.* 1985;32:261–266

American College of Obstetricians and Gynecologists. ACOG committee opinion. Condom availability for adolescents. Number 154-April 1995. Committee on Adolescent Health Care. American College of Obstetricians and Gynecologists. *Int J Gynaecol Obstet.* 1995;49:347–351

American College of Obstetricians and Gynecologists. The intrauterine device. ACOG technical bulletin number 164—February 1992. *Int J Gynaecol Obstet.* 1993;41:189–193

American College of Obstetricians and Gynecologists. Breastfeeding: Maternal and Infant Aspects. ACOG educational bulletin number 258—July 2000. *Obstet Gynecol.* 1999;96

Campbell OM, Gray RH. Characteristics and determinants of postpartum ovarian function in women in the United States. *Am J Obstet Gynecol.* 1993;169: 55–60

Chi IC, Potts M, Wilkens LR, Champion CB. Performance of the copper T-380A intrauterine device in breastfeeding women. *Contraception.* 1989;39: 603–618

Chi IC, Wilkens LR, Champion CB, Machemer RE, Rivera R. Insertional pain and other IUD insertion-related rare events for breastfeeding and non-breastfeeding women: a decade's experience in developing countries. *Adv Contracept.* 1989;5:101–119

Trussell J, Hatcher RA, Cates W Jr, Stewart FH, Kost K. Contraceptive failure in the United States: an update. *Stud Fam Plann.* 1990;21:51–54

Chapter 14

Breastfeeding Infants
With Special Needs

The benefits of human milk can be extended to neonates with special needs, including multiple birth. Infants with medical problems, such as prematurity, may require special assistance with breastfeeding or nutrient supplements to their mother's milk to ensure adequate growth and development. Feeding expressed human milk, modified as necessary, allows high-risk neonates to receive nutritive and nonnutritive beneficial properties from human milk. There are some circumstances when the delivery of a high-risk neonate is known beforehand, and an appropriate consultation with a neonatal specialist should include discussing the use of human milk and maintenance of milk supply. Milk expression and storage are discussed in detail in Chapter 11.

I. Very Low Birth Weight Infants

Even if the intent was for formula feeding, many mothers of high-risk infants will provide their milk when encouraged by their health care professional, even for short-term feeding. In these circumstances, breastfeeding means initiating and maintaining a method of milk expression. Centers caring for high-risk neonates should have trained staff readily available to assist the mother in methods of milk expression and optimal milk production (Chapter 11), and assist the dyad with breastfeeding sessions. Although the following discussion focuses on very low birth weight (VLBW) infants, those weighing less than 1,500 g at birth, the same issues may be pertinent to all premature and full-term hospitalized infants. The benefits of breastfeeding this special population should be discussed. (See Chapter 3.)

A. **Fortification of Human Milk**

1. *Rationale.* Delayed onset of feedings, volume restriction of enteral feedings, and variable composition of mother's milk are but a few of the factors posing limitations in the use of unsupplemented human milk for VLBW infants. A rapid rate of postnatal growth is necessary to compare with intrauterine rates. Thus, nutrient requirements to meet these growth needs are greater than at any other time in life. The nutrient content of human milk cannot meet all the needs imposed by this rapid rate of growth, especially in VLBW infants.

   Protein inadequacy (as evidenced by low blood urea nitrogen and albumin values) has been observed in VLBW infants fed unfortified human milk. Biochemical (as evidenced by low serum phosphorus and high serum calcium concentrations, and high serum alkaline phosphatase activity) and radiological rickets also are observed in VLBW infants fed unfortified human milk. Hyponatremia as well as vitamin inadequacy also are described in VLBW infants fed unfortified human milk. The feeding of human milk fortified with protein and minerals is associated with improved growth (weight, length, and head circumference), bone mineralization, and nutrient balance compared with unfortified human milk. Importantly, the use of fortified human milk is not associated with any increases in either feeding intolerance, necrotizing enterocolitis, or sepsis.

2. *Who should receive human milk fortification?* All infants with a birth weight less than 1,500 g should receive fortified human milk until they achieve a body weight of approximately 2,000 g if they are still in the hospital. Other infants may need human milk fortifiers if they require tube feeding and have a restricted fluid intake. Some form of nutrient supplementation of human milk after hospital discharge should be considered in selected infants.

3. *Approach to Fortification.* In usual circumstances, human milk fortifier is added to human milk once the infant has attained a feeding volume of approximately 100 mL/kg/day. The maximum concentration listed by manufacturers should be followed (the US products suggest 4 packets per

100 mL human milk). Powdered fortifiers are preferred because they do not dilute the milk itself but fortify nutrients already present. Liquid fortifiers or preterm formulas have been used when mothers have low milk production (as a mixture of formula with human milk in 1:1 or 1:2 proportion). Alternatively, if there is inadequate mother's milk to fortify for an entire day's feeding, preterm formula has been alternated with feedings of fortified human milk.

4. *Milk Fat Content.* Fat content is the most variable of all nutrients in human milk. The variance among women, through lactation and during the course of the day, probably is less than the variance from losses due to fat separation from the milk and/or its adherence to collection containers and feeding devices. Lack of ability to predict milk fat content, and therefore energy content, is a concern for caregivers of VLBW infants because fat is the major determinant of milk calorie content. Thus an occasional VLBW infant manifests a low rate of weight gain despite human milk fortification.

5. *Hindmilk.* It is well known that the fat content of human milk rises during a single milk expression. The arbitrary terms foremilk and hindmilk refer to milk collected at the beginning and toward the end of a single milk expression, respectively. Some clinicians have used the higher-fat hindmilk to augment the energy intake of the infant. Hindmilk feedings may enhance growth by supplying 2 to 3 times more fat, and therefore calories, than foremilk. Although differing in fat and energy contents, foremilk and hindmilk fractions have similar contents of protein and minerals. Mothers of high-risk infants with more than adequate milk production (approximately 130% of what is needed by the infant) can be taught to fractionate their milk into foremilk and hindmilk. An arbitrary practice is to collect all milk produced in the first 3 to 5 minutes of pumping as foremilk and collect the remaining milk separately as hindmilk. Hindmilk usually is used in conjunction with human milk fortifiers. Hindmilk alone should be used with caution because it may result in an imbalanced protein/calorie ratio and a dilution of needed minerals and vitamins.

6. *Too Much Foremilk?* If a mother limits the feeding time, but nurses her full-term infant more frequently, the calorie density of the milk is lower (less fat is ingested); weight gain may be adversely affected; and in some cases, the infant's hunger may not be satiated. In that scenario, the infant wishes to feed sooner and the frequency of nursing increases. This stimulates more milk production but the infant appears hungry despite good volume and milk transfer. Lengthening the nursing period to ensure adequate draining of the breast often solves the problem. Incomplete breast draining during mechanical milk expression also might not provide sufficient fat from the hindmilk component, a problem of special concern in hospitalized premature infants.

B. **Oral Feeding Issues.** Many VLBW infants and other high-risk infants require tube feeding because they are unable to latch onto the breast and/or fatigue easily with oral feeding. Tube-feeding techniques should be modified to provide human milk without any nutrient losses (Chapter 11). Infants who have been given bottle feedings may become accustomed to immediate milk flow, unlike the process of breastfeeding (which often requires 60–90 seconds of nonnutritive suckling before let-down and milk flow occurs). These differences between breastfeeding and bottle-feeding may lead to nipple or flow confusion and cause frustration for the mother and infant. Thus oral feeding must be tailored to the specific needs of the VLBW infant. The following steps can be taken to progress from tube-feeding to breastfeeding.

1. *Skin-to-skin contact* between a VLBW infant and its mother can be a first step toward oral feeding. First established as a method to improve survival of home-reared premature infants in Bogota, Colombia, the technique of placing the infant skin-to-skin upright between the mother's breasts has gained much support in neonatal intensive care nurseries. Skin-to-skin or "kangaroo" care is associated with beneficial effects on thermoregulation, heart rate stability, oxygen saturation, periodic breathing, and weight gain. Skin-to-skin care provides psychological

benefits to the mother and physical benefits to the infant. Mothers who practice kangaroo care have increased milk production and enhanced confidence in their ability to actually breastfeed. When the mother holds her infant skin-to-skin, she is exposed to the same skin and respiratory "environment" as her infant, and thus may provide specific antibodies against nursery-acquired pathogens.

2. *Pacifiers.* Contrary to the advice given for healthy term infants, pacifiers may have a role in the neonatal intensive care unit. Pacifiers are used to comfort infants in pain or those who cannot be fed. Pacifiers facilitate the development and strengthening of muscles used for sucking, and the nonnutritive sucking provides a training effect for future oral feeding. Some studies suggest that when given a pacifier during tube feeding, premature infants have better weight gain and reduced hospital length of stay.

3. *The transition from tube to oral feeding* usually begins with skin-to-skin contact. Eventually the infant can be encouraged to suckle at the mother's breast and/or smell or lick the milk on her nipple. Suck-swallow-breathe coordination may begin around 32 weeks' postmenstrual age, but considerable variability is observed in achieving this milestone, and some infants achieve complete oral feeding much earlier. Premature infants who are allowed to suckle at the "empty" breast have longer, sustained breastfeeding than infants who began suckling once they could "suck well." This suggests that practicing breastfeeding encourages suck-swallow coordination. Early oral feedings should be initiated for oral-motor training as well as to gauge readiness to feed.

4. *Assessments of readiness to breastfeed* should be performed serially and include assessments of signs of sucking, such as sucking on the hand, nipple, tube, or pacifier. In addition, signs of rooting behavior, ability of the infant to latch and stay on the breast, sucking ability, duration of suck, behavioral state, skin color changes, vital signs, and the infant's comfort level during the feeding are some factors that are evaluated.

5. *Early Breastfeeding.* A mother who has a strong let-down reflex, with copious milk flow, may need to pump prior to an early breastfeeding session. This reduces the infant's risk of choking on high milk flow. Some infants require feeding devices, nipple shields, and test weighing to optimize oral feeding. (See Chapter 11.) If possible, bottle-feeding should be avoided until mother and infant have a secure, confident breastfeeding technique. Tube feeding given during early attempts at breastfeeding is particularly helpful. It is best to begin breastfeeding when the infant is alert and hungry, not frantic or overstimulated. The mother should be seated in a comfortable chair with an upright back with the infant on a nursing pillow, which allows the infant to be closer to the mother and at the level of her breast.

   a. *Positioning* of the infant is essential for each breast-feeding session. The infant may be placed in the typical holds discussed in Chapter 6. The mother may have to modify her hold from a C-hold to a U-hold to ensure that the weight of her breast does not interfere with the infant's ability to suckle. In the latter hold the hand can provide additional jaw support. The U-hold is achieved by placing the thumb on one side of the breast behind the areola, with other fingers placed on the opposite side.

   b. *Behavioral cues* should be used to identify times for feeding sessions when the infant is awake and alert. If the infant continually falls asleep during attempts at breastfeeding, the mother may try switching to the opposite breast or using a feeding device to reduce fatigue during suckling. If the infant does not initiate suckling, the mother can express some milk onto her nipple so that her infant tastes her milk when she places her nipple and areola into the infant's mouth. Usually, if the infant suckles for a short period, the mother should pump afterward to drain her breasts and maintain her milk supply.

C. **Nutritional monitoring** of growth and biochemical indices is important in managing the human milk-fed VLBW infant.

Growth parameters should be monitored serially (daily weight and weekly length and head circumference). Weight gain greater than 15 g/kg/day (or 20 g/day if body weight is >2,000 g) is adequate. Length and head circumference should increase by approximately 1 cm/week. Biochemical evaluation of nutritional status generally includes serial measurements of electrolytes (sodium declines through lactation and acidosis due to reduced buffering capacity of fortified human milk has been observed); urea nitrogen (to assess short-term protein adequacy); albumin (to assess long-term protein adequacy); and calcium, phosphorus, and alkaline phosphatase (to assess bone mineral status). These biochemical evaluations might be obtained every 2 weeks, and more frequently if abnormalities are observed.

D. **Discharge planning** must be ongoing, initiated well in advance of the actual date of hospital discharge, and include parent input. The projected date should be regularly updated at multidisciplinary caregiver discharge planning rounds. Nutritional factors are prominent in the discharge plans (sustained pattern of weight gain of sufficient duration, nutritional risks assessed and treated, competent oral feeding without cardiopulmonary compromise). By discharge, it must be clear that the infant is capable of oral feeding ad libitum (approximately 180 mL/kg/day if test weighing is used) and continues to gain weight adequately (approximately 20 g/day). Abnormalities in biochemical measurements should be noted (eg, elevated alkaline phosphatase and decreased serum phosphorus, urea nitrogen, and albumin).

1. *Exclusive breastfeeding* should be encouraged post-discharge if there are no concerns with adequacy of intake, growth, or biochemical measurements. Usually exclusive breastfeeding means a combination of breastfeeding and/or feedings of expressed human milk. After discharge the use of expressed milk is reduced as breastfeeding sessions increase.

2. *A combination of breastfeeding and formula* is desirable post-discharge if there are concerns of inadequate intake, poor weight gain, and/or persistent biochemical abnormalities. There are a variety of ways to provide multinutrient

supplementation for the breastfeeding infant in the post-discharge period. One strategy is to add feedings of enriched post-discharge formula. Enriched formulas (22 kcal/oz) provide a nutrient composition that ranges between a term and a preterm formula. These formulas are available as powders so, if necessary, they can be concentrated (to 24 or 30 kcal/oz). Mothers should be encouraged to continue to breastfeed with the addition of 2 or 3 of the supplemental formula feedings per day. This plan allows nearly full breastfeeding. There are, however, no data to assess this practical approach for post-discharge breastfeeding with supplementation. If supplemental feedings are used, however, to obtain the best outcomes, some experts recommend continuing the supplementation for a minimum of 6 months after discharge.

3. *Multivitamin* (1 mL/day) *and iron supplementation* (2 mg/kg/day) are suggested if the premature infant is exclusively breastfed or fed expressed human milk in the post-discharge period. There also are case reports suggesting a risk of zinc deficiency in exclusively breastfed premature infants after hospital discharge. If growth is slow, poor feeding is noted, and perioral or perianal rashes are present, zinc deficiency should be considered. In these cases, zinc supplementation of 1 mg/kg/day should be considered.

   If the infant is receiving formula as a supplement to breastfeeding, the dose of multivitamin and iron supplementation should be reduced. Some clinicians suggest that each be given at half the usual dose. These supplements can be adjusted based on the proportion of formula fed to the infant.

4. *Monitoring* of growth and biochemical indices should be done 1 week after discharge and repeated at monthly intervals until normalized. This monitoring may help to gauge when to add or withdraw some of the formula supplements.

II. Cleft Lip and Cleft Palate

Oral feeding is a major problem for infants with congenital oral malformations. The cleft malformations prevent an effective seal around the nipple to facilitate oral feeding.

A. **The benefits of breastfeeding for infants with cleft lip and/or palate** include promotion of oral and facial muscular development, allowance for a better seal at the lip defect due to the pliability of the breast, reduced otitis media, and the provision of comfort and pleasure by nonnutritive sucking, even for the infant who cannot accomplish nutritive sucking. Mothers of these infants should be instructed in milk expression techniques so that milk is available if the infant is ineffective at the breast.

B. **Infants with cleft hard palate** are unable to generate negative sucking pressure in the oral cavity, resulting in an excessive intake of air. They commonly have nasal regurgitation of milk and often fatigue during prolonged attempts to breastfeed. These obstacles result in major feeding problems, inadequate milk intake, and poor weight gain during the first months after birth. If some negative pressure can be generated, breastfeeding may succeed. If not, then a soft artificial nipple with a large opening or direct delivery of milk into the mouth is used. Palatal prostheses are available to improve the ability to generate negative sucking pressure.

C. **Isolated cleft lip** malformation is more likely to be associated with breastfeeding success. The infants are capable of generating negative pressure, providing occlusion of the lip is maintained. This can be accomplished by using the thumb of the hand supporting the breast in the C-hold to fill in the cleft and form a seal.

D. **Infants with cleft lip and palate** are least likely to breastfeed because the malformation adversely affects all aspects of oral feeding. They cannot generate negative pressure and usually have poor oral-motor function. These infants usually require an individual feeding plan that uses human milk provided by special feeding devices (Chapter 11). Techniques to assist the mother in breastfeeding an infant with cleft palate and/or lip are outlined in Table 14-1. Meanwhile, the mother can express her milk to maintain an adequate supply.

TABLE 14-1. BREASTFEEDING TECHNIQUES FOR INFANTS WITH CLEFT LIP AND/OR PALATE

1. Feed frequently (every 2–3 hours) and know techniques to allow milk let-down and latch-on.

2. Hold the breast with the C-hold or palmar grasp technique (thumb above and fingers below areola). The U-hold from under the breast can also be used.

3. Hold the infant at breast level. For hypotonic infants, their trunk and head should be placed at the same level as the breast with pillows.

4. Use positions such as the clutch, or football, hold to avoid nasal regurgitation and airway occlusion.

5. Use the straddle position (infant sits upright on the mother's lap and straddles her abdomen), for infants with bilateral cleft lip and palate to promote gravity delivery of milk and decreased nasal regurgitation and aspiration.

6. Massage the breast rhythmically to enhance milk delivery.

Adapted from Wagner C. Personal Communication.

   E. **Surgical repair** of cleft lip usually occurs in the first few months after birth while the palate is repaired at approximately 9 to 12 months. The timing of the lip repair may interfere with breastfeeding. Historically, infants with cleft lip repair were denied breastfeeding; the baby was fed with a cup, dropper, or spoon. Recent studies demonstrate enhanced recovery in infants allowed to breastfeed post–cleft lip repair. Six weeks after surgery, one study found that breastfed infants, when compared with device-fed infants, had better weight gain, shortened postoperative hospital stay, decreased use of analgesia and sedation, and less need for intravenous fluid. Thus, in some cases, breastfeeding should resume as soon as possible in the postoperative period.

III. The Pierre Robin sequence includes oral abnormalities that affect feeding ability and may produce feeding problems: micrognathia, glossoptosis, and cleft palate. Infants with Pierre Robin sequence may have higher than average caloric needs, as a result of increased breathing difficulties, and chronic airway obstruction. Some will be able to achieve adequate caloric intake through modified breastfeeding and modified nipple-feeding techniques. Those who are unable to tolerate oral feedings will need tube feedings to provide adequate nutrition.

A. **Sucking and swallowing dysfunction** is a major cause of feeding difficulties in the initial newborn period. Micrognathia leads to problems with latch. The cleft palate creates sucking problems. The tongue is displaced posteriorly. Infants are unable to stroke the nipple efficiently, so they have difficulty propelling the milk into the oropharynx. Other swallowing difficulties result from the tongue deformity. The infants typically produce a few rapid sucks then stop to breathe. They usually cannot perform the 2 processes together. During oral feeding, milk gets into the nasopharynx, which, together with swallowing dysfunction and abnormal tongue position, creates an increased risk of aspiration. In cases in which the tongue has been tacked down anteriorly (glossopexy) to prevent choking and aspiration, infants still encounter difficulty with latch and have tongue mobility problems and ongoing swallowing difficulties.

B. **Human milk is advantageous** for these infants because they have an increased risk of aspiration and associated respiratory infections. The use of human milk is associated with a decrease in otitis media and upper respiratory infection, which is a particular concern because these infants are at increased risk for otitis media and hearing deficits.

IV. **Infants with Down syndrome** often require special interventions to ensure successful breastfeeding. Their oral structures may include a variety of abnormalities that affect feeding: macroglossia, micrognathia, high-arched palate, cleft palate, midfacial hypoplasia, and generalized hypotonia. Infants with Down syndrome exhibit ineffective suckling or tongue thrusting of their large, flattened tongues, which causes difficulty with latch-on. The infant cannot form a trough with the tongue around the areola, allowing milk to go down the side of the mouth instead of into the back of the mouth to be swallowed. Feeding behavior usually improves as the generalized tone improves. See Table 14-2 for suggested techniques for breastfeeding the infant with Down syndrome.

TABLE 14-2. BREASTFEEDING TECHNIQUES FOR INFANTS WITH DOWN SYNDROME

1. Feed at frequent, short intervals (every 2–3 hours).

2. Place the infant's trunk and head at the same level while supporting the head to facilitate head control.

3. Positioning

   a. The C-hold with the thumb on top and fingers below the areola helps to control the nipple.

   b. Support the infant's jaw from below with a finger. The index finger can be used to provide additional support for the jaw or to provide gentle downward pressure on the chin to open the baby's mouth wider.

   c. For hypotonic infants, the U-hold supports the breast and the infant's chin, allowing the mandible to rest within the interdigital space.

4. In cases of frequent choking and gulping air, place the back of the head superior to the nipple. The mother can lean back (such as in a recliner) so that the baby's throat is higher than the nipple. If this is effective, combine with frequent burping.

5. For infants with macroglossia, assist them in opening their mouths and latch. The C- and U-holds can be helpful.

6. To overcome the tongue thrusting

   a. Breastfeed with infant's chin pointing downward, almost touching the infant's chest.

   b. Gently stroke the infant's cheek toward his mouth, brushing his lips a few times.

   c. Use a clean index finger with well-trimmed nail to massage the outside of the infant's gums. Begin at the midline of the gum and move toward the sides of the gum.

   d. As the infant's mouth opens, press down firmly on the tongue tip with the tip of the index finger and count 1-2-3.

   e. Release the pressure, and move back on the tongue repeating this 1 or 2 more times. Avoid gagging the infant.

   f. Repeat this procedure 3 or 4 times prior to each breastfeeding session.

7. A nipple shield may be useful in hypotonic or weak infants as a transition to breastfeeding. (See Chapter 11.)

Adapted from Wagner C. Personal Communication.

V. **Breastfeeding multiples,** including twins and triplets, can be done successfully, and in many cases without the need for supplementation. Breastfeeding multiples, however, requires additional time and creates additional nutritional needs for the mother. One estimate is that mothers of twins require a total of 1,500 kcal/day above their requirement if they were neither pregnant nor lactating. There are a variety of ways that a mother can nurse multiple infants. Some mothers breastfeed exclusively, others do a combination of breastfeeding, mechanical milk expression, and bottle-feeding or other device feeding. Encouraging the father or extended family members to help with feedings alleviates some of the stress.

VI. **Tandem nursing** refers to continuation of breastfeeding into the next pregnancy and after delivery of the next child. A normal pregnancy is not an indication for immediate weaning, but preterm labor usually precludes continued breastfeeding. Some cultures mandate weaning when pregnancy is confirmed based on cultural, religious, or social tenets. A review of breastfeeding during pregnancy practices found that 69% of breastfeeding children wean spontaneously when the mother becomes pregnant, probably because of changes in the taste of the milk (increase in salt content, changes in hormone concentrations). The main reason for mother-initiated weaning is breast and nipple pain (related to hormonal changes and breast enlargement during pregnancy) and the arrival of the newborn. Weaning also may occur because of a decline in the milk supply or the disappearance of the mother's lap as the pregnancy progresses. Psychological support of the weaning or weaned toddler is important.

Care must be taken to ensure that the new infant has priority at the breast and that milk intake and growth are not compromised. Often the previously breastfeeding older child will be nursing only for comfort and to assert a continuing claim on the mother. Some studies demonstrate slower weight gain in newborns whose mothers are tandem nursing. The mother will produce milk at the same rate that it is removed; if she is nursing 2 or more infants, she will produce greater amounts of milk. This increased rate of milk synthesis and secretion places metabolic and nutritional demands on the mother.

VII. **Adoptive nursing,** or breastfeeding an adopted infant, is possible, and may be accomplished following preparation of the breasts to induce milk production. In the absence of the hormonal stimuli of pregnancy, over a period the nonpregnant mammary gland may undergo changes in response to the physical stimulation of suckling or pumping the breast. If the breast is stimulated, prolactin may be secreted, and milk may be produced. The increase in prolactin and milk production, however, is variable. A key component to successful lactation is let-down, directly dependent on adequate levels of circulating oxytocin. Let-down may be facilitated by exogenous oxytocin. Milk production may take from 1 to 6 weeks, on average about 4 weeks, after beginning pumping or nursing. Galactagogues often are used, but their efficacy is unproven. (See Chapter 12.) Clinicians advise beginning this process well before the arrival of the adopted baby because the adoption process can be stressful and may interfere with milk production. It is useful for the adoptive mother to use a supplemental feeding device and skin-to-skin contact. These techniques allow the infant to receive nutrition while suckling.

VIII. **Relactation** may be desired for mothers who initiated lactation but chose to stop because their infant was too sick to nurse, or because they themselves were too sick to nurse. Compared with mothers who initiate lactation to nurse an adopted infant, mothers who have previously lactated have the psychological advantage that they previously made milk. With renewed stimulation to the nipple, the neuroendocrine loop is reactivated, and milk production ensues. Successful relactation occurs in about 50% of women who initiate the process.

Selected References

Black RF, Jarman L, Simpson JB. *The Process of Breastfeeding. Lactation Specialist Self-Study Series.* Sudbury, MA: Jones and Bartlett Publishers, Inc; 1998: 207–208

Bu'Lock F, Woolridge MW, Baum JD. Development of coordination of sucking, swallowing and breathing: ultrasound study of term and preterm infants. *Dev Med Child Neurol.* 1990;32:669–678

Clarren S, Anderson B, Wolf LS. Feeding infants with cleft lip, cleft palate, or cleft lip and palate. *Cleft Palate J.* 1987;24:244–249

Cruz MJ, Kerschner JE, Beste DJ, Conley SF. Pierre Robin sequence: secondary respiratory difficulties and intrinsic feeding abnormalities. *Laryngoscope.* 1999;109:1632–1636

Darzi MA, Chowdri NA, Bhat AN. Breast feeding or spoon feeding after cleft lip repair: a prospective randomised study. *Br J Plast Surg.* 1996;49:24–26

Habel A, Sell D, Mars M. Management of cleft lip and palate. *Arch Dis Child.* 1996;74:360–366

Hurst NM, Valentine CJ, Renfro L, Burns P, Ferlic L. Skin-to-skin holding in the neonatal intensive care influences maternal milk volume. *J Perinatol.* 1997; 17:213–217

Kanamori G, Witter M, Brown J, Williams-Smith L. Otolaryngologic manifestations of Down syndrome. *Otolaryngol Clin North Am.* 2000;33:1285–1292

Kirschner E, LaRossa D. Cleft lip and palate. *Otolaryngol Clin North Am.* 2000; 33:1191–1215

Kirsten GF, Bergman NJ, Hann FM. Kangaroo mother care in the nursery. *Pediatr Clin North Am.* 2001;48:443–452

Lehman JA, Fishman JR, Neiman GS. Treatment of cleft palate associated with Robin sequence: appraisal of risk factors. *Cleft Palate Craniofac J.* 1995;32: 25–30

Meier PP. Breastfeeding in the special care nursery: prematures and infants with medical problems. *Pediatr Clin North Am.* 2001;48:425–442

Narayanan I, Mehta R, Choudhury DK, Jain BK. Sucking on the 'emptied' breast: non-nutritive sucking with a difference. *Arch Dis Child.* 1991;66:241–244

Nyqvist KH, Rubertsson C, Ewald U, Sjoden PO. Development of the preterm infant breastfeeding behavior scale (PIBBS): a study of nurse-mother agreement. *J Hum Lact.* 1996;12:207–219

Powers NG. Slow weight gain and low milk supply in the breastfeeding dyad. *Clin Perinatol.* 1999;26:399–430

Schanler RJ. The use of human milk for premature infants. *Pediatr Clin North Am.* 2001;48:207–219

Simpson C, Schanler RJ, Lau C. Early introduction of oral feeding in preterm infants. *Pediatrics.* 2002;110:517–522

Skinner J, Arvedson JC, Jones G, Spinner C, Rockwood J. Post-operative feeding strategies for infants with cleft lip. *Int J Pediatr Otorhinolaryngol.* 1997;42: 169–178

■ Chapter 15 ■

The Breastfeeding-Friendly Medical Office

The medical home, whether a partnership between the family and pediatric, obstetric, or family health care professionals, should establish a breastfeeding-friendly environment that encourages breastfeeding in the office setting. Office medical practices should be directed to support the goals of Healthy People 2010 to increase the percentage of mothers who breastfeed and the duration of breastfeeding. In addition, the entire office staff, professional and nonprofessional, should be educated about the value and implementation of breastfeeding and how t
port the breastfeeding dyad during the visit.

I. A Breastfeeding-Friendly Environment

The medical office presents a valuable opportunity to demonstrate that the health care staff believe that breastfeeding is the optimal form of nutrition for all babies. It is enlightening to walk through a clinical setting, critically observing the environment, and ask, "What message does the environment of this medical office convey to families?" The decor, advertising literature, and attention to the needs of breastfeeding mothers reflect the values of the office. Transforming the physician's office into a setting where breastfeeding is the societal norm will create an influential educational experience for parents and children.

A. Elements of a Breastfeeding-Friendly Environment

1. *Posters or enlarged photographs* of breastfeeding mothers and babies from a variety of ethnic and cultural backgrounds should be displayed throughout the office to encourage breastfeeding mothers to nurse their babies.

2. *Mother's Room and Waiting Room.* A private area equipped with a comfortable chair, a changing table, an electric breast pump and, ideally, a small refrigerator can become a breastfeeding room where mothers (including staff members) go to breastfeed in private or to express milk. The area will emphasize that breastfeeding is encouraged and supported in the practice. Breastfeeding in the waiting room itself should never be discouraged.

3. *Discourage Formula Marketing.* As reported, prenatal packs containing formula undermine breastfeeding success. Gifts from formula companies reflect the beliefs and values of the staff and should be reviewed and discussed. If breastfeeding is important to the practice, accepting formula marketing and similar gifts may be counterproductive. Careful thought should be given to magazines and other materials in the waiting room. Prenatal or postnatal formula company gifts for mothers or sign-up forms for formula company–sponsored "new mothers clubs" should not be encouraged in the office practice. When women sign up for such clubs, they will probably receive free formula either before or after the baby's birth.

4. *Track breastfeeding rates in the practice* to determine the effectiveness of breastfeeding promotion, support, and optimal clinical management. This allows the practice to see how it measures up against national breastfeeding goals and impresses on parents and staff that breastfeeding is important. In addition, analyzing breastfeeding initiation and duration trends in the patient population can help pinpoint critical periods when more support for breastfeeding at well-child visits can make a significant difference in breastfeeding success. Information can be gathered through the use of office surveys, periodic chart reviews, focus groups, and key informant interviews.

5. *Give encouragement* and assume that all women are still breastfeeding at each visit.

B. **Staff Education.** The key to providing breastfeeding care is effectively integrating relevant information and skills into existing daily routines without increasing the time required to provide a given service. Physicians and all staff should be educated in the basics of breastfeeding management to ensure that the practice communicates a consistent message and does not confuse families with conflicting information. Physicians and staff also should develop skills and comfort in evaluating breastfeeding through appropriate history and physical assessments. Excellent resources are available.

1. **Physician education** should occur during medical school and residency training. Many myths and personal beliefs affect breastfeeding attitudes and advice. Unless they are educated, health care professionals frequently offer advice based on personal experience. Clinician education through reputable breastfeeding courses, conferences, books, and on the Internet can introduce the novice to the basics of breastfeeding and can expand knowledge of management and diagnosis for the more sophisticated physician. It is important that physicians provide age-appropriate breastfeeding intervention and anticipatory guidance as part of every routine health screening visit for mother and baby. (See Chapter 8.)

2. **Nursing staff** often can attend breastfeeding courses or conferences offering continuing education units or can be required to complete a course on breastfeeding competency. Shorter educational presentations can be offered to non-nursing staff on-site, such as a slide show covering the health benefits of breastfeeding and discussion of breastfeeding-related issues specific to the employees' type of patient interaction. It is important to emphasize that office breastfeeding facilities should also be available to all staff.

3. **Support staff,** such as nursing assistants, laboratory technicians, receptionists, housekeeping, and administrative staff, should be included in educational presentations because they interact with breastfeeding mothers. The staff also should be encouraged to use breastfeeding facilities within the office. Employees also may share a cultural or linguistic background with patients. Leadership should assess the educational gaps of staff and develop strategies to fill those

gaps. Strategies may include holding in-house meetings or sending staff to conferences.

4. *Lactation specialists* may be used in a practice. Some physicians prefer to select a lactation specialist who has been certified as an IBCLC by the International Board of Lactation Consultant Examiners. Certification involves meeting specific requirements, and passing a written examination, and it is open to physicians, registered nurses, and other qualified individuals who have experience helping breastfeeding women. Some practices may choose to hire lactation specialists to handle their breastfeeding educational needs. Another option is to hire a lactation specialist on a case-by-case basis or to choose one in private or hospital practice who can handle referrals on a regular basis. Physicians should be aware of appropriate resources in their community.

C. **Patient Education.** Most women make their feeding choice early. In fact, one study reported that 78% of women made their feeding decision before the pregnancy or during the first trimester. (See Chapter 5.)

1. *Offering prenatal classes* that incorporate breastfeeding, breastfeeding classes for new mothers, or support groups for new mothers who are breastfeeding will provide accurate information and social support for families.

2. *A telephone support line,* either specifically dedicated to breastfeeding or incorporated within the practice telephone triage system, is beneficial as long as a health care professional with an appropriate level of breastfeeding knowledge handles the calls. The content of telephone calls should be recorded in the medical record. While it is often tempting to give breastfeeding guidance over the phone or via e-mail, if there is a question regarding the adequacy of breastfeeding and milk supply, it is best to evaluate the infant and mother in person (Chapter 8).

3. *Provide preventive monitoring,* including screening postpartum women for symptoms of depression. (See Chapter 9.)

4. *Peer counseling services,* available through La Leche League International, some Special Supplemental Nutrition Program for Women, Infants, and Children offices, and other breastfeeding support organizations can be offered to breastfeeding women. Many women feel more comfortable exchanging breastfeeding information with mothers from similar ethnic and cultural backgrounds.

5. *Community-based breastfeeding groups* may be a good resource for information. Examples include local La Leche League groups, peer counselors, and support groups offered through practices. Physicians can expand the network of support for breastfeeding by providing in-kind and financial support for local breastfeeding support groups.

6. *Printed materials* offered to women should be checked for accuracy and content and should be offered to families during first contact with a health care system. Excellent alternatives for literature from manufacturers include resources from the AAP, ACOG, AAFP, ABM, La Leche League International, Wellstart International, and childbirth organizations.

7. *Potential barriers to effective breastfeeding* should be anticipated and discouraged, especially those that may be encountered early in the postpartum period. New mothers often have questions about returning to work and using electric breast pumps. In one study, 1 of the top 3 reasons women gave for not breastfeeding was "could not breastfeed because had to return to work." Anticipating this concern and providing instruction about expression and storage assistance and support could improve breastfeeding duration. See Chapters 10 and 11 for a discussion on employment and the use of breast pumps. Physicians can encourage employers in their community to adopt workplace practices that support breastfeeding.

D. **National Initiatives.** The Breastfeeding Promotion in Pediatric Office Practices (BPPOP) program provided pediatricians with the latest scientific information, educational materials, and strategies for increasing breastfeeding rates toward Healthy People 2010 national goals. The follow-up BPPOP programs expanded the educational outreach to include obstetricians, family physicians, public health representatives, and physicians' training programs with an emphasis on culturally effective breastfeeding promotion and support to families with racially and ethnically diverse backgrounds.

II. Strategies for Implementation

Providing support, time, and effort up front are valuable and cost-effective. The examples below are included to stimulate thinking about possibilities in the hospital and office practice.

A. **Hospital strategies** to promote breastfeeding at various hospitals have been successful (Tables 6-1 and 6-3).

B. **The day 3 to 5 follow-up visit** should be scheduled before hospital discharge. To ensure infants are brought to the office or clinic at 3 to 5 days, some physicians schedule an appointment at discharge and leave the cord clamp on until the visit. At that time, history, weight, and physical examination are completed; breastfeeding is observed; and the clamp is removed. If, after the routine visit between 3 and 5 days the physician has concerns about breastfeeding, a problem-focused visit can be scheduled before the next routine checkup, or referral is made to a qualified lactation specialist. (See Table 8-3.)

TABLE 15-1. SELECTED STRATEGIES USED TO ENCOURAGE BREASTFEEDING IN THE OFFICE

Work with family life educators and home health nurses to ensure that the same breastfeeding messages are given.

Offer prenatal classes beneficial for patients.

Employ lactation specialists in the practice under the team leadership of the physician.

Provide positive feedback to mothers (present a Certificate of Achievement for breastfeeding at each visit).

Develop and support office and community-based breastfeeding activities.

Encourage breastfeeding education in schools.

Introduce breastfeeding benefits during an adolescent's office visit.

C. **Office Visits.** Developing partnerships and a collaborative breastfeeding agenda with others in the community is an effective way to strengthen breastfeeding management (Table 15-1).

Selected References

American Academy of Pediatrics Medical Home Initiatives for Children With Special Needs Project Advisory Committee. The medical home. *Pediatrics.* 2002;110:184–186

Arora S, McJunkin C, Wehrer J, Kuhn P. Major factors influencing breastfeeding rates: mother's perception of father's attitude and milk supply. *Pediatrics.* 2000;106:e67

Freed GL, Clark SJ, Lohr JA, Sorenson JR. Pediatrician involvement in breast-feeding promotion: a national study of residents and practitioners. *Pediatrics.* 1995;96:490–494

Howard FM, Howard CR, Weitzman M. The physician as advertiser: the unintentional discouragement of breast-feeding. *Obstet Gynecol.* 1993;81:1048–1051

Howard C, Howard F, Lawrence R, Andresen E, DeBlieck E, Weitzman M. Office prenatal formula advertising and its effect on breastfeeding patterns. *Obstet Gynecol.* 2000;95:296–303

Merewood A, Philipp BL. Becoming Baby-Friendly: overcoming the issue of accepting free formula. *J Hum Lact.* 2000;16:279–282

Philipp BL. Every call is an opportunity. Supporting breastfeeding mothers over the telephone. *Pediatr Clin North Am.* 2001;48:525–532

Philipp BL, Cadwell K. Fielding questions about breastfeeding. *Contemp Pediatr.* 1999;16:149–164

Philipp BL, Merewood A, O'Brien S. Physicians and breastfeeding promotion in the United States: a call for action. *Pediatrics.* 2001;107:584–587

Schanler RJ, O'Connor KG, Lawrence RA. Pediatricians' practices and attitudes regarding breastfeeding promotion. *Pediatrics.* 1999;103:e35

US Department of Health and Human Services. *Healthy People 2010: Conference Edition.* Vols 1&2. Washington, DC: US Department of Health and Human Services, Public Health Service, Office of the Assistant Secretary for Health; 2000

Breastfeeding Resources

Publications

Breastfeeding: A Guide for the Medical Profession
Ruth A. Lawrence, MD, and Robert M. Lawrence, MD
6th edition, 2005
Mosby, Inc

Breastfeeding and Human Lactation
Jan Riordan, EdD, RN, IBCLC, FAAN
3rd edition, 2005
Jones and Bartlett Publishers
800/832-0034
978/443-8000
www.jbpub.com

The Breastfeeding Answer Book
Nancy Mohrbacher, IBCLC, and Julie Stock, MA, IBCLC
Revised edition, 2003
La Leche League International
847/519-7730
847-519-0035 (fax)
www.lalecheleague.org

Breastfeeding Health Supervision and *Checklists for Breastfeeding Health
   Supervision*
American Academy of Pediatrics
1999
American Academy of Pediatrics
888/227-1770
www.aap.org

Breastfeeding in the United States: A National Agenda
United States Breastfeeding Committee
2001
US Department of Health and Human Services, Health Resources and
  Services Administration, Maternal and Child Health Bureau

Breastfeeding Triage Tool
Sandra Jolley
4th edition, 1998
Seattle-King County Department of Public Health
www.metrokc.gov/health/breastfeeding/factsheets.htm

*Bright Futures Guidelines for Health Supervision of Infants, Children, and
  Adolescents*
Morris Green, MD, and Judith S Palfrey, MD, eds
2nd edition, 2000
National Center for Education in Maternal and Child Health

Clinical Therapy in Breastfeeding Patients
Thomas Hale, RPh, PhD
2nd edition, 2002
Pharmasoft Publishing
800/378-1317
806/376-9901 (fax)
www.ibreastfeeding.com

*Drugs in Pregnancy and Lactation: A Reference Guide to Fetal and Neonatal
  Risk*
Gerald G. Briggs, B Pharm, Roger K Freeman, MD, and Sumner J. Yaffe,
  MD
7th edition, 2005
Lippincott Williams & Wilkins
800/683-3030
www.lww.com

Encounters with Children: Pediatric Behavior and Development
Suzanne D. Dixon, MD, MPH, and Martin T. Stein, MD
3rd edition, 2000
Mosby, Inc.

Family Physicians Supporting Breastfeeding
AAFP Breastfeeding Advisory Committee
Fall 2001
http://www.aafp.org/x6633.xml
Available online and as a printed document.

Guidelines for Health Supervision III
American Academy of Pediatrics Committee on Psychosocial Aspects of
 Child and Family Health
3rd edition, 2000
American Academy of Pediatrics
888/227-1770
www.aap.org

Guidelines for Perinatal Care
American Academy of Pediatrics, American College of Obstetricians and
 Gynecologists
5th edition, 2002
American Academy of Pediatrics, American College of Obstetricians and
 Gynecologists
888/227-1770
www.aap.org

Guidelines for the Care of Migrant Farmworkers' Children
American Academy of Pediatrics
2000
American Academy of Pediatrics
888/227-1770
www.aap.org

HHS Blueprint for Action on Breastfeeding
Department of Health and Human Services Office on Women's
 Health
2000
Department of Health and Human Services Office on Women's
 Health
800/994-WOMAN
www.4woman.gov

Medications and Mothers' Milk
Thomas Hale, RPh, PhD
11th edition, 2004
Pharmasoft Publishing
800/378-1317
806/376-9901 (fax)
www.ibreastfeeding.com

Pediatric Nutrition Handbook
American Academy of Pediatrics Committee on Nutrition
5th edition, 2003
American Academy of Pediatrics
888/227-1770
www.aap.org

Physicians' Breastfeeding Support Kit
Best Start Social Marketing, Inc.
1998
800/277-4975

Supporting Breastfeeding Mothers as They Return to Work
Marianne Neifert, MD
2000
American Academy of Pediatrics
www.aap.org/advocacy/bf/bfarticle.pdf

Ten Steps to Support Parents' Choice to Breastfeed Their Baby
Breastfeeding Promotion in Physicians' Office Practices
2003
American Academy of Pediatrics
www.aap.org/advocacy/bf/tensteps.pdf

Books for Parents

Amy Spangler's Breastfeeding: A Parent's Guide
Amy Spangler, RN, MN, IBCLC
7th edition, 2000
Abby Drue, Inc
817/594-5079
817/599-8924 (fax)
www.mommybabysite.com/books/parents_guide.htm

Breastfeeding Pure and Simple
Gwen Gotsch
Revised edition, 2000
La Leche League International
847/519-7730
847/519-0035 (fax)
www.lalecheleague.org

Breastfeeding Your Baby: Answers to Common Questions
American Academy of Pediatrics
2005
American Academy of Pediatrics
888/227-1770
www.aap.org

The Complete Book of Breastfeeding
Marvin S. Eiger, MD, and Sally Wendkos Olds
3rd edition, 1999
Workman Publishing Company, Inc

Dr Mom's Guide to Breastfeeding
Marianne Neifert, MD
1998
Plume, Penguin Putnam Inc

New Mother's Guide to Breastfeeding
American Academy of Pediatrics
2002
Bantam
888/227-1770
www.aap.org

The Nursing Mother's Companion
Kathleen Huggins, RN, MS
Revised edition, 1999
Harvard Common Press

The Nursing Mother's Problem Solver
Claire Martin, Nancy Funnemark Krebs, MD, MS, RD (editor)
2000
Simon & Schuster

The Womanly Art of Breastfeeding
La Leche League International
7th edition, 2004
La Leche League International
847/519-7730
847/519-0035 (fax)
www.lalecheleague.org

Working & Breastfeeding: Can You Do It? Yes, You Can!
Healthy Mothers, Healthy Babies Coalition
1997
703/836-6110
www.hmhb.org

Internet Resources

Academy of Breastfeeding Medicine	www.bfmed.org
American Academy of Family Physicians	www.aafp.org
	familydoctor.org
American Academy of Pediatrics	www.aap.org
American College of Obstetricians and Gynecologists	www.acog.org
Baby Friendly USA	www.babyfriendlyusa.org
Baby Milk Action	www.babymilkaction.org
Breastfeeding Federal Legislative Updates	
	www.house.gov/maloney/issues/breastfeeding/stateleg.htm
Breastfeeding Promotion in Physicians' Office Practices	
	www.aap.org/advocacy/bf/bppop-phaseII.htm
Breastfeeding Task Force of Greater Los Angeles	
	www.breastfeedingtaskforla.org
California Perinatal Quality Care Collaborative	www.cpqcc.org
Centers for Disease Control and Prevention	www.cdc.gov
Childrens Defense Fund	www.childrensdefense.org
Coalition for Improving Maternity Services	www.motherfriendly.org

Connect for Kids   www.connectforkids.org

DHHS Office on Women's Health: The National Women's Health
   Information Center   www.4woman.gov/breastfeeding

Dr Hale's Breastfeeding Pharmacology Page
                                       http://neonatal.ttuhsc.edu/lact/

Food and Drug Administration   www.fda.gov

Healthy People 2010 (National Objectives)
                                       http://www.HealthyPeople.gov

Human Milk Banking Association of North America
                                              www.hmbana.org

INFACT Canada: Infant Feeding Action Coalition
                                              www.infactcanada.ca

International Baby Food Action Network   www.ibfan.org

International Board of Lactation Consultant Examiners   www.iblce.org

International Childbirth Education Association   www.icea.org

International Code of Marketing of Breast-milk Substitutes
                       www.who.int/nut/documents/code_english.pdf

International Lactation Consultant Association   www.ilca.org

International Society for Research in Human Milk
   and Lactation   www.isrhml.org

La Leche League International   www.lalecheleague.org

Linkages   www.linkagesproject.org

Medela   www.medela.com

National Healthy Mothers, Healthy Babies Coalition   www.hmhb.org

National Institutes of Health   www.nih.gov

National Library of Medicine   www.nlm.nih.gov

National WIC Association   www.nwica.org

New York State Department of Health
               www.health.state.ny.us/nysdoh/b_feed/index.htm

Pediatrics (AAP professional journal)	www.pediatrics.org
San Diego County Breastfeeding Coalition	www.breastfeeding.org
United Nation Children's Fund	www.unicef.org
United States—National Library of Medicine	www.nlm.nih.gov
US Breastfeeding Committee	www.usbreastfeeding.org
US Department of Health and Human Services	www.dhhs.gov
US Food and Drug Administration	www.fda.gov/medwatch
USDA Food and Nutrition Service	www.fns.usda.gov/wic
World Alliance for Breastfeeding Action	www.waba.org.my

Please note: Inclusion in this publication does not imply an endorsement by the AAP or ACOG. The AAP and ACOG are not responsible for the content of the resources mentioned. Addresses, phone numbers, and Web site addresses are as current as possible, but may change at any time.

AMERICAN ACADEMY OF PEDIATRICS

POLICY STATEMENT
Organizational Principles to Guide and Define the Child Health Care System and/or Improve the Health of All Children

Section on Breastfeeding

Breastfeeding and the Use of Human Milk

ABSTRACT. Considerable advances have occurred in recent years in the scientific knowledge of the benefits of breastfeeding, the mechanisms underlying these benefits, and in the clinical management of breastfeeding. This policy statement on breastfeeding replaces the 1997 policy statement of the American Academy of Pediatrics and reflects this newer knowledge and the supporting publications. The benefits of breastfeeding for the infant, the mother, and the community are summarized, and recommendations to guide the pediatrician and other health care professionals in assisting mothers in the initiation and maintenance of breastfeeding for healthy term infants and high-risk infants are presented. The policy statement delineates various ways in which pediatricians can promote, protect, and support breastfeeding not only in their individual practices but also in the hospital, medical school, community, and nation. *Pediatrics* 2005;115:496–506; *breast, breastfeeding, breast milk, human milk, lactation.*

ABBREVIATIONS. AAP, American Academy of Pediatrics; WIC, Supplemental Nutrition Program for Women, Infants, and Children; CMV, cytomegalovirus; G6PD, glucose-6-phosphate dehydrogenase.

INTRODUCTION

Extensive research using improved epidemiologic methods and modern laboratory techniques documents diverse and compelling advantages for infants, mothers, families, and society from breastfeeding and use of human milk for infant feeding.[1] These advantages include health, nutritional, immunologic, developmental, psychologic, social, economic, and environmental benefits. In 1997, the American Academy of Pediatrics (AAP) published the policy statement *Breastfeeding and the Use of Human Milk.*[2] Since then, significant advances in science and clinical medicine have occurred. This revision cites substantial new research on the importance of breastfeeding and sets forth principles to guide pediatricians and other health care professionals in assisting women and children in the initiation and maintenance of breastfeeding. The ways pediatricians can protect, promote, and support breastfeeding in their individual practices, hospitals, medical schools, and communities are delineated, and the central role of the pediatrician in coordinating breastfeeding management and providing a medical home for the child is emphasized.[3] These recommenda-

tions are consistent with the goals and objectives of *Healthy People 2010,*[4] the Department of Health and Human Services' *HHS Blueprint for Action on Breastfeeding,*[5] and the United States Breastfeeding Committee's *Breastfeeding in the United States: A National Agenda.*[6]

This statement provides the foundation for issues related to breastfeeding and lactation management for other AAP publications including the *New Mother's Guide to Breastfeeding*[7] and chapters dealing with breastfeeding in the AAP/American College of Obstetricians and Gynecologists *Guidelines for Perinatal Care,*[8] the *Pediatric Nutrition Handbook,*[9] the *Red Book,*[10] and the *Handbook of Pediatric Environmental Health.*[11]

THE NEED

Child Health Benefits

Human milk is species-specific, and all substitute feeding preparations differ markedly from it, making human milk uniquely superior for infant feeding.[12] Exclusive breastfeeding is the reference or normative model against which all alternative feeding methods must be measured with regard to growth, health, development, and all other short- and long-term outcomes. In addition, human milk-fed premature infants receive significant benefits with respect to host protection and improved developmental outcomes compared with formula-fed premature infants.[13–22] From studies in preterm and term infants, the following outcomes have been documented.

Infectious Diseases

Research in developed and developing countries of the world, including middle-class populations in developed countries, provides strong evidence that human milk feeding decreases the incidence and/or severity of a wide range of infectious diseases[23] including bacterial meningitis,[24,25] bacteremia,[25,26] diarrhea,[22,33] respiratory tract infection,[22,33–40] necrotizing enterocolitis,[20,21] otitis media,[27,41–45] urinary tract infection,[46,47] and late-onset sepsis in preterm infants.[17,20] In addition, postneonatal infant mortality rates in the United States are reduced by 21% in breastfed infants.[48]

Other Health Outcomes

Some studies suggest decreased rates of sudden infant death syndrome in the first year of life[49–55] and reduction in incidence of insulin-dependent (type 1) and non–insulin-dependent (type 2) diabetes melli-

doi:10.1542/peds.2004-2491
PEDIATRICS (ISSN 0031 4005). Copyright © 2005 by the American Academy of Pediatrics.

tus,[56-59] lymphoma, leukemia, and Hodgkin disease,[60-62] overweight and obesity,[19,63-70] hypercholesterolemia,[71] and asthma[36-39] in older children and adults who were breastfed, compared with individuals who were not breastfed. Additional research in this area is warranted.

Neurodevelopment

Breastfeeding has been associated with slightly enhanced performance on tests of cognitive development.[14,15,72-80] Breastfeeding during a painful procedure such as a heel-stick for newborn screening provides analgesia to infants.[81,82]

Maternal Health Benefits

Important health benefits of breastfeeding and lactation are also described for mothers.[83] The benefits include decreased postpartum bleeding and more rapid uterine involution attributable to increased concentrations of oxytocin,[84] decreased menstrual blood loss and increased child spacing attributable to lactational amenorrhea,[85] earlier return to prepregnancy weight,[86] decreased risk of breast cancer,[87-92] decreased risk of ovarian cancer,[93] and possibly decreased risk of hip fractures and osteoporosis in the postmenopausal period.[94-96]

Community Benefits

In addition to specific health advantages for infants and mothers, economic, family, and environmental benefits have been described. These benefits include the potential for decreased annual health care costs of $3.6 billion in the United States[97,98]; decreased costs for public health programs such as the Special Supplemental Nutrition Program for Women, Infants, and Children (WIC)[99]; decreased parental employee absenteeism and associated loss of family income; more time for attention to siblings and other family matters as a result of decreased infant illness; decreased environmental burden for disposal of formula cans and bottles; and decreased energy demands for production and transport of artificial feeding products.[100-102] These savings for the country and for families would be offset to some unknown extent by increased costs for physician and lactation consultations, increased office-visit time, and cost of breast pumps and other equipment, all of which should be covered by insurance payments to providers and families.

CONTRAINDICATIONS TO BREASTFEEDING

Although breastfeeding is optimal for infants, there are a few conditions under which breastfeeding may not be in the best interest of the infant. Breastfeeding is contraindicated in infants with classic galactosemia (galactose 1-phosphate uridyltransferase deficiency)[103]; mothers who have active untreated tuberculosis disease or are human T-cell lymphotropic virus type I– or II–positive[104,105]; mothers who are receiving diagnostic or therapeutic radioactive isotopes or have had exposure to radioactive materials (for as long as there is radioactivity in the milk)[106-108]; mothers who are receiving antimetabolites or chemotherapeutic agents or a small number of other medications until they clear the milk[109,110];

mothers who are using drugs of abuse ("street drugs"); and mothers who have herpes simplex lesions on a breast (infant may feed from other breast if clear of lesions). Appropriate information about infection-control measures should be provided to mothers with infectious diseases.[111]

In the United States, mothers who are infected with human immunodeficiency virus (HIV) have been advised not to breastfeed their infants.[112] In developing areas of the world with populations at increased risk of other infectious diseases and nutritional deficiencies resulting in increased infant death rates, the mortality risks associated with artificial feeding may outweigh the possible risks of acquiring HIV infection.[113,114] One study in Africa detailed in 2 reports[115,116] found that exclusive breastfeeding for the first 3 to 6 months after birth by HIV-infected mothers did not increase the risk of HIV transmission to the infant, whereas infants who received mixed feedings (breastfeeding with other foods or milks) had a higher rate of HIV infection compared with infants who were exclusively formula-fed. Women in the United States who are HIV-positive should not breastfeed their offspring. Additional studies are needed before considering a change from current policy recommendations.

CONDITIONS THAT ARE NOT CONTRAINDICATIONS TO BREASTFEEDING

Certain conditions have been shown to be compatible with breastfeeding. Breastfeeding is not contraindicated for infants born to mothers who are hepatitis B surface antigen–positive,[111] mothers who are infected with hepatitis C virus (persons with hepatitis C virus antibody or hepatitis C virus-RNA–positive blood),[111] mothers who are febrile (unless cause is a contraindication outlined in the previous section),[117] mothers who have been exposed to low-level environmental chemical agents,[118,119] and mothers who are seropositive carriers of cytomegalovirus (CMV) (not recent converters if the infant is term).[111] Decisions about breastfeeding of very low birth weight infants (birth weight <1500 g) by mothers known to be CMV-seropositive should be made with consideration of the potential benefits of human milk versus the risk of CMV transmission.[120,121] Freezing and pasteurization can significantly decrease the CMV viral load in milk.[122]

Tobacco smoking by mothers is not a contraindication to breastfeeding, but health care professionals should advise all tobacco-using mothers to avoid smoking within the home and to make every effort to wean themselves from tobacco as rapidly as possible.[110]

Breastfeeding mothers should avoid the use of alcoholic beverages, because alcohol is concentrated in breast milk and its use can inhibit milk production. An occasional celebratory single, small alcoholic drink is acceptable, but breastfeeding should be avoided for 2 hours after the drink.[123]

For the great majority of newborns with jaundice and hyperbilirubinemia, breastfeeding can and should be continued without interruption. In rare instances of severe hyperbilirubinemia, breastfeed-

TABLE 1.   Breastfeeding Rates for Infants in the United States: Any (Exclusive)

	Actual: 2001			Healthy People 2010 Goals[4]		
	Initiation[125]	6 mo[125]	1 y[132]	Initiation	6 mo	1 y
All women	70% (46%)	33% (17%)	18%	75%	50%	25%
Black	53% (27%)	22% (11%)	12%			
Hispanic	73% (36%)	33% (16%)	18%			
Asian	NA	NA	NA			
White	72% (53%)	34% (19%)	18%			

NA indicates that the data are not available.

ing may need to be interrupted temporarily for a brief period.[124]

THE CHALLENGE

Data indicate that the rate of initiation and duration of breastfeeding in the United States are well below the *Healthy People 2010* goals (see Table 1).[4,125] Furthermore, many of the mothers counted as breastfeeding were supplementing their infants with formula during the first 6 months of the infant's life.[5,126] Although breastfeeding initiation rates have increased steadily since 1990, exclusive breastfeeding initiation rates have shown little or no increase over that same period of time. Similarly, 6 months after birth, the proportion of infants who are exclusively breastfed has increased at a much slower rate than that of infants who receive mixed feedings.[125] The AAP Section on Breastfeeding, American College of Obstetricians and Gynecologists, American Academy of Family Physicians, Academy of Breastfeeding Medicine, World Health Organization, United Nations Children's Fund, and many other health organizations recommend exclusive breastfeeding for the first 6 months of life.‡[2,127–130] Exclusive breastfeeding is defined as an infant's consumption of human milk with no supplementation of any type (no water, no juice, no nonhuman milk, and no foods) except for vitamins, minerals, and medications.[131] Exclusive breastfeeding has been shown to provide improved protection against many diseases and to increase the likelihood of continued breastfeeding for at least the first year of life.

Obstacles to initiation and continuation of breastfeeding include insufficient prenatal education about breastfeeding[132,133]; disruptive hospital policies and practices[134]; inappropriate interruption of breastfeeding[135]; early hospital discharge in some populations[136]; lack of timely routine follow-up care and postpartum home health visits[137]; maternal employment[138,139] (especially in the absence of workplace facilities and support for breastfeeding)[140]; lack of family and broad societal support[141]; media portrayal of bottle feeding as normative[142]; commercial promotion of infant formula through distribution of hospital discharge packs, coupons for free or discounted formula, and some television and general magazine advertising[143,144]; misinformation; and

lack of guidance and encouragement from health care professionals.[135,145,146]

RECOMMENDATIONS ON BREASTFEEDING FOR HEALTHY TERM INFANTS

1. Pediatricians and other health care professionals should recommend human milk for all infants in whom breastfeeding is not specifically contraindicated and provide parents with complete, current information on the benefits and techniques of breastfeeding to ensure that their feeding decision is a fully informed one.[147–149]
   - When direct breastfeeding is not possible, expressed human milk should be provided.[150,151] If a known contraindication to breastfeeding is identified, consider whether the contraindication may be temporary, and if so, advise pumping to maintain milk production. Before advising against breastfeeding or recommending premature weaning, weigh the benefits of breastfeeding against the risks of not receiving human milk.

2. Peripartum policies and practices that optimize breastfeeding initiation and maintenance should be encouraged.
   - Education of both parents before and after delivery of the infant is an essential component of successful breastfeeding. Support and encouragement by the father can greatly assist the mother during the initiation process and during subsequent periods when problems arise. Consistent with appropriate care for the mother, minimize or modify the course of maternal medications that have the potential for altering the infant's alertness and feeding behavior.[152,153] Avoid procedures that may interfere with breastfeeding or that may traumatize the infant, including unnecessary, excessive, and overvigorous suctioning of the oral cavity, esophagus, and airways to avoid oropharyngeal mucosal injury that may lead to aversive feeding behavior.[154,155]

3. Healthy infants should be placed and remain in direct skin-to-skin contact with their mothers immediately after delivery until the first feeding is accomplished.[156–158]
   - The alert, healthy newborn infant is capable of latching on to a breast without specific assistance within the first hour after birth.[156] Dry the infant, assign Apgar scores, and perform the initial physical assessment while the infant

‡ There is a difference of opinion among AAP experts on this matter. The Section on Breastfeeding acknowledges that the Committee on Nutrition supports introduction of complementary foods between 4 and 6 months of age when safe and nutritious complementary foods are available.

is with the mother. The mother is an optimal heat source for the infant.[159,160] Delay weighing, measuring, bathing, needle-sticks, and eye prophylaxis until after the first feeding is completed. Infants affected by maternal medications may require assistance for effective latch-on.[156] Except under unusual circumstances, the newborn infant should remain with the mother throughout the recovery period.[161]

4. Supplements (water, glucose water, formula, and other fluids) should not be given to breastfeeding newborn infants unless ordered by a physician when a medical indication exists.[148,162–165]

5. Pacifier use is best avoided during the initiation of breastfeeding and used only after breastfeeding is well established.[166–168]
   - In some infants early pacifier use may interfere with establishment of good breastfeeding practices, whereas in others it may indicate the presence of a breastfeeding problem that requires intervention.[169]
   - This recommendation does not contraindicate pacifier use for nonnutritive sucking and oral training of premature infants and other special care infants.

6. During the early weeks of breastfeeding, mothers should be encouraged to have 8 to 12 feedings at the breast every 24 hours, offering the breast whenever the infant shows early signs of hunger such as increased alertness, physical activity, mouthing, or rooting.[170]
   - Crying is a late indicator of hunger.[171] Appropriate initiation of breastfeeding is facilitated by continuous rooming-in throughout the day and night.[172] The mother should offer both breasts at each feeding for as long a period as the infant remains at the breast.[173] At each feed the first breast offered should be alternated so that both breasts receive equal stimulation and draining. In the early weeks after birth, nondemanding infants should be aroused to feed if 4 hours have elapsed since the beginning of the last feeding.
   - After breastfeeding is well established, the frequency of feeding may decline to approximately 8 times per 24 hours, but the infant may increase the frequency again with growth spurts or when an increase in milk volume is desired.

7. Formal evaluation of breastfeeding, including observation of position, latch, and milk transfer, should be undertaken by trained caregivers at least twice daily and fully documented in the record during each day in the hospital after birth.[174,175]
   - Encouraging the mother to record the time and duration of each breastfeeding, as well as urine and stool output during the early days of breastfeeding in the hospital and the first weeks at home, helps to facilitate the evaluation process. Problems identified in the hospital should be addressed at that time, and a documented plan for management should be clearly communicated to both parents and to the medical home.

8. All breastfeeding newborn infants should be seen by a pediatrician or other knowledgeable and experienced health care professional at 3 to 5 days of age as recommended by the AAP.[124,176,177]
   - This visit should include infant weight; physical examination, especially for jaundice and hydration; maternal history of breast problems (painful feedings, engorgement); infant elimination patterns (expect 3–5 urines and 3–4 stools per day by 3–5 days of age; 4–6 urines and 3–6 stools per day by 5–7 days of age); and a formal, observed evaluation of breastfeeding, including position, latch, and milk transfer. Weight loss in the infant of greater than 7% from birth weight indicates possible breastfeeding problems and requires more intensive evaluation of breastfeeding and possible intervention to correct problems and improve milk production and transfer.

9. Breastfeeding infants should have a second ambulatory visit at 2 to 3 weeks of age so that the health care professional can monitor weight gain and provide additional support and encouragement to the mother during this critical period.

10. Pediatricians and parents should be aware that exclusive breastfeeding is sufficient to support optimal growth and development for approximately the first 6 months of life‡ and provides continuing protection against diarrhea and respiratory tract infection.[30,34,128,178–184] Breastfeeding should be continued for at least the first year of life and beyond for as long as mutually desired by mother and child.[185]
    - Complementary foods rich in iron should be introduced gradually beginning around 6 months of age.[186–187] Preterm and low birth weight infants and infants with hematologic disorders or infants who had inadequate iron stores at birth generally require iron supplementation before 6 months of age.[148,188–192] Iron may be administered while continuing exclusive breastfeeding.
    - Unique needs or feeding behaviors of individual infants may indicate a need for introduction of complementary foods as early as 4 months of age, whereas other infants may not be ready to accept other foods until approximately 8 months of age.[193]
    - Introduction of complementary feedings before 6 months of age generally does not increase total caloric intake or rate of growth and only substitutes foods that lack the protective components of human milk.[194]
    - During the first 6 months of age, even in hot climates, water and juice are unnecessary for breastfed infants and may introduce contaminants or allergens.[195]
    - Increased duration of breastfeeding confers significant health and developmental benefits for the child and the mother, especially in delaying return of fertility (thereby promoting optimal intervals between births).[196]

228

- There is no upper limit to the duration of breastfeeding and no evidence of psychologic or developmental harm from breastfeeding into the third year of life or longer.[197]
- Infants weaned before 12 months of age should not receive cow's milk but should receive iron-fortified infant formula.[198]

11. All breastfed infants should receive 1.0 mg of vitamin K_1 oxide intramuscularly after the first feeding is completed and within the first 6 hours of life.[199]
  - Oral vitamin K is not recommended. It may not provide the adequate stores of vitamin K necessary to prevent hemorrhage later in infancy in breastfed infants unless repeated doses are administered during the first 4 months of life.[200]

12. All breastfed infants should receive 200 IU of oral vitamin D drops daily beginning during the first 2 months of life and continuing until the daily consumption of vitamin D-fortified formula or milk is 500 mL.[201]
  - Although human milk contains small amounts of vitamin D, it is not enough to prevent rickets. Exposure of the skin to ultraviolet B wavelengths from sunlight is the usual mechanism for production of vitamin D. However, significant risk of sunburn (short-term) and skin cancer (long-term) attributable to sunlight exposure, especially in younger children, makes it prudent to counsel against exposure to sunlight. Furthermore, sunscreen decreases vitamin D production in skin.

13. Supplementary fluoride should not be provided during the first 6 months of life.[202]
  - From 6 months to 3 years of age, the decision whether to provide fluoride supplementation should be made on the basis of the fluoride concentration in the water supply (fluoride supplementation generally is not needed unless the concentration in the drinking water is <0.3 ppm) and in other food, fluid sources, and toothpaste.

14. Mother and infant should sleep in proximity to each other to facilitate breastfeeding.[203]

15. Should hospitalization of the breastfeeding mother or infant be necessary, every effort should be made to maintain breastfeeding, preferably directly, or pumping the breasts and feeding expressed milk if necessary.

ADDITIONAL RECOMMENDATIONS FOR HIGH-RISK INFANTS

- Hospitals and physicians should recommend human milk for premature and other high-risk infants either by direct breastfeeding and/or using the mother's own expressed milk.[13] Maternal support and education on breastfeeding and milk expression should be provided from the earliest possible time. Mother-infant skin-to-skin contact and direct breastfeeding should be encouraged as early as feasible.[204,205] Fortification of expressed human milk is indicated for many very low birth weight infants.[13] Banked human milk may be a suitable feeding alternative for infants whose mothers are unable or unwilling to provide their own milk. Human milk banks in North America adhere to national guidelines for quality control of screening and testing of donors and pasteurize all milk before distribution.[206–208] Fresh human milk from unscreened donors is not recommended because of the risk of transmission of infectious agents.
- Precautions should be followed for infants with glucose-6-phosphate dehydrogenase (G6PD) deficiency. G6PD deficiency has been associated with an increased risk of hemolysis, hyperbilirubinemia, and kernicterus.[209] Mothers who breastfeed infants with known or suspected G6PD deficiency should not ingest fava beans or medications such as nitrofurantoin, primaquine phosphate, or phenazopyridine hydrochloride, which are known to induce hemolysis in deficient individuals.[210,211]

ROLE OF PEDIATRICIANS AND OTHER HEALTH CARE PROFESSIONALS IN PROTECTING, PROMOTING, AND SUPPORTING BREASTFEEDING

Many pediatricians and other health care professionals have made great efforts in recent years to support and improve breastfeeding success by following the principles and guidance provided by the AAP,[2] the American College of Obstetricians and Gynecologists,[127] the American Academy of Family Physicians,[128] and many other organizations.[5,6,8,130,133,142,162] The following guidelines summarize these concepts for providing an optimal breastfeeding environment.

General

- Promote, support, and protect breastfeeding enthusiastically. In consideration of the extensively published evidence for improved health and developmental outcomes in breastfed infants and their mothers, a strong position on behalf of breastfeeding is warranted.
- Promote breastfeeding as a cultural norm and encourage family and societal support for breastfeeding.
- Recognize the effect of cultural diversity on breastfeeding attitudes and practices and encourage variations, if appropriate, that effectively promote and support breastfeeding in different cultures.

Education

- Become knowledgeable and skilled in the physiology and the current clinical management of breastfeeding.
- Encourage development of formal training in breastfeeding and lactation in medical schools, in residency and fellowship training programs, and for practicing pediatricians.
- Use every opportunity to provide age-appropriate breastfeeding education to children and adults in the medical setting and in outreach programs for student and parent groups.

Clinical Practice

- Work collaboratively with the obstetric community to ensure that women receive accurate and sufficient information throughout the perinatal period to make a fully informed decision about infant feeding.

- Work collaboratively with the dental community to ensure that women are encouraged to continue to breastfeed and use good oral health practices. Infants should receive an oral health-risk assessment by the pediatrician between 6 months and 1 year of age and/or referred to a dentist for evaluation and treatment if at risk of dental caries or other oral health problems.[212]
- Promote hospital policies and procedures that facilitate breastfeeding. Work actively toward eliminating hospital policies and practices that discourage breastfeeding (eg, promotion of infant formula in hospitals including infant formula discharge packs and formula discount coupons, separation of mother and infant, inappropriate infant feeding images, and lack of adequate encouragement and support of breastfeeding by all health care staff). Encourage hospitals to provide in-depth training in breastfeeding for all health care staff (including physicians) and have lactation experts available at all times.
- Provide effective breast pumps and private lactation areas for all breastfeeding mothers (patients and staff) in ambulatory and inpatient areas of the hospital.[213]
- Develop office practices that promote and support breastfeeding by using the guidelines and materials provided by the AAP Breastfeeding Promotion in Physicians' Office Practices program.[214]
- Become familiar with local breastfeeding resources (eg, WIC clinics, breastfeeding medical and nursing specialists, lactation educators and consultants, lay support groups, and breast-pump rental stations) so that patients can be referred appropriately.[215] When specialized breastfeeding services are used, the essential role of the pediatrician as the infant's primary health care professional within the framework of the medical home needs to be clarified for parents.
- Encourage adequate, routine insurance coverage for necessary breastfeeding services and supplies, including the time required by pediatricians and other licensed health care professionals to assess and manage breastfeeding and the cost for the rental of breast pumps.
- Develop and maintain effective communication and coordination with other health care professionals to ensure optimal breastfeeding education, support, and counseling. AAP and WIC breastfeeding coordinators can facilitate collaborative relationships and develop programs in the community and in professional organizations for support of breastfeeding.
- Advise mothers to continue their breast self-examinations on a monthly basis throughout lactation and to continue to have annual clinical breast examinations by their physicians.

Society
- Encourage the media to portray breastfeeding as positive and normative.

- Encourage employers to provide appropriate facilities and adequate time in the workplace for breastfeeding and/or milk expression.
- Encourage child care providers to support breastfeeding and the use of expressed human milk provided by the parent.
- Support the efforts of parents and the courts to ensure continuation of breastfeeding in separation and custody proceedings.
- Provide counsel to adoptive mothers who decide to breastfeed through induced lactation, a process requiring professional support and encouragement.
- Encourage development and approval of governmental policies and legislation that are supportive of a mother's choice to breastfeed.

Research
- Promote continued basic and clinical research in the field of breastfeeding. Encourage investigators and funding agencies to pursue studies that further delineate the scientific understandings of lactation and breastfeeding that lead to improved clinical practice in this medical field.[216]

CONCLUSIONS
Although economic, cultural, and political pressures often confound decisions about infant feeding, the AAP firmly adheres to the position that breastfeeding ensures the best possible health as well as the best developmental and psychosocial outcomes for the infant. Enthusiastic support and involvement of pediatricians in the promotion and practice of breastfeeding is essential to the achievement of optimal infant and child health, growth, and development.

Section on Breastfeeding, 2003–2004
*Lawrence M. Gartner, MD, Chairperson
Jane Morton, MD
Ruth A. Lawrence, MD
Audrey J. Naylor, MD, DrPH
Donna O'Hare, MD
Richard J. Schanler, MD

*Arthur I. Eidelman, MD
  Policy Committee Chairperson

Liaisons
Nancy F. Krebs, MD
  Committee on Nutrition
Alice Lenihan, MPH, RD, LPN
  National WIC Association
John Queenan, MD
  American College of Obstetricians and Gynecologists

Staff
Betty Crase, IBCLC, RLC

*Lead authors

REFERENCES
1. Kramer MS, Chalmers B, Hodnett ED, et al. Promotion of Breastfeeding Intervention Trial (PROBIT): a randomized trial in the Republic of Belarus. *JAMA.* 2001;285:413–420
2. American Academy of Pediatrics, Work Group on Breastfeeding. Breastfeeding and the use of human milk. *Pediatrics.* 1997;100:1035–1039

3. American Academy of Pediatrics, Medical Home Initiatives for Children With Special Needs Project Advisory Committee. The medical home. *Pediatrics.* 2002;110:184–186
4. US Department of Health and Human Services. *Healthy People 2010: Conference Edition—Volumes I and II.* Washington, DC: US Department of Health and Human Services, Public Health Service, Office of the Assistant Secretary for Health; 2000:47–48
5. US Department of Health and Human Services. *HHS Blueprint for Action on Breastfeeding.* Washington, DC: US Department of Health and Human Services, Office on Women's Health; 2000
6. United States Breastfeeding Committee. *Breastfeeding in the United States: A National Agenda.* Rockville, MD: US Department of Health and Human Services, Health Resources and Services Administration, Maternal and Child Health Bureau; 2001
7. American Academy of Pediatrics. *New Mother's Guide to Breastfeeding.* Meek JY, ed. New York, NY: Bantam Books; 2002
8. American Academy of Pediatrics, American College of Obstetricians and Gynecologists. *Guidelines for Perinatal Care.* Gilstrap LC, Oh W, eds. 5th ed. Elk Grove Village, IL: American Academy of Pediatrics; 2002
9. American Academy of Pediatrics, Committee on Nutrition. *Pediatric Nutrition Handbook.* Kleinman RE, ed. 5th ed. Elk Grove Village, IL: American Academy of Pediatrics; 2004
10. American Academy of Pediatrics. *Red Book: 2003 Report of the Committee on Infectious Diseases.* Pickering LK, ed. 26th ed. Elk Grove Village, IL: American Academy of Pediatrics; 2003
11. American Academy of Pediatrics, Committee on Environmental Health. *Handbook of Pediatric Environmental Health.* Etzel RA, Balk SJ, eds. 2nd ed. Elk Grove Village, IL: American Academy of Pediatrics; 2003
12. Hambraeus L, Forsum E, Lönnerdal B. Nutritional aspects of breast milk and cow's milk formulas. In: Hambraeus L, Hanson L, MacFarlane H, eds. *Symposium on Food and Immunology.* Stockholm, Sweden: Almqvist and Wiksell; 1975
13. Schanler RJ. The use of human milk for premature infants. *Pediatr Clin North Am.* 2001;48:207–219
14. Lucas A, Morley R, Cole TJ. Randomised trial of early diet in preterm babies and later intelligence quotient. *BMJ.* 1998;317:1481–1487
15. Horwood LJ, Darlow BA, Mogridge N. Breast milk feeding and cognitive ability at 7–8 years. *Arch Dis Child Fetal Neonatal Ed.* 2001;84: F23–F27
16. Amin SB, Merle KS, Orlando MS, Dalzell LE, Guillet R. Brainstem maturation in premature infants as a function of enteral feeding type. *Pediatrics.* 2000;106:318–322
17. Hylander MA, Strobino DM, Dhanireddy R. Human milk feedings and infection among very low birth weight infants. *Pediatrics.* 1998;102(3). Available at: www.pediatrics.org/cgi/content/full/102/3/e38
18. Hylander MA, Strobino DM, Pezzullo JC, Dhanireddy R. Association of human milk feedings with a reduction in retinopathy of prematurity among very low birthweight infants. *J Perinatol.* 2001; 21:356–362
19. Singhal A, Farooqi IS, O'Rahilly S, Cole TJ, Fewtrell M, Lucas A. Early nutrition and leptin concentrations in later life. *Am J Clin Nutr.* 2002; 75:993–999
20. Schanler RJ, Shulman RJ, Lau C. Feeding strategies for premature infants: beneficial outcomes of feeding fortified human milk versus preterm formula. *Pediatrics.* 1999;103:1150–1157
21. Lucas A, Cole TJ. Breast milk and neonatal necrotising enterocolitis. *Lancet.* 1990;336:1519–1523
22. Blaymore Bier J, Oliver T, Ferguson A, Vohr BR. Human milk reduces outpatient upper respiratory symptoms in premature infants during their first year of life. *J Perinatol.* 2002;22:354–359
23. Heinig MJ. Host defense benefits of breastfeeding for the infant. Effect of breastfeeding duration and exclusivity. *Pediatr Clin North Am.* 2001; 48:105–123, ix
24. Cochi SL, Fleming DW, Hightower AW, et al. Primary invasive *Haemophilus influenzae* type b disease: a population-based assessment of risk factors. *J Pediatr.* 1986;108:887–896
25. Istre GR, Conner JS, Broome CV, Hightower A, Hopkins RS. Risk factors for primary invasive *Haemophilus influenzae* disease: increased risk from day care attendance and school-aged household members. *J Pediatr.* 1985;106:190–195
26. Takala AK, Eskola J, Palmgren J, et al. Risk factors of invasive *Haemophilus influenzae* type b disease among children in Finland. *J Pediatr.* 1989;115:694–701
27. Dewey KG, Heinig MJ, Nommsen-Rivers LA. Differences in morbidity between breast-fed and formula-fed infants. *J Pediatr.* 1995;126:696–702

28. Howie PW, Forsyth JS, Ogston SA, Clark A, Florey CD. Protective effect of breast feeding against infection. *BMJ.* 1990;300:11–16
29. Kramer MS, Guo T, Platt RW, et al. Infant growth and health outcomes associated with 3 compared with 6 mo of exclusive breastfeeding. *Am J Clin Nutr.* 2003;78:291–295
30. Popkin BM, Adair L, Akin JS, Black R, Briscoe J, Flieger W. Breastfeeding and diarrheal morbidity. *Pediatrics.* 1990;86:874–882
31. Beaudry M, Dufour R, Marcoux S. Relation between infant feeding and infections during the first six months of life. *J Pediatr.* 1995;126: 191–197
32. Bhandari N, Bahl R, Mazumdar S, Martines J, Black RE, Bhan MK. Effect of community-based promotion of exclusive breastfeeding on diarrhoeal illness and growth: a cluster randomized controlled trial. Infant Feeding Study Group. *Lancet.* 2003;361:1418–1423
33. Lopez-Alarcon M, Villalpando S, Fajardo A. Breast-feeding lowers the frequency and duration of acute respiratory infection and diarrhea in infants under six months of age. *J Nutr.* 1997;127:436–443
34. Bachrach VR, Schwarz E, Bachrach LR. Breastfeeding and the risk of hospitalization for respiratory disease in infancy: a meta-analysis. *Arch Pediatr Adolesc Med.* 2003;157:237–243
35. Oddy WH, Sly PD, de Klerk NH, et al. Breast feeding and respiratory morbidity in infancy: a birth cohort study. *Arch Dis Child.* 2003;88: 224–228
36. Chulada PC, Arbes SJ Jr, Dunson D, Zeldin DC. Breast-feeding and the prevalence of asthma and wheeze in children: analyses from the Third National Health and Nutrition Examination Survey, 1988–1994. *J Allergy Clin Immunol.* 2003;111:328–336
37. Oddy WH, Peat JK, de Klerk NH. Maternal asthma, infant feeding, and the risk of asthma in childhood. *J Allergy Clin Immunol.* 2002;110:65–67
38. Gdalevich M, Mimouni D, Mimouni M. Breast-feeding and the risk of bronchial asthma in childhood: a systematic review with meta-analysis of prospective studies. *J Pediatr.* 2001;139:261–266
39. Oddy WH, Holt PG, Sly PD, et al. Association between breast feeding and asthma in 6 year old children: findings of a prospective birth cohort study. *BMJ.* 1999;319:815–819
40. Wright AL, Holberg CJ, Taussig LM, Martinez FD. Relationship of infant feeding to recurrent wheezing at age 6 years. *Arch Pediatr Adolesc Med.* 1995;149:758–763
41. Saarinen UM. Prolonged breast feeding as prophylaxis for recurrent otitis media. *Acta Paediatr Scand.* 1982;71:567–571
42. Duncan B, Ey J, Holberg CJ, Wright AL, Martinez FD, Taussig LM. Exclusive breast-feeding for at least 4 months protects against otitis media. *Pediatrics.* 1993;91:867–872
43. Owen MJ, Baldwin CD, Swank PR, Pannu AK, Johnson DL, Howie VM. Relation of infant feeding practices, cigarette smoke exposure, and group child care to the onset and duration of otitis media with effusion in the first two years of life. *J Pediatr.* 1993;123:702–711
44. Paradise JL, Elster BA, Tan L. Evidence in infants with cleft palate that breast milk protects against otitis media. *Pediatrics.* 1994;94:853–860
45. Aniansson G, Alm B, Andersson B, et al. A prospective cohort study on breast-feeding and otitis media in Swedish infants. *Pediatr Infect Dis J.* 1994;13:183–188
46. Pisacane A, Graziano L, Mazzarella G, Scarpellino B, Zona G. Breastfeeding and urinary tract infection. *J Pediatr.* 1992;120:87–89
47. Marild S, Hansson S, Jodal U, Oden A, Svedberg K. Protective effect of breastfeeding against urinary tract infection. *Acta Paediatr.* 2004;93: 164–168
48. Chen A, Rogan WJ. Breastfeeding and the risk of postneonatal death in the United States. *Pediatrics.* 2004;113(5). Available at: www.pediatrics.org/cgi/content/full/113/5/e435
49. Horne RS, Parslow PM, Ferens D, Watts AM, Adamson TM. Comparison of evoked arousability in breast and formula fed infants. *Arch Dis Child.* 2004;89(1):22–25
50. Ford RPK, Taylor BJ, Mitchell EA, et al. Breastfeeding and the risk of sudden infant death syndrome. *Int J Epidemiol.* 1993;22:885–890
51. Mitchell EA, Taylor BJ, Ford RPK, et al. Four modifiable and other major risk factors for cot death: the New Zealand study. *J Paediatr Child Health.* 1992;28(suppl 1):S3–S8
52. Scragg LK, Mitchell EA, Tonkin SL, Hassall IB. Evaluation of the cot death prevention programme in South Auckland. *N Z Med J.* 1993;106: 8–10
53. Alm B, Wennergren G, Norvenius SG, et al. Breast feeding and the sudden infant death syndrome in Scandinavia, 1992–95. *Arch Dis Child.* 2002;86:400–402
54. McVea KL, Turner PD, Peppler DK. The role of breastfeeding in sudden infant death syndrome. *J Hum Lact.* 2000;16:13–20

231

55. Mosko S, Richard C, McKenna J. Infant arousals during mother-infant bed sharing: implications for infant sleep and sudden infant death syndrome research. *Pediatrics*. 1997;100:841–849

56. Gerstein HC. Cow's milk exposure and type 1 diabetes mellitus. A critical overview of the clinical literature. *Diabetes Care*. 1994;17:13–19

57. Kostraba JN, Cruickshanks KJ, Lawler-Heavner J, et al. Early exposure to cow's milk and solid foods in infancy, genetic predisposition, and the risk of IDDM. *Diabetes*. 1993;42:288–295

58. Pettit DJ, Forman MR, Hanson RL, Knowler WC, Bennett PH. Breast-feeding and the incidence of non-insulin-dependent diabetes mellitus in Pima Indians. *Lancet*. 1997;350:166–168

59. Perez-Bravo E, Carrasco E, Guitierrez-Lopez MD, Martinez MT, Lopez G, de los Rios MG. Genetic predisposition and environmental factors leading to the development of insulin-dependent diabetes mellitus in Chilean children. *J Mol Med*. 1996;74:105–109

60. Davis MK. Review of the evidence for an association between infant feeding and childhood cancer. *Int J Cancer Suppl*. 1998;11:29–33

61. Smulevich VB, Solionova LG, Belyakova SV. Parental occupation and other factors and cancer risk in children: I. Study methodology and non-occupational factors. *Int J Cancer*. 1999;83:712–717

62. Bener A, Denic S, Galadari S. Longer breast-feeding and protection against childhood leukaemia and lymphomas. *Eur J Cancer*. 2001;37:234–238

63. Armstrong J, Reilly JJ, Child Health Information Team. Breastfeeding and lowering the risk of childhood obesity. *Lancet*. 2002;359:2003–2004

64. Dewey KG, Heinig MJ, Nommsen LA, Peerson JM, Lonnerdal B. Breast-fed infants are leaner than formula-fed infants at 1 year of age: the DARLING study. *Am J Clin Nutr*. 1993;57:140–145

65. Arenz S, Ruckerl R, Koletzko B, Von Kries R. Breast-feeding and childhood obesity—a systematic review. *Int J Obes Relat Metab Disord*. 2004;28:1247–1256

66. Grummer-Strawn LM, Mei Z. Does breastfeeding protect against pediatric overweight? Analysis of longitudinal data from the Centers for Disease Control and Prevention Pediatric Nutrition Surveillance System. *Pediatrics*. 2004;113(2). Available at: www.pediatrics.org/cgi/content/full/113/2/e81

67. Stettler N, Zemel BS, Kumanyika S, Stallings VA. Infant weight gain and childhood overweight status in a multicenter, cohort study. *Pediatrics*. 2002;109:194–199

68. Gillman MW, Rifas-Shiman SL, Camargo CA, et al. Risk of overweight among adolescents who were breastfed as infants. *JAMA*. 2001;285:2461–2467

69. Toschke AM, Vignerova J, Lhotska L, Osancova K, Koletzko B, von Kries R. Overweight and obesity in 6- to 14-year old Czech children in 1991: protective effect of breast-feeding. *J Pediatr*. 2002;141:764–769

70. American Academy of Pediatrics, Committee on Nutrition. Prevention of pediatric overweight and obesity. *Pediatrics*. 2003;112:424–430

71. Owen CG, Whincup PH, Odoki K, Gilg JA, Cook DG. Infant feeding and blood cholesterol: a study in adolescents and a systematic review. *Pediatrics*. 2002;110:597–608

72. Horwood LJ, Fergusson DM. Breastfeeding and later cognitive and academic outcomes. *Pediatrics*. 1998;101(1). Available at: www.pediatrics.org/cgi/content/full/101/1/e9

73. Anderson JW, Johnstone BM, Remley DT. Breast-feeding and cognitive development: a meta-analysis. *Am J Clin Nutr*. 1999;70:525–535

74. Jacobson SW, Chiodo LM, Jacobson JL. Breastfeeding effects on intelligence quotient in 4- and 11-year-old children. *Pediatrics*. 1999;103(5). Available at: www.pediatrics.org/cgi/content/full/103/5/e71

75. Reynolds A. Breastfeeding and brain development. *Pediatr Clin North Am*. 2001;48:159–171

76. Mortensen EL, Michaelsen KF, Sanders SA, Reinisch JM. The association between duration of breastfeeding and adult intelligence. *JAMA*. 2002;287:2365–2371

77. Batstra L, Neeleman J, Hadders-Algra M. Can breast feeding modify the adverse effects of smoking during pregnancy on the child's cognitive development? *J Epidemiol Community Health*. 2003;57:403–404

78. Rao MR, Hediger ML, Levine RJ, Naficy AB, Vik T. Effect of breast-feeding on cognitive development of infants born small for gestational age. *Acta Paediatr*. 2002;91:267–274

79. Bier JA, Oliver T, Ferguson AE, Vohr BR. Human milk improves cognitive and motor development of premature infants during infancy. *J Hum Lact*. 2002;18:361–367

80. Feldman R, Eidelman AI. Direct and indirect effects of breast-milk on the neurobehavioral and cognitive development of premature infants. *Dev Psychobiol*. 2003;43:109–119

81. Gray L, Miller LW, Phillip BL, Blass EM. Breastfeeding is analgesic in healthy newborns. *Pediatrics*. 2002;109:590–593

82. Carbajal R, Veerapen S, Couderc S, Jugie M, Ville Y. Analgesic effect of breast feeding in term neonates: randomized controlled trial. *BMJ*. 2003;326:13

83. Labbok MH. Effects of breastfeeding on the mother. *Pediatr Clin North Am*. 2001;48:143–158

84. Chua S, Arulkumaran S, Lim I, Selamat N, Ratnam SS. Influence of breastfeeding and nipple stimulation on postpartum uterine activity. *Br J Obstet Gynaecol*. 1994;101:804–805

85. Kennedy KI, Labbok MH, Van Look PF. Lactational amenorrhea method for family planning. *Int J Gynaecol Obstet*. 1996;54:55–57

86. Dewey KG, Heinig MJ, Nommsen LA. Maternal weight-loss patterns during prolonged lactation. *Am J Clin Nutr*. 1993;58:162–166

87. Newcomb PA, Storer BE, Longnecker MP, et al. Lactation and a reduced risk of premenopausal breast cancer. *N Engl J Med*. 1994;330:81–87

88. Collaborative Group on Hormonal Factors in Breast Cancer. Breast cancer and breastfeeding: collaborative reanalysis of individual data from 47 epidemiological studies in 30 countries, including 50302 women with breast cancer and 96973 women without the disease. *Lancet*. 2002;360:187–195

89. Lee SY, Kim MT, Kim SW, Song MS, Yoon SJ. Effect of lifetime lactation on breast cancer risk: a Korean women's cohort study. *Int J Cancer*. 2003;105:390–393

90. Tryggvadottir L, Tulinius H, Eyfjord JE, Sigurvinsson T. Breastfeeding and reduced risk of breast cancer in an Icelandic cohort study. *Am J Epidemiol*. 2001;154:37–42

91. Enger SM, Ross RK, Paganini-Hill A, Bernstein L. Breastfeeding experience and breast cancer risk among postmenopausal women. *Cancer Epidemiol Biomarkers Prev*. 1998;7:365–369

92. Jernstrom H, Lubinski J, Lynch HT, et al. Breast-feeding and the risk of breast cancer in BRCA1 and BRCA2 mutation carriers. *J Natl Cancer Inst*. 2004;96:1094–1098

93. Rosenblatt KA, Thomas DB. Lactation and the risk of epithelial ovarian cancer. WHO Collaborative Study of Neoplasia and Steroid contraceptives. *Int J Epidemiol*. 1993;22:192–197

94. Cumming RG, Klineberg RJ. Breastfeeding and other reproductive factors and the risk of hip fractures in elderly women. *Int J Epidemiol*. 1993;22:684–691

95. Lopez JM, Gonzalez G, Reyes V, Campino C, Diaz S. Bone turnover and density in healthy women during breastfeeding and after weaning. *Osteoporos Int*. 1996;6:153–159

96. Paton LM, Alexander JL, Nowson CA, et al. Pregnancy and lactation have no long-term deleterious effect on measures of bone mineral in healthy women: a twin study. *Am J Clin Nutr*. 2003;77:707–714

97. Weimer J. *The Economic Benefits of Breast Feeding: A Review and Analysis*. Food Assistance and Nutrition Research Report No. 13. Washington, DC: Food and Rural Economics Division, Economic Research Service, US Department of Agriculture; 2001

98. Ball TM, Wright AL. Health care cost of formula-feeding in the first year of life. *Pediatrics*. 1999;103:870–876

99. Tuttle CR, Dewey KG. Potential cost savings for Medi-Cal, AFDC, food stamps, and WIC programs associated with increasing breast-feeding among low-income Hmong women in California. *J Am Diet Assoc*. 1996;96:885–890

100. Cohen R, Mrtek MB, Mrtek RG. Comparison of maternal absenteeism and infant illness rates among breast-feeding and formula-feeding women in two corporations. *Am J Health Promot*. 1995;10:148–153

101. Jarosz LA. Breast-feeding versus formula: cost comparison. *Hawaii Med J*. 1993;52:14–18

102. Levine RE, Huffman SL, Center to Prevent Childhood Malnutrition. *The Economic Value of Breastfeeding, the National, Public Sector, Hospital and Household Levels: A Review of the Literature*. Washington, DC: Social Sector Analysis Project, Agency for International Development; 1990

103. Chen Y-T. Defects in galactose metabolism. In: Behrman RE, Kliegman RM, Jenson HB, eds. *Nelson Textbook of Pediatrics*. 16th ed. Philadelphia, PA: W. B. Saunders; 2000:413–414

104. Ando Y, Saito K, Nakano S, et al. Bottle-feeding can prevent transmission of HTLV-I from mothers to their babies. *J Infect*. 1989;19:25–29

105. Centers for Disease Control and Prevention and USPHS Working Group. Guidelines for counseling persons infected with human T-lymphotropic virus type I (HTLV-1) and type II (HTLV-II). *Ann Intern Med*. 1993;118:448–454

106. Gori G, Cama G, Guerresi E, et al. Radioactivity in breastmilk and placenta after Chernobyl accident [letter]. *Am J Obstet Gynecol*. 1988;158:1243–1244

107. Robinson PS, Barker P, Campbell A, Henson P, Surveyor I, Young PR. Iodine-131 in breast milk following therapy for thyroid carcinoma. *J Nucl Med.* 1994;35:1797–1801

108. Bakheet SM, Hammami MM. Patterns of radioiodine uptake by the lactating breast. *Eur J Nucl Med.* 1994;21:604–608

109. Egan PC, Costanza ME, Dodion P, Egorin MJ, Bachur NR. Doxorubicin and cisplatin excretion into human milk. *Cancer Treat Rep.* 1985;69:1387–1389

110. American Academy of Pediatrics, Committee on Drugs. Transfer of drugs and other chemicals into human milk. *Pediatrics.* 2001;108:776–789

111. American Academy of Pediatrics. Transmission of infectious agents via human milk. In: Pickering LK, ed. *Red Book: 2003 Report of the Committee on Infectious Diseases.* 26th ed. Elk Grove Village, IL: American Academy of Pediatrics; 2003:118–121

112. Read JS; American Academy of Pediatrics, Committee on Pediatric AIDS. Human milk, breastfeeding, and transmission of human immunodeficiency virus type 1 in the United States. *Pediatrics.* 2003;112:1196–1205

113. World Health Organization. *HIV and Infant Feeding: A Guide for Health Care Managers and Supervisors.* Publication Nos. WHO/FRH/NUT/98.2, UNAIDS/98.4, UNICEF/PD/NUT/(J)98.2. Geneva, Switzerland: World Health Organization; 1998

114. Kourtis AP, Buteera S, Ibegbu C, Belec L, Duerr A. Breast milk and HIV-1: vector of transmission or vehicle of protection? *Lancet Infect Dis.* 2003;3:786–793

115. Coutsoudis A, Pillay K, Spooner E, Kuhn L, Coovadia HM. Influence of infant-feeding patterns on early mother-to-child transmission of HIV-1 in Durban, South Africa: a prospective cohort study. South African Vitamin A Study Group. *Lancet.* 1999;354:471–476

116. Coutsoudis A, Rollins N. Breast-feeding and HIV transmission: the jury is still out. *J Pediatr Gastroenterol Nutr.* 2003;36:434–442

117. Lawrence RA, Lawrence RM. Appendix E. Precautions and breastfeeding recommendations for selected maternal infections. In: *Breastfeeding: A Guide for the Medical Profession.* 5th ed. St Louis, MO: Mosby Inc; 1999:868–885

118. Berlin CM Jr, LaKind JS, Sonawane BR, et al. Conclusions, research needs, and recommendations of the expert panel: Technical Workshop on Human Milk Surveillance and Research for Environmental Chemicals in the United States. *J Toxicol Environ Health A.* 2002;65:1929–1935

119. Ribas-Fito N, Cardo E, Sala M, et al. Breastfeeding, exposure to organochlorine compounds, and neurodevelopment in infants. *Pediatrics.* 2003;111(5). Available at: www.pediatrics.org/cgi/content/full/111/5/e580

120. Hamprecht K, Maschmann J, Vochem M, Dietz K, Speer CP, Jahn G. Epidemiology of transmission of cytomegalovirus from mother to preterm infant by breastfeeding. *Lancet.* 2001;357:513–518

121. Yasuda A, Kimura H, Hayakawa M, et al. Evaluation of cytomegalovirus infections transmitted via breast milk in preterm infants with a real-time polymerase chain reaction assay. *Pediatrics.* 2003;111:1333–1336

122. Friis H, Andersen HK. Rate of inactivation of cytomegalovirus in raw banked milk during storage at −20 degrees C and pasteurisation. *Br Med J (Clin Res Ed).* 1982;285:1604–1605

123. Anderson PO. Alcohol and breastfeeding. *J Hum Lact.* 1995;11:321–323

124. American Academy of Pediatrics, Subcommittee on Hyperbilirubinemia. Management of hyperbilirubinemia in the newborn infant 35 or more weeks of gestation. *Pediatrics.* 2004;114:297–316

125. Ryan AS, Wenjun Z, Acosta A. Breastfeeding continues to increase into the new millennium. *Pediatrics.* 2002;110:1103–1109

126. Polhamus B, Dalenius K, Thompson D, et al. *Pediatric Nutrition Surveillance 2001 Report.* Atlanta, GA: US Department of Health and Human Services, Centers for Disease Control and Prevention; 2003

127. American College of Obstetricians and Gynecologists. Breastfeeding: maternal and infant aspects. *ACOG Educational Bulletin Number 258.* Washington, DC: American College of Obstetricians and Gynecologists; 2000

128. American Academy of Family Physicians. *AAFP Policy Statement on Breastfeeding.* Leawood, KS: American Academy of Family Physicians; 2001

129. Fifty-Fourth World Health Assembly. *Global Strategy for Infant and Young Child Feeding. The Optimal Duration of Exclusive Breastfeeding.* Geneva, Switzerland: World Health Organization; 2001

130. United Nations Children's Fund. *Breastfeeding: Foundation for a Healthy Future.* New York, NY: United Nations Children's Fund; 1999

131. Institute of Medicine, Committee on Nutritional Status During Pregnancy and Lactation. *Nutrition During Lactation.* Washington, DC: National Academy Press; 1991:24–25, 161–171, 197–200

132. The Ross Mothers Survey. *Breastfeeding Trends Through 2002.* Abbott Park, IL: Ross Products Division, Abbot Laboratories; 2002

133. World Health Organization and United Nations Children's Fund. *Protecting, Promoting and Supporting Breast-Feeding: The Special Role of Maternity Services.* Geneva, Switzerland: World Health Organization; 1989:13–18

134. Powers NG, Naylor AJ, Wester RA. Hospital policies: crucial to breastfeeding success. *Semin Perinatol.* 1994;18:517–524

135. Freed GL, Clark SJ, Sorenson J, Lohr JA, Cefalo R, Curtis P. National assessment of physicians' breast-feeding knowledge, attitudes, training, and experience. *JAMA.* 1995;273:472–476

136. Braveman P, Egerter S, Pearl M, Marchi K, Miller C. Problems associated with early discharge of newborn infants. *Pediatrics.* 1995;96:716–726

137. Williams LR, Cooper MK. Nurse-managed postpartum home care. *J Obstet Gynecol Neonatal Nurs.* 1993;22:25–31

138. Gielen AC, Faden RR, O'Campo P, Brown CH, Paige DM. Maternal employment during the early postpartum period: effects on initiation and continuation of breast-feeding. *Pediatrics.* 1991;87:298–305

139. Ryan AS, Martinez GA. Breast-feeding and the working mother: a profile. *Pediatrics.* 1989;83:524–531

140. Frederick IB, Auerback KG. Maternal-infant separation and breastfeeding. The return to work or school. *J Reprod Med.* 1985;30:523–526

141. Spisak S, Gross SS. *Second Followup Report: The Surgeon General's Workshop on Breastfeeding and Human Lactation.* Washington, DC: National Center for Education in Maternal and Child Health; 1991

142. World Health Assembly. *International Code of Marketing of Breast-Milk Substitutes.* Resolution of the 34th World Health Assembly. No. 34.22, Geneva, Switzerland: World Health Organization; 1981

143. Howard CR, Howard FM, Weitzman ML. Infant formula distribution and advertising in pregnancy: a hospital survey. *Birth.* 1994;21:14–19

144. Howard FM, Howard CR, Weitzman M. The physician as advertiser: the unintentional discouragement of breast-feeding. *Obstet Gynecol.* 1993;81:1048–1051

145. Freed GL, Jones TM, Fraley JK. Attitudes and education of pediatric house staff concerning breast-feeding. *South Med J.* 1992;85:483–485

146. Williams EL, Hammer LD. Breastfeeding attitudes and knowledge of pediatricians-in-training. *Am J Prev Med.* 1995;11:26–33

147. Gartner LM. Introduction. Breastfeeding in the hospital. *Semin Perinatol.* 1994;18:475

148. American Academy of Pediatrics, Committee on Nutrition. Breastfeeding. In: Kleinman RE, ed. *Pediatric Nutrition Handbook.* 5th ed. Elk Grove Village, IL: American Academy of Pediatrics; 2004:55–85

149. American Dietetic Association. Position of the American Dietetic Association: breaking the barriers to breastfeeding. *J Am Diet Assoc.* 2001;101:1213–1220

150. Schanler RJ, Hurst NM. Human milk for the hospitalized preterm infant. *Semin Perinatol.* 1994;18:476–484

151. Lemons P, Stuart M, Lemons JA. Breast-feeding the premature infant. *Clin Perinatol.* 1986;13:111–122

152. Kron RE, Stein M, Goddard KE. Newborn sucking behavior affected by obstetric sedation. *Pediatrics.* 1966;37:1012–1016

153. Ransjo-Arvidson AB, Matthiesen AS, Lilja G, Nissen E, Widstrom AM, Uvnas-Moberg K. Maternal analgesia during labor disturbs newborn behavior: effects on breastfeeding, temperature, and crying. *Birth.* 2001;28:5–12

154. Widstrom A-M, Thingstrom-Paulsson J. The position of the tongue during rooting reflexes elicited in newborn infants before the first suckle. *Acta Paediatr.* 1993;82:281–283

155. Wolf L, Glass RP. *Feeding and Swallowing Disorders in Infancy: Assessment and Management.* San Antonio, TX: Harcourt Assessment, Inc; 1992

156. Righard L, Alade MO. Effect of delivery room routine on success of first breast-feed. *Lancet.* 1990;336:1105–1107

157. Wiberg B, Humble K, de Chateau P. Long-term effect on mother-infant behavior of extra contact during the first hour post partum. V. Follow-up at three years. *Scand J Soc Med.* 1989;17:181–191

158. Mikiel-Kostyra K, Mazur J, Boltruszko I. Effect of early skin-to-skin contact after delivery on duration of breastfeeding: a prospective cohort study. *Acta Paediatr.* 2002;91:1301–1306

159. Christensson K, Siles C, Moreno L, et al. Temperature, metabolic adaptation and crying in healthy, full-term newborns cared for skin-to-skin or in a cot. *Acta Paediatr.* 1992;81:488–493

233

160. Van Den Bosch CA, Bullough CH. Effect of early suckling on term neonates' core body temperature. *Ann Trop Paediatr.* 1990;10: 347–353

161. Sosa R, Kennell JH, Klaus M, Urrutia JJ. The effect of early mother-infant contact on breast feeding, infection and growth. In: Lloyd JL, ed. *Breast-feeding and the Mother.* Amsterdam, Netherlands: Elsevier; 1976: 179–193

162. American Academy of Pediatrics, American College of Obstetricians and Gynecologists. Care of the neonate. In: Gilstrap LC, Oh W, eds. *Guidelines for Perinatal Care.* 5th ed. Elk Grove Village, IL: American Academy of Pediatrics; 2002:222

163. Shrago L. Glucose water supplementation of the breastfed infant during the first three days of life. *J Hum Lact.* 1987;3:82–86

164. Goldberg NM, Adams E. Supplementary water for breast-fed babies in a hot and dry climate—not really a necessity. *Arch Dis Child.* 1983;58: 73–74

165. Eidelman AI. Hypoglycemia in the breastfed neonate. *Pediatr Clin North Am.* 2001;48:377–387

166. Howard CR, Howard FM, Lamphear B, de Blieck EA, Eberly S, Lawrence RA. The effects of early pacifier use on breastfeeding duration. *Pediatrics.* 1999;103(3). Available at: www.pediatrics.org/cgi/content/full/103/3/e33

167. Howard CR, Howard FM, Lanphear B, et al. Randomized clinical trial of pacifier use and bottle-feeding or cupfeeding and their effect on breastfeeding. *Pediatrics.* 2003;111:511–518

168. Schubiger G, Schwarz U, Tonz O. UNICEF/WHO Baby-Friendly Hospital Initiative: does the use of bottles and pacifiers in the neonatal nursery prevent successful breastfeeding? Neonatal Study Group. *Eur J Pediatr.* 1997;156:874–877

169. Kramer MS, Barr RG, Dagenais S, et al. Pacifier use, early weaning, and cry/fuss behavior: a randomized controlled trial. *JAMA.* 2001;286: 322–326

170. Gunther M. Instinct and the nursing couple. *Lancet.* 1955;1:575–578

171. Klaus MH. The frequency of suckling. A neglected but essential ingredient of breast-feeding. *Obstet Gynecol Clin North Am.* 1987;14: 623–633

172. Procianoy RS, Fernandes-Filho PH, Lazaro L, Sartori NC, Drebes S. The influence of rooming-in on breastfeeding. *J Trop Pediatr.* 1983;29: 112–114

173. Anderson GC. Risk in mother-infant separation postbirth. *Image J Nurs Sch.* 1989;21:196–199

174. Riordan J, Bibb D, Miller M, Rawlins T. Predicting breastfeeding duration using the LATCH breastfeeding assessment tool. *J Hum Lact.* 2001;17:20–23

175. Hall RT, Mercer AM, Teasley SL, et al. A breast-feeding assessment score to evaluate the risk for cessation of breast-feeding by 7 to 10 days of age. *J Pediatr.* 2002;141:659–664

176. American Academy of Pediatrics, Committee on Practice and Ambulatory Medicine. Recommendations for preventive pediatric health care. *Pediatrics.* 2000;105:645–646

177. American Academy of Pediatrics, Committee on Fetus and Newborn. Hospital stay for healthy term newborns. *Pediatrics.* 1995;96:788–790

178. Ahn CH, MacLean WC Jr. Growth of the exclusively breast-fed infant. *Am J Clin Nutr.* 1980;33:183–192

179. Brown KH, Dewey KG, Allen LH. *Complementary Feeding of Young Children in Developing Countries: A Review of Current Scientific Knowledge.* Publication No. WHO/NUT/98.1. Geneva, Switzerland: World Health Organization; 1998

180. Heinig MJ, Nommsen LA, Peerson JM, Lonnerdal B, Dewey KG. Intake and growth of breast-fed and formula-fed infants in relation to the timing of introduction of complementary foods: the DARLING study. Davis Area Research on Lactation, Infant Nutrition, and Growth. *Acta Paediatr.* 1993;82:999–1006

181. Kramer MS, Kakuma R. *The Optimal Duration of Exclusive Breastfeeding. A Systematic Review.* Geneva, Switzerland: World Health Organization; 2002

182. Chantry CJ, Howard CR, Auinger P. Breastfeeding fully for 6 months vs. 4 months decreases risk of respiratory tract infection [abstract 1114]. *Pediatr Res.* 2002;51:191A

183. Dewey KG, Cohen RJ, Brown KH, Rivera LL. Effects of exclusive breastfeeding for four versus six months on maternal nutritional status and infant motor development: results of two randomized trials in Honduras. *J Nutr.* 2001;131:262–267

184. Butte NF, Lopez-Alarcon MG, Garza C. *Nutrient Adequacy of Exclusive Breastfeeding for the Term Infant During the First Six Months of Life.* Geneva, Switzerland: World Health Organization; 2002

185. Sugarman M, Kendall-Tackett KA. Weaning ages in a sample of American women who practice extended breastfeeding. *Clin Pediatr (Phila).* 1995;34:642–647

186. Dallman PR. Progress in the prevention of iron deficiency in infants. *Acta Paediatr Scand Suppl.* 1990;365:28–37

187. Domellof M, Lonnerdal B, Abrams SA, Hernell O. Iron absorption in breast-fed infants: effects of age, iron status, iron supplements, and complementary foods. *Am J Clin Nutr.* 2002;76:198–204

188. American Academy of Pediatrics, Committee on Fetus and Newborn and American College of Obstetricians and Gynecologists. Nutritional needs of preterm neonates. In: *Guidelines for Perinatal Care.* 5th ed. Washington, DC: American Academy of Pediatrics, American College of Obstetricians and Gynecologists; 2002:259–263

189. American Academy of Pediatrics, Committee on Nutrition. Nutritional needs of the preterm infant. In: Kleinman RE, ed. *Pediatric Nutrition Handbook.* 5th ed. Elk Grove Village, IL: American Academy of Pediatrics; 2004:23–54

190. Pisacane A, De Vizia B, Valiante A, et al. Iron status in breast-fed infants. *J Pediatr.* 1995;127:429–431

191. Griffin IJ, Abrams SA. Iron and breastfeeding. *Pediatr Clin North Am.* 2001;48:401–413

192. Dewey KG, Cohen RJ, Rivera LL, Brown KH. Effects of age of introduction of complementary foods on iron status of breastfed infants in Honduras. *Am J Clin Nutr.* 1998;67:878–884

193. Naylor AJ, Morrow AL. *Developmental Readiness of Normal Full Term Infants to Progress From Exclusive Breastfeeding to the Introduction of Complementary Foods: Reviews of the Relevant Literature Concerning Infant Immunologic, Gastrointestinal, Oral Motor and Maternal Reproductive and Lactational Development.* Washington, DC: Wellstart International and the LINKAGES Project/Academy of Educational Development; 2001

194. Cohen RJ, Brown KH, Canahuati J, Rivera LL, Dewey KG. Determinants of growth from birth to 12 months among breast-fed Honduran infants in relation to age of introduction of complementary foods. *Pediatrics.* 1995;96:504–510

195. Ashraf RN, Jalil F, Aperia A, Lindblad BS. Additional water is not needed for healthy breast-fed babies in a hot climate. *Acta Paediatr.* 1993;82:1007–1011

196. Huffman SL, Ford K, Allen H, Streble P. Nutrition and fertility in Bangladesh: breastfeeding and post partum amenorrhoea. *Popul Stud (Camb).* 1987;41:447–462

197. Dettwyler KA. A time to wean: the hominid blueprint for the natural age of weaning in modern human populations. In: Stuart-Macadam P, Dettwyler KA, eds. *Breastfeeding: Biocultural Perspectives.* Hawthorne, NY: Aldine de Gruyter; 1995:39–73

198. American Academy of Pediatrics, Committee on Nutrition. Iron fortification of infant formulas. *Pediatrics.* 1999;104:119–123

199. American Academy of Pediatrics, Committee on Fetus and Newborn. Controversies concerning vitamin K and the newborn. *Pediatrics.* 2003; 112:191–192

200. Hansen KN, Ebbesen F. Neonatal vitamin K prophylaxis in Denmark: three years' experience with oral administration during the first three months of life compared with one oral administration at birth. *Acta Paediatr.* 1996;85:1137–1139

201. Gartner LM, Greer FR; American Academy of Pediatrics, Section on Breastfeeding and Committee on Nutrition. Prevention of rickets and vitamin D deficiency: new guidelines for vitamin D intake. *Pediatrics.* 2003;111:908–910

202. Centers for Disease Control and Prevention. Recommendations for using fluoride to prevent and control dental caries in the United States. *MMWR Recomm Rep.* 2001;50(RR-14):1–42

203. Blair PS, Fleming PJ, Smith IJ, et al. Babies sleeping with parents: case-control study of factors influencing the risk of the sudden infant death syndrome. *BMJ.* 1999;319:1457–1462

204. Charpak N, Ruiz-Pelaez JG, Figueroa de C Z, Charpak Y. Kangaroo mother versus traditional care for newborn infants ≤2000 grams: a randomized, controlled trial. *Pediatrics.* 1997;100:682–688

205. Hurst N, Valentine CJ, Renfro L, Burns P, Ferlic L. Skin-to-skin holding in the neonatal intensive care influences maternal milk volume. *J Perinatol.* 1997;17:213–217

206. Hughes V. Guidelines for the establishment and operation of a human milk bank. *J Hum Lact.* 1990;6:185–186

207. Human Milk Banking Association of North America. *Guidelines for Establishment and Operation of a Donor Human Milk Bank.* Raleigh, NC: Human Milk Banking Association of North America Inc; 2003

208. Arnold LD. Clinical uses of donor milk. *J Hum Lact.* 1990;6:132–133

09. Kaplan M, Hammerman C. Severe neonatal hyperbilirubinemia: a potential complication of glucose-6-phosphate dehydrogenase deficiency. *Clin Perinatol.* 1998;25:575–590, viii

10. Kaplan M, Vreman HJ, Hammerman C, Schimmel MS, Abrahamov A, Stevenson DK. Favism by proxy in nursing glucose-6-dehydrogenase-deficient neonates. *J Perinatol.* 1998;18:477–479

11. Gerk PM, Kuhn RJ, Desai NS, McNamara PJ. Active transport of nitrofurantoin into human milk. *Pharmacotherapy.* 2001;21:669–675

12. American Academy of Pediatrics, Section on Pediatric Dentistry. Oral health risk assessment timing and establishment of the dental home. *Pediatrics.* 2003;111:1113–1116

13. Fewtrell MS, Lucas P, Collier S, Singhal A, Ahluwalia JS, Lucas A. Randomized trial comparing the efficacy of a novel manual breast pump with a standard electric breast pump in mothers who delivered preterm infants. *Pediatrics.* 2001;107:1291–1297

214. American Academy of Pediatrics, Breastfeeding Promotion in Physicians' Office Practices Program. Elk Grove Village, IL: American Academy of Pediatrics; 2001, 2004

215. Freed GL, Clark SJ, Lohr JA, Sorenson JR. Pediatrician involvement in breast-feeding promotion: a national study of residents and practitioners. *Pediatrics.* 1995;96:490–494

216. Brown LP, Bair AH, Meier PP. Does federal funding for breastfeeding research target our national health objectives? *Pediatrics.* 2003;111(4). Available at: www.pediatrics.org/cgi/content/full/111/4/e360

All policy statements from the American Academy of Pediatrics automatically expire 5 years after publication unless reaffirmed, revised, or retired at or before that time.

AMERICAN ACADEMY OF PEDIATRICS

Committee on Drugs

The Transfer of Drugs and Other Chemicals Into Human Milk

ABSTRACT. The American Academy of Pediatrics places emphasis on increasing breastfeeding in the United States. A common reason for the cessation of breastfeeding is the use of medication by the nursing mother and advice by her physician to stop nursing. Such advice may not be warranted. This statement is intended to supply the pediatrician, obstetrician, and family physician with data, if known, concerning the excretion of drugs into human milk. Most drugs likely to be prescribed to the nursing mother should have no effect on milk supply or on infant well-being. This information is important not only to protect nursing infants from untoward effects of maternal medication but also to allow effective pharmacologic treatment of breastfeeding mothers. Nicotine, psychotropic drugs, and silicone implants are 3 important topics reviewed in this statement.

INTRODUCTION

A statement on the transfer of drugs and chemicals into human milk was first published in 1983,[1] with revisions in 1989[2] and 1994.[3] Information continues to become available. The current statement is intended to revise the lists of agents transferred into human milk and describe their possible effects on the infant or on lactation, if known (Tables 1–7). If a pharmacologic or chemical agent does not appear in the tables, it does not mean that it is not transferred into human milk or that it does not have an effect on the infant; it only indicates that there were no reports found in the literature. These tables should assist the physician in counseling a nursing mother regarding breastfeeding when the mother has a condition for which a drug is medically indicated.

BREASTFEEDING AND SMOKING

In the previous edition of this statement, the Committee on Drugs placed nicotine (smoking) in Table 2, "Drugs of Abuse-Contraindicated During Breastfeeding." The reasons for placing nicotine and, thus, smoking in Table 2 were documented decrease in milk production and weight gain in the infant of the smoking mother and exposure of the infant to environmental tobacco smoke as demonstrated by the presence of nicotine and its primary metabolite, cotinine, in human milk.[4–12] There is controversy regarding the effects of nicotine on infant size at 1 year of age.[13,14] There are hundreds of compounds in tobacco smoke; however, nicotine and its metabolite acotinine are most often used as markers of tobacco

exposure. Nicotine is not necessarily the only component that might cause an increase in respiratory illnesses (including otitis media) in the nursing infant attributable to both transmammary secretion of compounds and environmental exposure. Nicotine is present in milk in concentrations between 1.5 and 3.0 times the simultaneous maternal plasma concentration,[15] and elimination half-life is similar—60 to 90 minutes in milk and plasma.[7] There is no evidence to document whether this amount of nicotine presents a health risk to the nursing infant.

The Committee on Drugs wishes to support the emphasis of the American Academy of Pediatrics on increasing breastfeeding in the United States. Pregnancy and lactation are ideal occasions for physicians to urge cessation of smoking. It is recognized that there are women who are unable to stop smoking cigarettes. One study reported that, among women who continue to smoke throughout breastfeeding, the incidence of acute respiratory illness is decreased among their infants, compared with infants of smoking mothers who are bottle fed.[16] It may be that breastfeeding and smoking is less detrimental to the child than bottle feeding and smoking. The Committee on Drugs awaits more data on this issue. The Committee on Drugs therefore has not placed nicotine (and thus smoking) in any of the Tables but hopes that the interest in breastfeeding by a smoking woman will serve as a point of discussion about smoking cessation between the pediatrician and the prospective lactating woman or nursing mother. Alternate (oral, transcutaneous) sources of nicotine to assist with smoking cessation, however, have not been studied sufficiently for the Committee on Drugs to make a recommendation for or against them in breastfeeding women.

PSYCHOTROPIC DRUGS

Anti-anxiety drugs, antidepressants, and neuroleptic drugs have been placed in Table 4, "Drugs for Which the Effect on Nursing Infants Is Unknown but May Be of Concern." These drugs appear in low concentrations (usually with a milk-to-plasma ratio of 0.5–1.0) in milk after maternal ingestion. Because of the long half-life of these compounds and some of their metabolites, nursing infants may have measurable amounts in their plasma and tissues, such as the brain. This is particularly important in infants during the first few months of life, with immature hepatic and renal function. Nursing mothers should be informed that if they take one of these drugs, the infant will be exposed to it. Because these drugs affect neurotransmitter function in the developing central

The recommendations in this statement do not indicate an exclusive course of treatment or serve as a standard of medical care. Variations, taking into account individual circumstances, may be appropriate.

ervous system, it may not be possible to predict long-term neurodevelopmental effects.

SILICONE BREAST IMPLANTS AND BREASTFEEDING

Approximately 800 000 to 1 million women in the United States have received breast implants containing silicone (elemental silicon with chemical bonds to oxygen) in the implant envelope or in the envelope and the interior gel. Concern has been raised about the possible effects to the nursing infant if mothers with implants breastfeed. This concern was initially raised in reports that described esophageal dysfunction in 11 children whose mothers had implants.[17,18] This finding has not been confirmed by other reports. Silicone chemistry is extremely complex; the polymer involved in the covering and the interior of the breast implant consists of a polymer of alternating silicon and oxygen atoms with methyl groups attached to the oxygen groups (methyl polydimethylsiloxane).[19] The length of the polymer determines whether it is a solid, gel, or liquid. There are only a few instances of the polymer being assayed in the milk of women with implants; the concentrations are not elevated over control samples.[20] There is no evidence at the present time that this polymer is directly toxic to human tissues; however, concern also exists that toxicity may be mediated through an immunologic mechanism. This has yet to be confirmed in humans. Except for the study cited above, there have been no other reports of clinical problems in infants of mothers with silicone breast implants.[21] It is unlikely that elemental silicon causes difficulty, because silicon is present in higher concentrations in cow milk and formula than in milk of humans with implants.[22] The anticolic compound simethicone is a silicone and has a structure very similar to the methyl polydimethylsiloxane in breast implants. Simethicone has been used for decades in this country and Europe without any evidence of toxicity to infants. The Committee on Drugs does not feel that the evidence currently justifies classifying silicone implants as a contraindication to breastfeeding.

DRUG THERAPY OF THE LACTATING WOMAN

The following should be considered before prescribing drugs to lactating women:

1. Is drug therapy really necessary? If drugs are required, consultation between the pediatrician and the mother's physician can be most useful in determining what options to choose.
2. The safest drug should be chosen, for example, acetaminophen rather than aspirin for analgesia.
3. If there is a possibility that a drug may present a risk to the infant, consideration should be given to measurement of blood concentrations in the nursing infant.
4. Drug exposure to the nursing infant may be minimized by having the mother take the medication just after she has breastfed the infant or just before the infant is due to have a lengthy sleep period.

Data have been obtained from a search of the medical literature. Because methodologies used to quantitate drugs in milk continue to improve, this information will require frequent updating. Drugs cited in Tables 1 through 7 are listed in alphabetical order by generic name; brand names are available from the current *Physicians' Desk Reference*,[23] *USP DI 2001: Drug Information for the Health Care Professional, Volume I*,[24] and *USP Dictionary of USAN and International Drug Names*.[25] The reference list is not inclusive of all articles published on the topic.

Physicians who encounter adverse effects in infants who have been receiving drug-contaminated human milk are urged to document these effects in a communication to the Food and Drug Administration (http://www.fda.gov/medwatch/index.html) and to the Committee on Drugs. This communication should include the generic and brand names of the drug, the maternal dose and mode of administration, the concentration of the drug in milk and maternal and infant blood in relation to the time of ingestion, the method used for laboratory identification, the age of the infant, and the adverse effects. Such reports may substantially increase the pediatric community's fund of knowledge regarding drug transfer into human milk and the potential or actual risk to the infant.

TABLE 1. Cytotoxic Drugs That May Interfere With Cellular Metabolism of the Nursing Infant

Drug	Reason for Concern, Reported Sign or Symptom in Infant, or Effect on Lactation	Reference No.
Cyclophosphamide	Possible immune suppression; unknown effect on growth or association with carcinogenesis; neutropenia	26, 27
Cyclosporine	Possible immune suppression; unknown effect on growth or association with carcinogenesis	28, 29
Doxorubicin*	Possible immune suppression; unknown effect on growth or association with carcinogenesis	30
Methotrexate	Possible immune suppression; unknown effect on growth or association with carcinogenesis; neutropenia	31

* Drug is concentrated in human milk.

TABLE 2. Drugs of Abuse for Which Adverse Effects on the Infant During Breastfeeding Have Been Reported*

Drug	Reported Effect or Reasons for Concern	Reference No.
Amphetamine†	Irritability, poor sleeping pattern	32
Cocaine	Cocaine intoxication: irritability, vomiting, diarrhea, tremulousness, seizures	33
Heroin	Tremors, restlessness, vomiting, poor feeding	34
Marijuana	Only 1 report in literature; no effect mentioned; very long half-life for some components	35
Phencyclidine	Potent hallucinogen	36

* The Committee on Drugs strongly believes that nursing mothers should not ingest drugs of abuse, because they are hazardous to the nursing infant and to the health of the mother.
† Drug is concentrated in human milk.

TABLE 3. Radioactive Compounds That Require Temporary Cessation of Breastfeeding*

Compound	Recommended Time for Cessation of Breastfeeding	Reference No.
Copper 64 (^{64}Cu)	Radioactivity in milk present at 50 h	37
Gallium 67 (^{67}Ga)	Radioactivity in milk present for 2 wk	38
Indium 111 (^{111}In)	Very small amount present at 20 h	39
Iodine 123 (^{123}I)	Radioactivity in milk present up to 36 h	40, 41
Iodine 125 (^{125}I)	Radioactivity in milk present for 12 d	42
Iodine 131 (^{131}I)	Radioactivity in milk present 2–14 d, depending on study	43–46
Iodine^{131}	If used for treatment of thyroid cancer, high radioactivity may prolong exposure to infant	47, 48
Radioactive sodium	Radioactivity in milk present 96 h	49
Technetium 99m (^{99m}Tc), ^{99m}Tc macroaggregates, ^{99m}Tc O$_4$	Radioactivity in milk present 15 h to 3 d	41, 50–55

* Consult nuclear medicine physician before performing diagnostic study so that radionuclide that has the shortest excretion time in breast milk can be used. Before study, the mother should pump her breast and store enough milk in the freezer for feeding the infant; after study, the mother should pump her breast to maintain milk production but discard all milk pumped for the required time that radioactivity is present in milk. Milk samples can be screened by radiology departments for radioactivity before resumption of nursing.

Drug	Reported or Possible Effect	Reference No.
Anti-anxiety		
Alprazolam	None	57
Diazepam	None	58–62
Lorazepam	None	63
Midazolam	—	64
Perphenazine	None	65
Prazepam†	None	66
Quazepam	None	67
Temazepam	—	68
Antidepressants		
Amitriptyline	None	69, 70
Amoxapine	None	71
Bupropion	None	72
Clomipramine	None	73
Desipramine	None	74, 75
Dothiepin	None	76, 77
Doxepin	None	78
Fluoxetine	Colic, irritability, feeding and sleep disorders, slow weight gain	79–87
Fluvoxamine	—	88
Imipramine	None	74
Nortriptyline	None	89, 90
Paroxetine	None	91
Sertraline†	None	92, 93
Trazodone	None	94
Antipsychotic		
Chlorpromazine	Galactorrhea in mother; drowsiness and lethargy in infant; decline in developmental scores	95–98
Chlorprothixene	None	99
Clozapine†	None	100
Haloperidol	Decline in developmental scores	101–104
Mesoridazine	None	105
Trifluoperazine	None	104
OTHERS		
Amiodarone	Possible hypothyroidism	106
Chloramphenicol	Possible idiosyncratic bone marrow suppression	107, 108
Clofazimine	Potential for transfer of high percentage of maternal dose; possible increase in skin pigmentation	109
Lamotrigine	Potential therapeutic serum concentrations in infant	110
Metoclopramide†	None described; dopaminergic blocking agent	111, 112
Metronidazole	In vitro mutagen; may discontinue breastfeeding for 12–24 h to allow excretion of dose when single-dose therapy given to mother	113, 114
Tinidazole	See metronidazole	115

* Psychotropic drugs, the compounds listed under anti-anxiety, antidepressant, and antipsychotic categories, are of special concern when given to nursing mothers for long periods. Although there are very few case reports of adverse effects in breastfeeding infants, these drugs do appear in human milk and, thus, could conceivably alter short-term and long-term central nervous system function.[56] See discussion in text of psychotropic drugs.
† Drug is concentrated in human milk relative to simultaneous maternal plasma concentrations.

Drug	Reported Effect	Reference No.
Acebutolol	Hypotension; bradycardia; tachypnea	116
5-Aminosalicylic acid	Diarrhea (1 case)	117–119
Atenolol	Cyanosis; bradycardia	120–124
Bromocriptine	Suppresses lactation; may be hazardous to the mother	125, 126
Aspirin (salicylates)	Metabolic acidosis (1 case)	127–129
Clemastine	Drowsiness, irritability, refusal to feed, high-pitched cry, neck stiffness (1 case)	130
Ergotamine	Vomiting, diarrhea, convulsions (doses used in migraine medications)	131
Lithium	One-third to one-half therapeutic blood concentration in infants	132–134
Phenindione	Anticoagulant: increased prothrombin and partial thromboplastin time in 1 infant; not used in United States	135
Phenobarbital	Sedation; infantile spasms after weaning from milk containing phenobarbital, methemoglobinemia (1 case)	136–140
Primidone	Sedation, feeding problems	136, 137
Sulfasalazine (salicylazosulfapyridine)	Bloody diarrhea (1 case)	141

* Blood concentration in the infant may be of clinical importance.

TABLE 6. Maternal Medication Usually Compatible With Breastfeeding*

Drug	Reported Sign or Symptom in Infant or Effect on Lactation	Reference No.
Acetaminophen	None	142–144
Acetazolamide	None	145
Acitretin	—	146
Acyclovir†	None	147, 148
Alcohol (ethanol)	With large amounts, drowsiness, diaphoresis, deep sleep, weakness, decrease in linear growth, abnormal weight gain; maternal ingestion of 1 g/kg daily decreases milk ejection reflex	4, 149–152
Allopurinol	—	153
Amoxicillin	None	154
Antimony	—	155
Atropine	None	156
Azapropazone (apazone)	—	157
Aztreonam	None	158
B₁ (thiamin)	None	159
B₆ (pyridoxine)	None	160–162
B₁₂	None	163
Baclofen	None	164
Barbiturate	See Table 5	
Bendroflumethiazide	Suppresses lactation	165
Bishydroxycoumarin (dicumarol)	None	166
Bromide	Rash, weakness, absence of cry with maternal intake of 5.4 g/d	167
Butorphanol	None	168
Caffeine	Irritability, poor sleeping pattern, excreted slowly; no effect with moderate intake of caffeinated beverages (2–3 cups per day)	169–174
Captopril	None	175
Carbamazepine	None	176, 177
Carbetocin	None	178
Carbimazole	Goiter	83, 179, 180
Cascara	None	181
Cefadroxil	None	154
Cefazolin	None	182
Cefotaxime	None	183
Cefoxitin	None	183
Cefprozil	—	184
Ceftazidime	None	185
Ceftriaxone	None	186
Chloral hydrate	Sleepiness	187
Chloroform	None	188
Chloroquine	None	189–191
Chlorothiazide	None	192, 193
Chlorthalidone	Excreted slowly	194
Cimetidine†	None	195, 196
Ciprofloxacin	None	197, 198
Cisapride	None	199
Cisplatin	Not found in milk	30
Clindamycin	None	200
Clogestone	None	201
Codeine	None	144, 156, 202
Colchicine	—	203–205
Contraceptive pill with estrogen/progesterone	Rare breast enlargement; decrease in milk production and protein content (not confirmed in several studies)	206–213
Cycloserine	None	214
D (vitamin)	None; follow up infant's serum calcium level if mother receives pharmacologic doses	215–217
Danthron	Increased bowel activity	218
Dapsone	None; sulfonamide detected in infant's urine	191, 219
Dexbrompheniramine maleate with d-isoephedrine	Crying, poor sleeping patterns, irritability	220
Diatrizoate	None	221
Digoxin	None	222, 223
Diltiazem	None	224
Dipyrone	None	225
Disopyramide	None	226, 227
Domperidone	None	228
Dyphylline†	None	229
Enalapril	—	230
Erythromycin†	None	231
Estradiol	Withdrawal, vaginal bleeding	232
Ethambutol	None	214
Ethanol (cf. alcohol)	—	

Drug	Reported Sign or Symptom in Infant or Effect on Lactation	Reference No.
Ethosuximide	None, drug appears in infant serum	176, 233
Fentanyl	—	234
Fexofenadine	None	235
Flecainide	—	236, 237
Fleroxacin	One 400-mg dose given to nursing mothers; infants not given breast milk for 48 h	238
Fluconazole	None	239
Flufenamic acid	None	240
Fluorescein	—	241
Folic acid	None	242
Gadopentetic (Gadolinium)	None	243
Gentamicin	None	244
Gold salts	None	245–249
Halothane	None	250
Hydralazine	None	251
Hydrochlorothiazide	—	192, 193
Hydroxychloroquine†	None	252, 253
Ibuprofen	None	254, 255
Indomethacin	Seizure (1 case)	256–258
Iodides	May affect thyroid activity; see iodine	259
Iodine	Goiter	259
Iodine (povidone-iodine, eg, in a vaginal douche)	Elevated iodine levels in breast milk, odor of iodine on infant's skin	259
Iohexol	None	97
Iopanoic acid	None	260
Isoniazid	None; acetyl (hepatotoxic) metabolite secreted but no hepatotoxicity reported in infants	214, 261
Interferon-α	—	262
Ivermectin	None	263, 264
K₁ (vitamin)	None	265, 266
Kanamycin	None	214
Ketoconazole	None	267
Ketorolac	—	268
Labetalol	None	269, 270
Levonorgestrel	—	271–274
Levothyroxine	None	275
Lidocaine	None	276
Loperamide	—	277
Loratadine	None	278
Magnesium sulfate	None	279
Medroxyprogesterone	None	201, 280
Mefenamic acid	None	281
Meperidine	None	61, 282
Methadone	None	283–287
Methimazole (active metabolite of carbimazole)	None	288, 289
Methohexital	None	61
Methyldopa	None	290
Methyprylon	Drowsiness	291
Metoprolol†	None	120
Metrizamide	None	292
Metrizoate	None	97
Mexiletine	None	293, 294
Minoxidil	None	295
Morphine	None; infant may have measurable blood concentration	282, 296–298
Moxalactam	None	299
Nadolol†	None	300
Nalidixic acid	Hemolysis in infant with glucose-6-phosphate dehydrogenase (G-6-PD) deficiency	301
Naproxen	—	302
Nefopam	None	303
Nifedipine	—	304
Nitrofurantoin	Hemolysis in infant with G-6-PD deficiency	305
Norethynodrel	None	306
Norsteroids	None	307
Noscapine	None	308
Ofloxacin	None	198
Oxprenolol	None	309, 310
Phenylbutazone	None	311
Phenytoin	Methemoglobinemia (1 case)	138, 176, 312
Piroxicam	None	313
Prednisolone	None	314, 315
Prednisone	None	316

TABLE 6.   Continued

Drug	Reported Sign or Symptom in Infant or Effect on Lactation	Reference No.
Procainamide	None	317
Progesterone	None	318
Propoxyphene	None	319
Propranolol	None	320–322
Propylthiouracil	None	323
Pseudoephedrine†	None	324
Pyridostigmine	None	325
Pyrimethamine	None	326
Quinidine	None	191, 327
Quinine	None	296
Riboflavin	None	159
Rifampin	None	214
Scopolamine	—	156
Secobarbital	None	328
Senna	None	329
Sotalol	—	237, 330
Spironolactone	None	331
Streptomycin	None	214
Sulbactam	None	332
Sulfapyridine	Caution in infant with jaundice or G-6-PD deficiency and ill, stressed, or premature infant; appears in infant's milk	333, 334
Sulfisoxazole	Caution in infant with jaundice or G-6-PD deficiency and ill, stressed, or premature infant; appears in infant's milk	335
Sumatriptan	None	336
Suprofen	None	337
Terbutaline	None	338
Terfenadine	None	235
Tetracycline	None; negligible absorption by infant	339, 340
Theophylline	Irritability	169, 341
Thiopental	None	139, 342
Thiouracil	None mentioned; drug not used in United States	343
Ticarcillin	None	344
Timolol	None	310
Tolbutamide	Possible jaundice	345
Tolmetin	None	346
Trimethoprim/sulfamethoxazole	None	347, 348
Triprolidine	None	324
Valproic acid	None	176, 349, 350
Verapamil	None	351
Warfarin	None	352
Zolpidem	None	353

* Drugs listed have been reported in the literature as having the effects listed or no effect. The word "none" means that no observable change was seen in the nursing infant while the mother was ingesting the compound. Dashes indicate no mention of clinical effect on the infant. It is emphasized that many of the literature citations concern single case reports or small series of infants.
† Drug is concentrated in human milk.

TABLE 7.   Food and Environmental Agents: Effects on Breastfeeding

Agent	Reported Sign or Symptom in Infant or Effect on Lactation	Reference No.
Aflatoxin	None	354–356
Aspartame	Caution if mother or infant has phenylketonuria	357
Bromide (photographic laboratory)	Potential absorption and bromide transfer into milk; see Table 6	358
Cadmium	None reported	359
Chlordane	None reported	360
Chocolate (theobromine)	Irritability or increased bowel activity if excess amounts (≥16 oz/d) consumed by mother	169, 361
DDT, benzene hexachlorides, dieldrin, aldrin, hepatachlorepoxide	None	362–370
Fava beans	Hemolysis in patient with G-6-PD deficiency	371
Fluorides	None	372, 373
Hexachlorobenzene	Skin rash, diarrhea, vomiting, dark urine, neurotoxicity, death	374, 375
Hexachlorophene	None; possible contamination of milk from nipple washing	376
Lead	Possible neurotoxicity	377–380
Mercury, methylmercury	May affect neurodevelopment	381–383
Methylmethacrylate	None	384
Monosodium glutamate	None	385
Polychlorinated biphenyls and polybrominated biphenyls	Lack of endurance, hypotonia, sullen, expressionless facies	386–390
Silicone	Esophageal dysmotility	17–22
Tetrachloroethylene cleaning fluid (perchloroethylene)	Obstructive jaundice, dark urine	391
Vegetarian diet	Signs of B_{12} deficiency	392

ACKNOWLEDGMENT

The Committee on Drugs would like to thank Linda Watson for ⋯er work in reference identification, document retrieval, and ⋯anuscript preparation.

REFERENCES

1. American Academy of Pediatrics, Committee on Drugs. The transfer of drugs and other chemicals into human breast milk. *Pediatrics.* 1983;72: 375–383

2. American Academy of Pediatrics, Committee on Drugs. Transfer of drugs and other chemicals into human milk. *Pediatrics.* 1989;84: 924–936

3. American Academy of Pediatrics, Committee on Drugs. Transfer of drugs and other chemicals into human milk. *Pediatrics.* 1994;93:137–150

4. Bisdom W. Alcohol and nicotine poisoning in nurslings. *JAMA.* 1937; 109:178

5. Ferguson BB, Wilson DJ, Schaffner W. Determination of nicotine concentrations in human milk. *Am J Dis Child.* 1976;130:837–839

6. Luck W, Nau H. Nicotine and cotinine concentrations in the milk of smoking mothers: influence of cigarette consumption and diurnal variation. *Eur J Pediatr.* 1987;146:21–26

7. Luck W, Nau H. Nicotine and cotinine concentrations in serum and milk of nursing mothers. *Br J Clin Pharmacol.* 1984;18:9–15

8. Luck W, Nau H. Nicotine and cotinine concentrations in serum and urine of infants exposed via passive smoking or milk from smoking mothers. *J Pediatr.* 1985;107:816–820

9. Labrecque M, Marcoux S, Weber JP, Fabia J, Ferron L. Feeding and urine cotinine values in babies whose mothers smoke. *Pediatrics.* 1989; 83:93–97

10. Schwartz-Bickenbach D, Schulte-Hobein B, Abt S, Plum C, Nau H. Smoking and passive smoking during pregnancy and early infancy: effects on birth weight, lactation period, and cotinine concentrations in mother's milk and infant's urine. *Toxicol Lett.* 1987;35:73–81

11. Schulte-Hobein B, Schwartz-Bickenbach D, Abt S, Plum C, Nau H. Cigarette smoke exposure and development of infants throughout the first year of life: influence of passive smoking and nursing on cotinine levels in breast milk and infant's urine. *Acta Paediatr.* 1992;81:550–557

12. Hopkinson JM, Schanler RJ, Fraley JK, Garza C. Milk production by mothers of premature infants: influence of cigarette smoking. *Pediatrics.* 1992;90:934–938

13. Little RE, Lambert MD III, Worthington-Roberts B, Ervin CH. Maternal smoking during lactation: relation to infant size at one year of age. *Am J Epidemiol.* 1994;140:544–554

14. Boshuizen HC, Verkerk PH, Reerink JD, Herngreen WP, Zaadstra BM, Verloove-Vanhorick SP. Maternal smoking during lactation: relation to growth during the first year of life in a Dutch birth cohort. *Am J Epidemiol.* 1998;147:117–126

15. Steldinger R, Luck W, Nau H. Half lives of nicotine in milk of smoking mothers: implications for nursing. *J Perinat Med.* 1988;16:261–262

16. Woodward A, Douglas RM, Graham NM, Miles H. Acute respiratory illness in Adelaide children: breast feeding modifies the effect of passive smoking. *J Epidemiol Community Health.* 1990;44:224–230

17. Levine JJ, Ilowite NT. Sclerodermalike esophageal disease in children breast-fed by mothers with silicone breast implants. *JAMA.* 1994;271: 213–216

18. Levine JJ, Trachtman H, Gold DM, Pettei MJ. Esophageal dysmotility in children breast-fed by mothers with silicone breast implants: long-term follow-up and response to treatment. *Dig Dis Sci.* 1996;41: 1600–1603

19. LeVier RR, Harrison MC, Cook RR, Lane TH. What is silicone? *Plast Reconstr Surg.* 1993;92:163–167

20. Berlin CM Jr. Silicone breast implants and breast-feeding. *Pediatrics.* 1994;94:547–549

21. Kjoller K, Mclaughlin JK, Friis S, et al. Health outcomes in offspring of mothers with breast implants. *Pediatrics.* 1998;102:1112–1115

22. Semple JL, Lugowski SJ, Baines CJ, Smith DC, McHugh A. Breast milk contamination and silicone implants: preliminary results using silicon as a proxy measurement for silicone. *Plast Reconstr Surg.* 1998;102: 528–533

23. *Physicians' Desk Reference.* Montvale, NJ: Medical Economics Company; 2001

24. US Pharmacopeia. *USP DI 2001: Information for the Health Care Professional, Volume I.* Hutchinson TA, ed. Englewood, CO: Micromedex; 2001

25. US Pharmacopeia. *USP Dictionary of USAN and International Drug Names.* Rockville, MD: US Pharmacopeia; 2000

26. Wiernik PH, Duncan JH. Cyclophosphamide in human milk. *Lancet.* 1971;1:912

27. Amato D, Niblett JS. Neutropenia from cyclophosphamide in breast milk. *Med J Aust.* 1977;1:383–384

28. Flechner SM, Katz AR, Rogers AJ, Van Buren C, Kahan BD. The presence of cyclosporine in body tissue and fluids during pregnancy. *Am J Kidney Dis.* 1985;5:60–63

29. Nyberg G, Haljamae U, Frisenette-Fich C, Wennergren M, Kjellmer I. Breast-feeding during treatment with cyclosporine. *Transplantation.* 1998;65:253–255

30. Egan PC, Costanza ME, Dodion P, Egorin MJ, Bachur NR. Doxorubicin and cisplatin excretion into human milk. *Cancer Treat Rep.* 1985;69: 1387–1389

31. Johns DG, Rutherford LD, Leighton PC, Vogel CL. Secretion of methotrexate into human milk. *Am J Obstet Gynecol.* 1972;112:978–980

32. Steiner E, Villen T, Hallberg M, Rane A. Amphetamine secretion in breast milk. *Eur J Clin Pharmacol.* 1984;27:123–124

33. Chasnoff IJ, Lewis DE, Squires L. Cocaine intoxication in a breast-fed infant. *Pediatrics.* 1987;80:836–838

34. Cobrinik RW, Hood RT Jr, Chusid E. The effect of maternal narcotic addiction on the newborn infant: review of literature and report of 22 cases. *Pediatrics.* 1959;24:288–304

35. Perez-Reyes M, Wall ME. Presence of delta9-tetrahydrocannabinol in human milk. *N Engl J Med.* 1982;307:819–820

36. Kaufman KR, Petrucha RA, Pitts FN Jr, Weekes ME. PCP in amniotic fluid and breast milk: case report. *J Clin Psychiatry.* 1983;44:269–270

37. McArdle HJ, Danks DM. Secretion of copper 64 into breast milk following intravenous injection in a human subject. *J Trace Elem Exp Med.* 1991;4:81–84

38. Tobin RE, Schneider PB. Uptake of 67Ga in the lactating breast and its persistence in milk: case report. *J Nucl Med.* 1976;17:1055–1056

39. Butt D, Szaz KF. Indium-111 radioactivity in breast milk. *Br J Radiol.* 1986;59:80

40. Hedrick WR, Di Simone RN, Keen RL. Radiation dosimetry from breast milk excretion of radioiodine and pertechnetate. *J Nucl Med.* 1986;27:1569–1571

41. Rose MR, Prescott MC, Herman KJ. Excretion of iodine-123-hippuran, technetium-99 m-red blood cells, and technetium-99 m-macroaggregated albumin into breast milk. *J Nucl Med.* 1990;31:978–984

42. Palmer KE. Excretion of 125I in breast milk following administration of labelled fibrinogen. *Br J Radiol.* 1979;52:672–673

43. Honour AJ, Myant NB, Rowlands EN. Secretion of radioiodine in digestive juices and milk in man. *Clin Sci.* 1952;11:447–462

44. Karjalainen P, Penttila IM, Pystynen P. The amount and form of radioactivity in human milk after lung scanning, renography and placental localization by 131 I labelled tracers. *Acta Obstet Gynecol Scand.* 1971;50:357–361

45. Bland EP, Docker MF, Crawford JS, Farr RF. Radioactive iodine uptake by thyroid of breast-fed infants after maternal blood-volume measurements. *Lancet.* 1969;2:1039–1041

46. Nurnberger CE, Lipscomb A. Transmission of radioiodine (I131) to infants through human maternal milk. *JAMA.* 1952;150:1398–1400

47. Robinson PS, Barker P, Campbell A, Henson P, Surveyor I, Young PR. Iodine-131 in breast milk following therapy for thyroid carcinoma. *J Nucl Med.* 1994;35:1797–1801

48. Rubow S, Klopper J, Wasserman H, Baard B, van Niekerk M. The excretion of radiopharmaceuticals in human breast milk: additional data and dosimetry. *Eur J Nucl Med.* 1994;21:144–153

49. Pommerenke WT, Hahn PF. Secretion of radio-active sodium in human milk. *Proc Soc Exp Biol Med.* 1943;52:223–224

50. O'Connell ME, Sutton H. Excretion of radioactivity in breast milk following 99Tcm-Sn polyphosphate. *Br J Radiol.* 1976;49:377–379

51. Berke RA, Hoops EC, Kereiakes JC, Saenger EL. Radiation dose to breast-feeding. *J Nucl Med.* 1973;14:51–52

52. Vagenakis AG, Abreau CM, Braverman LE. Duration of radioactivity in the milk of a nursing mother following 99 mTc administration. *J Nucl Med.* 1971;12:188

53. Wyburn JR. Human breast milk excretion of radionuclides following administration of radiopharmaceuticals. *J Nucl Med.* 1973;14:115–117

54. Pittard WB III, Merkatz R, Fletcher BD. Radioactive excretion in human milk following administration of technetium Tc 99 m macroaggregated albumin. *Pediatrics.* 1982;70:231–234

55. Maisels MJ, Gilcher RO. Excretion of technetium in human milk. *Pediatrics.* 1983;71:841–842

56. American Academy of Pediatrics, Committee on Drugs. Psychotropic drugs in pregnancy and lactation. *Pediatrics.* 1982;69:241–244

57. Oo CY, Kuhn RJ, Desai N, Wright CE, McNamara PJ. Pharmacokinet-

ics in lactating women: prediction of alprazolam transfer into milk. *Br J Clin Pharmacol.* 1995;40:231–236

58. Patrick MJ, Tilstone WJH, Reavey P. Diazepam and breast-feeding. *Lancet.* 1972;1:542–543

59. Cole AP, Hailey DM. Diazepam and active metabolite in breast milk and their transfer to the neonate. *Arch Dis Child.* 1975;50:741–742

60. Dusci LJ, Good SM, Hall RW, Ilett KF. Excretion of diazepam and its metabolites in human milk during withdrawal from combination high dose diazepam and oxazepam. *Br J Clin Pharmacol.* 1990;29:123–126

61. Borgatta L, Jenny RW, Gruss L, Ong C, Barad D. Clinical significance of methohexital, meperidine, and diazepam in breast milk. *J Clin Pharmacol.* 1997;37:186–192

62. Dencker SJ, Johansson G, Milsom I. Quantification of naturally occurring benzodiazepine-like substances in human breast milk. *Psychopharmacology (Berl).* 1992;107:69–72

63. Summerfield RJ, Nielson MS. Excretion of lorazepam into breast milk. *Br J Anaesth.* 1985;57:1042–1043

64. Matheson I, Lunde PK, Bredesen JE. Midazolam and nitrazepam in the maternity ward: milk concentrations and clinical effects. *Br J Clin Pharmacol.* 1990;30:787–793

65. Olesen OV, Bartels U, Poulsen JH. Perphenazine in breast milk and serum. *Am J Psychiatry.* 1990;147:1378–1379

66. Brodie RR, Chasseaud LF, Taylor T. Concentrations of N-descyclopropylmethylprazepam in whole-blood, plasma, and milk after administration of prazepam to humans. *Biopharm Drug Dispos.* 1981;2:59–68

67. Hilbert JM, Gural RP, Symchowicz S, Zampaglione N. Excretion of quazepam into human breast milk. *J Clin Pharmacol.* 1984;24:457–462

68. Lebedevs TH, Wojnar-Horton RE, Yapp P, et al. Excretion of temazepam in breast milk. *Br J Clin Pharmacol.* 1992;33:204–206

69. Bader TF, Newman K. Amitriptyline in human breast milk and the nursing infant's serum. *Am J Psychiatry.* 1980;137:855–856

70. Erickson SH, Smith GH, Heidrich F. Tricyclics and breast feeding. *Am J Psychiatry.* 1979;136:1483–1484

71. Gelenberg AJ. Single case stuy. Amoxapine, a new antidepressant, appears in human milk. *J Nerv Ment Dis.* 1979;167:635–636

72. Briggs GG, Samson JH, Ambrose PJ, Schroeder DH. Excretion of bupropion in breast milk. *Ann Pharmacother.* 1993;27:431–433

73. Schimmell MS, Katz EZ, Shaag Y, Pastuszak A, Koren G. Toxic neonatal effects following maternal clomipramine therapy. *Clin Toxicol.* 1991;29:479–484

74. Sovner R, Orsulak PJ. Excretion of imipramine and desipramine in human breast milk. *Am J Psychiatry.* 1979;136:451–452

75. Stancer HC, Reed KL. Desipramine and 2-hydroxydesipramine in human breast milk and the nursery infant's serum. *Am J Psychiatry.* 1986;143:1597–1600

76. Rees JA, Glass RC, Sporne GA. Serum and breast-milk concentrations of dothiepin [letter]. *Practitioner.* 1976;217:686

77. Ilett KF, Lebedevs TH, Wojnar-Horton RE, et al. The excretion of dothiepin and its primary metabolites in breast milk. *Br J Clin Pharmacol.* 1992;33:635–639

78. Kemp J, Ilett KF, Booth J, Hackett LP. Excretion of doxepin and N-desmethyldoxepin in human milk. *Br J Clin Pharmacol.* 1985;20:497–499

79. Burch KJ, Wells BG. Fluoxetine/norfluoxetine concentrations in human milk. *Pediatrics.* 1992;89:676–677

80. Lester BM, Cucca J, Andreozzi L, Flanagan P, Oh W. Possible association between fluoxetine hydrochloride and colic in an infant. *J Am Acad Child Adolesc Psychiatry.* 1993;32:1253–1255

81. Burch KJ, Wells BG. Fluoxetine/norfluoxetine concentrations in human milk. *Pediatrics.* 1992;89:676–677

82. Taddio A, Ito S, Koren G. Excretion of fluoxetine and its metabolite, norfluoxetine, in human breast milk. *J Clin Pharmacol.* 1996;36:42–47

83. Brent NB, Wisner KL. Fluoxetine and carbamazepine concentrations in a nursing mother/infant pair. *Clin Pediatr (Phila).* 1998;37:41–44

84. Isenberg KE. Excretion of fluoxetine in human breast milk. *J Clin Psychiatry.* 1990;51:169

85. Nulman I, Koren G. The safety of fluoxetine during pregnancy and lactation. *Teratology.* 1996;53:304–308

86. Yoshida K, Smith B, Craggs M, Kumar RC. Fluoxetine in breast-milk and developmental outcome of breast-fed infants. *Br J Psychiatry.* 1998;172:175–178

87. Chambers CD, Anderson PO, Thomas RG, et al. Weight gain in infants breastfed by mothers who take fluoxetine. *Pediatrics.* 1999;104(5). Available at: http://www.pediatrics.org/cgi/content/full/104/5/e61. Accessed December 20, 2000

88. Wright S, Dawling S, Ashford JJ. Excretion of fluvoxamine in breast milk. *Br J Clin Pharmacol.* 1991;31:209

89. Wisner KL, Perel JM. Serum nortriptyline levels in nursing mothers and their infants. *Am J Psychiatry.* 1991;148:1234–1236

90. Wisner KL, Perel JM. Nortriptyline treatment of breast-feeding women. *Am J Psychiatry.* 1996;153:295

91. Stowe ZN, Cohen LS, Hostetter A, Ritchie JC, Owens MJ, Nemeroff CB. Paroxetine in human breast milk and nursing infants. *Am J Psychiatry* 2000;157:185–189

92. Epperson CN, Anderson GM, McDougle CJ. Sertraline and breast-feeding. *N Engl J Med.* 1997;336:1189–1190

93. Stowe ZN, Owens MJ, Landry JC, et al. Sertraline and desmethylsertraline in human breast milk and nursing infants. *Am J Psychiatry* 1997;154:1255–1260

94. Verbeeck RK, Ross SG, McKenna EA. Excretion of trazodone in breast milk. *Br J Clin Pharmacol.* 1986;22:367–370

95. Polishuk WZ, Kulcsar SA. Effects of chlorpromazine on pituitary function. *J Clin Endocrinol Metab.* 1956;16:292

96. Wiles DH, Orr MW, Kolakowska T. Chlorpromazine levels in plasma and milk of nursing mothers. *Br J Clin Pharmacol.* 1978;5:272–273

97. Nielsen ST, Matheson I, Rasmussen JN, Skinnemoen K, Andrew E, Hafsahl G. Excretion of iohexol and metrizoate in human breast milk. *Acta Radiol.* 1987;28:523–526

98. Ohkubo T, Shimoyama R, Sugawara K. Determination of chlorpromazine in human breast milk and serum by high-performance liquid chromatography. *J Chromatogr.* 1993;614:328–332

99. Matheson I, Evang A, Overo KF, Syversen G. Presence of chlorprothixene and its metabolites in breast milk. *Eur J Clin Pharmacol.* 1984 27:611–613

100. Barnas C, Bergant A, Hummer M, Saria A, Fleischhacker WW. Clozapine concentrations in maternal and fetal plasma, amniotic fluid, and breast milk. *Am J Psychiatry.* 1994;151:945

101. Stewart RB, Karas B, Springer PK. Haloperidol excretion in human milk. *Am J Psychiatry.* 1980;137:849–850

102. Whalley LJ, Blain PG, Prime JK. Haloperidol secreted in breast milk. *Br Med J (Clin Res Ed).* 1981;282:1746–1747

103. Ohkubo T, Shimoyama R, Sugawara K. Measurement of haloperidol in human breast milk by high-performance liquid chromatography. *J Pharm Sci.* 1992;81:947–949

104. Yoshida K, Smith B, Craggs M, Kumar RC. Neuroleptic drugs in breast milk: a study of pharmacokinetics and of possible adverse effects in breast-fed infants. *Psychol Med.* 1998;28:81–91

105. Ananth J. Side effects in the neonate from psychotropic agents excreted through breast-feeding. *Am J Psychiatry.* 1978;135:801–805

106. Plomp TA, Vulsma T, de Vijlder JJ. Use of amiodarone during pregnancy. *Eur J Obstet Gynecol Reprod Biol.* 1992;43:201–207

107. Havelka J, Hejzlar M, Popov V, Viktorinova D, Prochazka J. Excretion of chloramphenicol in human milk. *Chemotherapy.* 1968;13:204–211

108. Smadel JE, Woodward TE, Ley HL Jr, et al. Chloramphenicol (Chloromycetin) in the treatment of tsutsugamushi disease (scrub typhus). *J Clin Invest.* 1949;28:1196

109. Venkatesan K, Mathur A, Girdhar A, Girdhar BK. Excretion of clofazimine in human milk in leprosy patients. *Lepr Rev.* 1997;68:242–246

110. Tomson T, Ohman I, Vitols S. Lamotrigine in pregnancy and lactation a case report. *Epilepsia.* 1997;38:1039–1041

111. Gupta AP, Gupta PK. Metoclopramide as a lactogogue. *Clin Pediatr (Phila).* 1985;24:269–272

112. Kauppila A, Arvela P, Koivisto M, Kivinen S, Ylikorkala O, Pelkonen O. Metoclopramide and breast feeding: transfer into milk and the newborn. *Eur J Clin Pharmacol.* 1983;25:819–823

113. Erickson SH, Oppenheim GL, Smith GH. Metronidazole in breast milk. *Obstet Gynecol.* 1981;57:48–50

114. Heisterberg L, Branebjerg PE. Blood and milk concentrations of metronidazole in mothers and infants. *J Perinat Med.* 1983;11:114–120

115. Evaldson GR, Lindgren S, Nord CE, Rane AT. Tinidazole milk excretion and pharmacokinetics in lactating women. *Br J Clin Pharmacol.* 1985;19:503–507

116. Boutroy MJ, Bianchetti G, Dubruc C, Vert P, Morselli PL. To nurse when receiving acebutolol: is it dangerous for the neonate? *Eur J Clin Pharmacol.* 1986;30:737–739

117. Nelis GF. Diarrhoea due to 5-aminosalicylic acid in breast milk. *Lancet* 1989;1:383

118. Jenss H, Weber P, Hartmann F. 5-Aminosalicylic acid its metabolite in breast milk during lactation [letter]. *Am J Gastroenterol.* 1990;85:331

119. Klotz U, Harings-Kaim A. Negligible excretion of 5-aminosalicylic acid in breast milk. *Lancet.* 1993;342:618–619

120. Liedholm H, Melander A, Bitzen PO, et al. Accumulation of atenolol and metoprolol in human breast milk. *Eur J Clin Pharmacol.* 1981;20: 229–231

121. Schimmel MS, Eidelman AI, Wilschanski MA, Shaw D Jr, Ogilvie RJ,

Koren G. Toxic effects of atenolol consumed during breast feeding. *J Pediatr.* 1989;114:476–478

2. Thorley KJ, McAinsh J. Levels of the beta-blockers atenolol and propanolol in the breast milk of women treated for hypertension in pregnancy. *Biopharm Drug Dispos.* 1983;4:299–301

3. Kulas J, Lunell NO, Rosing U, Steen B, Rane A. Atenolol and metoprolol. A comparison of their excretion into human breast milk. *Acta Obstet Gynecol Scand Suppl.* 1984;118:65–69

4. White WB, Andreoli JW, Wong SH, Cohn RD. Atenolol in human plasma and breast milk. *Obstet Gynecol.* 1984;63:42S–44S

5. Kulski JK, Hartmann PE, Martin JD, Smith M. Effects of bromocriptine mesylate on the composition of the mammary secretion in non-breast-feeding women. *Obstet Gynecol.* 1978;52:38–42

6. Katz M, Kroll D, Pak I, Osimoni A, Hirsch M. Puerperal hypertension, stroke, and seizures after suppression of lactation with bromocriptine. *Obstet Gynecol.* 1985;66:822–824

7. Clark JH, Wilson WG. A 16-day-old breast-fed infant with metabolic acidosis caused by salicylate. *Clin Pediatr (Phila).* 1981;20:53–54

8. Levy G. Salicylate pharmacokinetics in the human neonate. In: Marselli PL, ed. *Basic and Therapeutic Aspects of Perinatal Pharmacology.* New York, NY: Raven Press; 1975:319

9. Jamali F, Keshavarz E. Salicylate excretion in breast milk. *Int J Pharm.* 1981;8:285–290

10. Kok TH, Taitz LS, Bennett MJ, Holt DW. Drowsiness due to clemastine transmitted in breast milk. *Lancet.* 1982;1:914–915

1. Fomina PI. Untersuchungen uber den Ubergang des aktiven agens des Mutterkorns in die milch stillender Mutter. *Arch Gynecol.* 1934;157:275

2. Schou M, Amdisen A. Lithium and pregnancy. 3. Lithium ingestion by children breast-fed by women on lithium treatment. *Br Med J.* 1973;2:138

3. Tunnessen WW Jr, Hertz CG. Toxic effects of lithium in newborn infants: a commentary. *J Pediatr.* 1972;81:804–807

4. Sykes PA, Quarrie J, Alexander FW. Lithium carbonate and breast-feeding. *Br Med J.* 1976;2:1299

5. Eckstein HB, Jack B. Breast-feeding and anticoagulant therapy. *Lancet.* 1970;1:672–673

6. Nau H, Rating D, Hauser I, Jager E, Koch S, Helge H. Placental transfer and pharmacokinetics of primidone and its metabolites phenobarbital, PEMA and hydroxyphenobarbital in neonates and infants of epileptic mothers. *Eur J Clin Pharmacol.* 1980;18:31–42

7. Kuhnz W, Koch S, Helge H, Nau H. Primidone and phenobarbital during lactation period in epileptic women: total and free drug serum levels in the nursed infants and their effects on neonatal behavior. *Dev Pharmacol Ther.* 1988;11:147–154

8. Finch E, Lorber J. Methaemoglobinaemia in newborn probably due to phenytoin excreted in human milk. *J Obstet Gynaecol Br Emp.* 1954;61:833–834

9. Tyson RM, Shrader EA, Perlman HH. Drugs transmitted through breast milk. II. Barbiturates. *J Pediatr.* 1938;13:86–90

10. Knott C, Reynolds F, Clayden G. Infantile spasms on weaning from breast milk containing anticonvulsants. *Lancet.* 1987;2:272–273

1. Branski D, Kerem E, Gross-Kieselstein E, Hurvitz H, Litt R, Abrahamov A. Bloody diarrhea—a possible complication of sulfasalazine transferred through human breast milk. *J Pediatr Gastroenterol Nutr.* 1986;5:316–317

2. Berlin CM Jr, Yaffe SJ, Ragni M. Disposition of acetaminophen in milk, saliva, and plasma of lactating women. *Pediatr Pharmacol (New York).* 1980;1:135–141

3. Bitzen PO, Gustafsson B, Jostell KG, Melander A, Wahlin-Boll E. Excretion of paracetamol in human breast milk. *Eur J Clin Pharmacol.* 1981;20:123–125

4. Findlay JW, DeAngelis RL, Kearney MF, Welch RM, Findlay JM. Analgesic drugs in breast milk and plasma. *Clin Pharmacol Ther.* 1981; 29:625–633

5. Soderman P, Hartvig P, Fagerlund C. Acetazolamide excretion into human breast milk. *Br J Clin Pharmacol.* 1984;17:599–600

6. Rollman O, Pihl-Lundin I. Acitretin excretion into human breast milk. *Acta Derm Venereol.* 1990;70:487–490

7. Lau RJ, Emery MG, Galinsky RE. Unexpected accumulation of acyclovir in breast milk with estimation of infant exposure. *Obstet Gynecol.* 1987;69:468–471

8. Meyer LJ, de Miranda P, Sheth N, Spruance S. Acyclovir in human breast milk. *Am J Obstet Gynecol.* 1988;158:586–588

9. Binkiewicz A, Robinson MJ, Senior B. Pseudo-Cushing syndrome caused by alcohol in breast milk. *J Pediatr.* 1978;93:965–967

10. Cobo E. Effect of different doses of ethanol on the milk-ejecting reflex in lactating women. *Am J Obstet Gynecol.* 1973;115:817–821

1. Kesaniemi YA. Ethanol and acetaldehyde in the milk and peripheral

blood of lactating women after ethanol administration. *J Obstet Gynaecol Br Commonw.* 1974;81:84–86

152. Little RE, Anderson KW, Ervin CH, Worthington-Roberts B, Clarren SK. Maternal alcohol use during breast-feeding and infant mental and motor development at one year. *N Engl J Med.* 1989;321:425–430

153. Kamilli I, Gresser U. Allopurinol and oxypurinol in human breast milk. *Clin Investig.* 1993;71:161–164

154. Kafetzis DA, Siafas CA, Georgakopoulos PA, Papadatos CJ. Passage of cephalosporins and amoxicillin into the breast milk. *Acta Paediatr Scand.* 1981;70:285–288

155. Berman JD, Melby PC, Neva FA. Concentration of Pentostam in human breast milk. *Trans R Soc Trop Med Hyg.* 1989;83:784–785

156. Sapeika N. Excretion of drugs in human milk: review. *J Obstet Gynaecol Br Emp.* 1947;54:426–431

157. Bald R, Bernbeck-Betthauser EM, Spahn H, Mutschler E. Excretion of azpropazone in human breast milk. *Eur J Clin Pharmacol.* 1990;39:271–273

158. Fleiss PM, Richwald GA, Gordon J, Stern M, Frantz M, Devlin RG. Aztreonam in human serum and breast milk. *Br J Clin Pharmacol.* 1985;19:509–511

159. Nail PA, Thomas MR, Eakin R. The effect of thiamin and riboflavin supplementation on the level of those vitamins in human breast milk and urine. *Am J Clin Nutr.* 1980;33:198–204

160. Roepke JL, Kirksey A. Vitamin B6 nutriture during pregnancy lactation. I. Vitamin B6 intake, levels of the vitamin in biological fluids, condition of the infant at birth. *Am J Clin Nutr.* 1979;32:2249–2256

161. West KD, Kirksey A. Influence of vitamin B6 intake on the content of the vitamin in human milk. *Am J Clin Nutr.* 1976;29:961–969

162. Greentree LB. Dangers of vitamin B6 in nursing mothers. *N Engl J Med.* 1979;300:141–142

163. Samson RR, McClelland DB. Vitamin B12 in human colostrum and milk. Quantitation of the vitamin and its binder and the uptake of bound vitamin B12 by intestinal bacteria. *Acta Paediatr Scand.* 1980;69:93–99

164. Eriksson G, Swahn CG. Concentrations of baclofen in serum and breast milk from a lactating woman. *Scand J Clin Lab Invest.* 1981;41:185–187

165. Healy M. Suppressing lactaton with oral diuretics. *Lancet.* 1961;1:1353

166. Brambel CE, Hunter RE. Effect of dicumarol on the nursing infant. *Am J Obstet Gynecol.* 1950;59:1153

167. Tyson RM, Shrader EA, Perlman HH. Drugs transmitted through breast milk. III. Bromides. *J Pediatr.* 1938;13:91–93

168. Pittman KA, Smyth RD, Losada M, Zighelboim I, Maduska AL, Sunshine A. Human perinatal distribution of butorphanol. *Am J Obstet Gynecol.* 1980;138:797–800

169. Berlin CM Jr. Excretion of the methylxanthines in human milk. *Semin Perinatol.* 1981;5:389–394

170. Tyrala EE, Dodson WE. Caffeine secretion into breast milk. *Arch Dis Child.* 1979;54:787–800

171. Hildebrandt R, Gundert-Remy U. Lack of pharmacological active saliva levels of caffeine in breast-fed infants. *Pediatr Pharmacol (New York).* 1983;3:237–244

172. Berlin CM Jr, Denson HM, Daniel CH, Ward RM. Disposition of dietary caffeine in milk, saliva, and plasma of lactating women. *Pediatrics.* 1984;73:59–63

173. Ryu JE. Caffeine in human milk and in serum of breast-fed infants. *Dev Pharmacol Ther.* 1985;8:329–337

174. Ryu JE. Effect of maternal caffeine consumption on heart rate and sleep time of breast-fed infants. *Dev Pharmacol Ther.* 1985;8:355–363

175. Devlin RG, Fleiss PM. Captopril in human blood and breast milk. *J Clin Pharmacol.* 1981;21:110–113

176. Nau H, Kuhnz W, Egger JH, Rating D, Helge H. Anticonvulsants during pregnancy and lactation. Transplacental, maternal and neonatal pharmacokinetics. *Clin Pharmacokinet.* 1982;7:508–543

177. Pynnonen S, Kanto J, Sillanpaa M, Erkkola R. Carbamazepine: placental transport, tissue concentrations in foetus and newborn, and level in milk. *Acta Pharmacol Toxicol (Copenh).* 1977;41:244–253

178. Silcox J, Schulz P, Horbay GL, Wassenaar W. Transfer of carbetocin into human breast milk. *Obstet Gynecol.* 1993;82:456–459

179. Cooper DS. Antithyroid drugs: to breast-feed or not to breast-feed. *Am J Obstet Gynecol.* 1987;157:234–235

180. Lamberg BA, Ikonen E, Osterlund K, et al. Antithyroid treatment of maternal hyperthyroidism during lactation. *Clin Endocrinol (Oxf).* 1984; 21:81–87

181. Tyson RM, Shrader EA, Perlman HH. Drugs transmitted through breast milk. I. Laxatives. *J Pediatr.* 1937;11:824–832

182. Yoshioka H, Cho K, Takimoto M, Maruyama S, Shimizu T. Transfer of cefazolin into human milk. *J Pediatr.* 1979;94:151–152

183. Dresse A, Lambotte R, Dubois M, Delapierre D, Kramp R. Transmam-

245

mary passage of cefoxitin: additional results. *J Clin Pharmacol.* 1983;23: 438–440

184. Shyu WC, Shah VR, Campbell DA, et al. Excretion of cefprozil into human breast milk. *Antimicrob Agents Chemother.* 1992;36:938–941

185. Blanco JD, Jorgensen JH, Castaneda YS, Crawford SA. Ceftazidime levels in human breast milk. *Antimicrob Agents Chemother.* 1983;23: 479–480

186. Bourget P, Quinquis-Desmaris V, Fernandez H. Ceftriaxone distribution and protein binding between maternal blood and milk postpartum. *Ann Pharmacother.* 1993;27:294–297

187. Lacey JH. Dichloralphenazone and breast milk. *Br Med J.* 1971;4:684

188. Reed CB. A study of the conditions that require the removal of the child from the breast. *Surg Gynecol Obstet.* 1908;6:514

189. Soares R, Paulini E, Pereira JP. Da concentracao e eliminacao da cloroquina atraves da circulacao placentaria e do leite materno, de pacientes sob regime do sal loroquinado. *Rev Bras Malariol Doencas Trop.* 1957;9:19

190. Ogunbona FA, Onyeji CO, Bolaji OO, Torimiro SE. Excretion of chloroquine and desethylchloroquine in human milk. *Br J Clin Pharmacol.* 1987;23:473–476

191. Edstein MD, Veenendaal JR, Newman K, Hyslop R. Excretion of chloroquine, dapsone and pyrimethamine in human milk. *Br J Clin Pharmacol.* 1986;22:733–735

192. Werthmann MW Jr, Krees SV. Excretion of chlorothiazide in human breast milk. *J Pediatr.* 1972;81:781–783

193. Miller EM, Cohn RD, Burghart PH. Hydrochlorothiazide disposition in a mother and her breast-fed infant. *J Pediatr.* 1982;101:789–791

194. Mulley BA, Parr GD, Pau WK, Rye RM, Mould JJ, Siddle NC. Placental transfer of chlorthalidone and its elimination in maternal milk. *Eur J Clin Pharmacol.* 1978;13:129–131

195. Somogyi A, Gugler R. Cimetidine excretion into breast milk. *Br J Clin Pharmacol.* 1979;7:627–629

196. Oo CY, Kuhn RJ, Desai N, McNamara PJ. Active transport of cimetidine into human milk. *Clin Pharmacol Ther.* 1995;58:548–555

197. Gardner DK, Gabbe SG, Harter C. Simultaneous concentrations of ciprofloxacin in breast milk and in serum in mother and breast-fed infant. *Clin Pharm.* 1992;11:352–354

198. Giamarellou H, Kolokythas E, Petrikkos G, Gazis J, Aravantinos D, Sfikakis P. Pharmacokinetics of three newer quinolones in pregnant and lactating women. *Am J Med.* 1989;87(suppl):49S–51S

199. Hofmeyr GJ, Sonnendecker EW. Secretion of the gastrokinetic agent cisapride in human milk. *Eur J Clin Pharmacol.* 1986;30:735–736

200. Smith JA, Morgan JR, Rachlis AR, Papsin FR. Clindamycin in human breast milk [letter]. *Can Med Assoc J.* 1975;112:806

201. Zacharias S, Aguilera E, Assenzo JR, Zanartu J. Effects of hormonal and nonhormonal contraceptives on lactation and incidence of pregnancy. *Contraception.* 1986;33:203–213

202. Meny RG, Naumburg EG, Alger LS, Brill-Miller JL, Brown S. Codeine and the breastfed neonate. *J Hum Lact.* 1993;9:237–240

203. Milunsky JM. Breast-feeding during colchicine therapy for familial Mediterranean fever [letter]. *J Pediatr.* 1991;119:164

204. Ben-Chetrit E, Scherrmann J-M, Levy M. Colchicine in breast milk of patients with familial Mediterranean fever. *Arthritis Rheum.* 1996;39: 1213–1217

205. Guillonneau M, Aigrain EJ, Galliot M, Binet MH, Darbois Y. Colchicine is excreted at high concentrations in human breast milk. *Eur J Obstet Gynecol Reprod Biol.* 1995;61:177–178

206. Nilsson S, Mellbin T, Hofvander Y, Sundelin C, Valentin J, Nygren KG. Long-term follow-up of children breast-fed by mothers using oral contraceptives. *Contraception.* 1986;34:443–457

207. Nilsson S, Nygren KG. Transfer of contraceptive steroids to human milk. *Res Reprod.* 1979;11:1–2

208. American Academy of Pediatrics, Committee on Drugs. Breast-feeding and contraception. *Pediatrics.* 1981;68:138–140

209. Barsivala VM, Virkar KD. The effect of oral contraceptives on concentration of various components of human milk. *Contraception.* 1973;7: 307–312

210. Borglin NE, Sandholm LE. Effect of oral contraceptives on lactation. *Fertil Steril.* 1971;22:39–41

211. Curtis EM. Oral-contraceptive feminization of a normal male infant: report of a case. *Obstet Gynecol.* 1964;23:295–296

212. Kora SJ. Effect of oral contraceptives on lactation. *Fertil Steril.* 1969;20: 419–423

213. Toaff R, Ashkenazi H, Schwartz A, Herzberg M. Effects of oestrogen and progestagen on the composition of human breast milk. *J Reprod Fertil.* 1969;19:475–482

214. Snider DE Jr, Powell KE. Should women taking antituberculosis drugs breast-feed? *Arch Intern Med.* 1984;144:589–590

215. Cancela L, Le Boulch N, Miravet L. Relationship between the vitamin D content of maternal milk and the vitamin D status of nursing women and breast-fed infants. *J Endocrinol.* 1986;110:43–50

216. Rothberg AD, Pettifor JM, Cohen DF, Sonnendecker EW, Ross FP. Maternal-infant vitamin D relationships during breast-feeding. *J Pediatr.* 1982;101:500–503

217. Greer FR, Hollis BW, Napoli JL. High concentrations of vitamin D2 in human milk associated with pharmacologic doses of vitamin D2. *J Pediatr.* 1984;105:61–64

218. Greenhalf JO, Leonard HS. Laxatives in the treatment of constipation in pregnant and breast-feeding mothers. *Practitioner.* 1973;210:259–263

219. Dreisbach JA. Sulphone levels in breast milk of mothers on sulphone therapy. *Lepr Rev.* 1952;23:101–106

220. Mortimer EA Jr. Drug toxicity from breast milk [letter]? *Pediatrics* 1977;60:780–781

221. FitzJohn TP, Williams DG, Laker MF, Owen JP. Intravenous urography during lactation. *Br J Radiol.* 1982;55:603–605

222. Loughnan PM. Digoxin excretion in human breast milk. *J Pediatr.* 1978;92:1019–1020

223. Levy M, Granit L, Laufer N. Excretion of drugs in human milk. *N Engl J Med.* 1977;297:789

224. Okada M, Inoue H, Nakamura Y, Kishimoto M, Suzuki T. Excretion of diltiazem in human milk [letter]. *N Engl J Med.* 1985;312:992–993

225. Zylber-Katz E, Linder N, Granit L, Levy M. Excretion of dipyrone metabolites in human breast milk. *Eur J Clin Pharmacol.* 1986;30: 359–361

226. MacKintosh D, Buchanan N. Excretion of disopyramide in human breast milk [letter]. *Br J Clin Pharmacol.* 1985;19:856–857

227. Hoppu K, Neuvonen PJ, Korte T. Disopyramide and breast feeding [letter]. *Br J Clin Pharmacol.* 1986;21:553

228. Hofmeyr GJ, van Idlekinge B. Domperidone and lactation [letter]. *Lancet.* 1983;1:647

229. Jorboe CH, Cook LN, Malesic I, Fleischaker J. Dyphylline elimination kinetics in lactating women: blood to milk transfer. *J Clin Pharmacol.* 1981;21:405–410

230. Redman CW, Kelly JG, Cooper WD. The excretion of enalapril and enalaprilat in human breast milk. *Eur J Clin Pharmacol.* 1990;38:99

231. Matsuda S. Transfer of antibiotics into maternal milk. *Biol Res Pregnancy Perinatol.* 1984;5:57–60

232. Nilsson S, Nygren KG, Johansson ED. Transfer of estradiol to human milk. *Am J Obstet Gynecol.* 1978;132:653–657

233. Koup JR, Rose JQ, Cohen ME. Ethosuximide pharmacokinetics in a pregnant patient and her newborn. *Epilepsia.* 1978;19:535–539

234. Steer PL, Biddle CJ, Marley WS, Lantz RK, Sulik PL. Concentration of fentanyl in colostrum after an analgesic dose. *Can J Anaesth.* 1992;39: 231–235

235. Lucas BD Jr, Purdy CY, Scarim SK, Benjamin S, Abel SR, Hilleman DE. Terfenadine pharmacokinetics in breast milk in lactating women. *Clin Pharmacol Ther.* 1995;57:398–402

236. McQuinn RL, Pisani A, Wafa S, et al. Flecainide excretion in human breast milk. *Clin Pharmacol Ther.* 1990;48:262–267

237. Wagner X, Jouglard J, Moulin M, Miller AM, Petitjean J, Pisapia A. Coadministration of flecainide acetate and sotalol during pregnancy: lack of teratogenic effects, passage across the placenta, and excretion in human breast milk. *Am Heart J.* 1990;119:700–702

238. Dan M, Weidekamm E, Sagiv R, Portmann R, Zakut H. Penetration of fleroxacin into breast milk and pharmacokinetics in lactating women. *Antimicrob Agents Chemother.* 1993;37:293–296

239. Force RW. Fluconazole concentrations in breast milk. *Pediatr Infect Dis J.* 1995;14:235–236

240. Buchanan RA, Eaton CJ, Koeff ST, Kinkel AW. The breast milk excretion of flufenamic acid. *Curr Ther Res Clin Exp.* 1969;11:533–538

241. Mattern J, Mayer PR. Excretion of fluorescein into breast milk. *Am J Ophthalmol.* 1990;109:598–599

242. Retief FP, Heyns AD, Oosthuizen M, Oelofse R, van Reenen OR. Aspects of folate metabolism in lactating women studied after ingestion of 14C-methylfolate. *Am J Med Sci.* 1979;277:281–288

243. Rofsky NM, Weinreb JC, Litt AW. Quantitative analysis of gadopentetate dimeglumine excreted in breast milk. *J Magn Reson Imaging.* 1993;3:131–132

244. Celiloglu M, Celiker S, Guven H, Tuncok Y, Demir N, Erten O. Gentamicin excretion and uptake from breast milk by nursing infants. *Obstet Gynecol.* 1994;84:263–265

245. Bell RA, Dale IM. Gold secretion in maternal milk [letter]. *Arthritis Rheum.* 1976;19:1374

246. Blau SP. Letter: metabolism of gold during lactation. *Arthritis Rheum.* 1973;16:777–778

247. Gottlieb NL. Suggested errata. *Arthritis Rheum.* 1974;17:1057

48. Ostensen M, Skavdal K, Myklebust G, Tomassen Y, Aarbakke J. Excretion of gold into human breast milk. *Eur J Clin Pharmacol.* 1986;31: 251–252

49. Bennett PN, Humphries SJ, Osborne JP, Clarke AK, Taylor A. Use of sodium aurothiomalate during lactation. *Br J Clin Pharmacol.* 1990;29: 777–779

50. Cote CJ, Kenepp NB, Reed SB, Strobel GE. Trace concentrations of halothane in human breast milk. *Br J Anaesth.* 1976;48:541–543

51. Liedholm H, Wahlin-Boll E, Hanson A, Ingemarsson I, Melander A. Transplacental passage and breast milk concentrations of hydralazine. *Eur J Clin Pharmacol.* 1982;21:417–419

52. Ostensen M, Brown ND, Chiang PK, Aarbakke J. Hydroxychloroquine in human breast milk. *Eur J Clin Pharmacol.* 1985;28:357

53. Nation RL, Hackett LP, Dusci LJ, Ilett KF. Excretion of hydroxychloroquine in human milk. *Br J Clin Pharmacol.* 1984;17:368–369

54. Townsend RJ, Benedetti T, Erickson SH, Gillespie WR, Albert KS. A study to evaluate the passage of ibuprofen into breast-milk. *Drug Intell Clin Pharm.* 1982;16:482–483

55. Townsend RJ, Benedetti TJ, Erickson SH, et al. Excretion of ibuprofen into breast milk. *Am J Obstet Gynecol.* 1984;149:184–186

56. Eeg-Olofsson O, Malmros I, Elwin CE, Steen B. Convulsions in a breast-fed infant after maternal indomethacin [letter]. *Lancet.* 1978;2: 215

57. Fairhead FW. Convulsions in a breast-fed infant after maternal indomethacin [letter]. *Lancet.* 1978;2:576

58. Lebedevs TH, Wojnar-Horton RE, Yapp P, et al. Excretion of indomethacin in breast milk. *Br J Clin Pharmacol.* 1991;32:751–754

59. Postellon DC, Aronow R. Iodine in mother's milk [letter]. *JAMA.* 1982;247:463

60. Holmdahl KH. Cholecystography during lactation. *Acta Radiol.* 1955; 45:305–307

61. Berlin CM, Lee C. Isoniazid and acetylisoniazid disposition in human milk, saliva and plasma [abstr]. *Fed Proc.* 1979;38:426

62. Kumar AR, Hale TW, Mock RE. Transfer of interferon alfa into human breast milk. *J Hum Lact.* 2000;16:226–228

63. Ogbuokiri JE, Ozumba BC, Okonkwo PO. Ivermectin levels in human breast milk. *Eur J Clin Pharmacol.* 1993;45:389–390

64. Ogbuokiri JE, Ozumba BC, Okonkwo PO. Ivermectin levels in human breast milk. *Eur J Clin Pharmacol.* 1994;46:89–90

65. Dyggve HV, Dam H, Sondergaard E. Influence on the prothrombin time of breast-fed newborn babies of one single dose of vitamin K1 or synkavit given to the mother within 2 hours after birth. *Acta Obstet Gynecol Scand.* 1956;35:440–444

66. Von Kries R, Shearer M, McCarthy PT, Haug M, Harzer G, Goebel U. Vitamin K-1 content of maternal milk: Influence of the stage of lactation, lipid composition, and vitamin K-1 supplements given to the mother. *Pediatr Res.* 1987;22:513–517

67. Moretti ME, Ito S, Koren G. Disposition of maternal ketoconazole in breast milk. *Am J Obstet Gynecol.* 1995;173:1625–1626

68. Wischnik A, Manth SM, Lloyd J, Bullingham R, Thompson JS. The excretion of ketorolac tromethamine into breast milk after multiple oral dosing. *Eur J Clin Pharmacol.* 1989;36:521–524

69. Lunell HO, Kulas J, Rane A. Transfer of labetalol into amniotic fluid and breast milk in lactating women. *Eur J Clin Pharmacol.* 1985;28: 597–599

70. Atkinson H, Begg EJ. Concentration of beta-blocking drugs in human milk [letter]. *J Pediatr.* 1990;116:156

71. Diaz S, Herreros C, Juez G, et al. Fertility regulation in nursing women: VII. Influence of Norplant levonorgestrel implants upon lactation and infant growth. *Contraception.* 1985;32:53–74

72. Shaaban MM, Odlind V, Salem HT, et al. Levonorgestrel concentrations in maternal and infant serum during use of subdermal levonorgestrel contraceptive implants, Norplant by nursing mothers. *Contraception.* 1986;33:357–363

73. Shikary ZK, Betrabet SS, Patel ZM, et al. ICMR task force study on hormonal contraception. Transfer of levonorgestrel (LNG) administered through different drug delivery systems from the maternal circulation into the newborn infant's circulation via breast milk. *Contraception.* 1987;35:477–486

74. McCann MF, Moggia AV, Higgins JE, Potts M, Becker C. The effects of a progestin-only oral contraceptive (levonorgestrel 0.03 mg) on breast-feeding. *Contraception.* 1989;40:635–648

75. Mizuta H, Amino N, Ichihara K, et al. Thyroid hormones in human milk and their influence on thyroid function of breast-fed babies. *Pediatr Res.* 1983;17:468–471

76. Zeisler JA, Gaarder TD, De Mesquita SA. Lidocaine excretion in breast milk. *Drug Intell Clin Pharm.* 1986;20:691–693

277. Nikodem VC, Hofmeyr GJ. Secretion of the antidiarrhoeal agent loperamide oxide in breast milk. *Eur J Clin Pharmacol.* 1992;42:695–696

278. Hilbert J, Radwanski E, Affrime MB, Perentesis G, Symchowicz S, Zampaglione N. Excretion of loratadine in human breast milk. *J Clin Pharmacol.* 1988;28:234–239

279. Cruikshank DP, Varner MW, Pitkin RM. Breast milk magnesium and calcium concentrations following magnesium sulfate treatment. *Am J Obstet Gynecol.* 1982;143:685

280. Hannon PR, Duggan AK, Serwint JR, Vogelhut JW, Witter F, DeAngelis C. The influence of medroxyprogesterone on the duration of breast-feeding in mothers in an urban community. *Arch Pediatr Adolesc Med.* 1997;151:490–496

281. Buchanan RA, Eaton CJ, Koeff ST, Kinkel AW. The breast milk excretion of mefenamic acid. *Curr Ther Res Clin Exp.* 1968;10:592–597

282. Wittels B, Scott DT, Sinatra RS. Exogenous opioids in human breast milk and acute neonatal neurobehavior: a preliminary study. *Anesthesiology.* 1990;73:864–869

283. Blinick G, Inturrisi CE, Jerez E, Wallach RC. Methadone assays in pregnant women and progeny. *Am J Obstet Gynecol.* 1975;121:617–621

284. Blinick G, Wallach RC, Jerez E, Ackerman BD. Drug addiction in pregnancy and the neonate. *Am J Obstet Gynecol.* 1976;125:135–142

285. Wojnar-Horton RE, Kristensen JH, Yapp P, Ilett KF, Dusci LJ, Hackett LP. Methadone distribution and excretion into breast milk of clients in a methadone maintenance programme. *Br J Clin Pharmacol.* 1997;44: 543–547

286. Geraghty B, Graham EA, Logan B, Weiss EL. Methadone levels in breast milk. *J Hum Lact.* 1997;13:227–230

287. McCarthy JJ, Posey BL. Methadone levels in human milk. *J Hum Lact.* 2000;16:115–120

288. Cooper DS, Bode HH, Nath B, Saxe V, Maloof F, Ridgway EC. Methimazole pharmacology in man: studies using or newly developed radioimmunoassay for methimazole. *J Clin Endocrinol Metab.* 1984;58: 473–479

289. Azizi F. Effect of methimazole treatment of maternal thyrotoxicosis on thyroid function in breast-feeding infants. *J Pediatr.* 1996;128:855–858

290. White WB, Andreoli JW, Cohn RD. Alpha-methyldopa disposition in mothers with hypertension and in their breast-fed infants. *Clin Pharmacol Ther.* 1985;37:387–390

291. Shore MF. Drugs can be dangerous during pregnancy and lactations. *Can Pharm J.* 1970;103:358

292. Ilett KF, Hackett LP, Paterson JW, McCormick CC. Excretion of metrizamide in milk. *Br J Radiol.* 1981;54:537–538

293. Lownes HE, Ives TJ. Mexiletine use in pregnancy and lactation. *Am J Obstet Gynecol.* 1987;157:446–447

294. Lewis AM, Patel L, Johnston A, Turner P. Mexiletine in human blood and breast milk. *Postgrad Med J.* 1981;57:546–547

295. Valdivieso A, Valdes G, Spiro TE, Westerman RL. Minoxidil in breast milk [letter]. *Ann Intern Med.* 1985;102:135

296. Terwilliger WG, Hatcher RA. The elimination of morphine and quinine in human milk. *Surg Gynecol Obstet.* 1934;58:823–826

297. Robieux I, Koren G, Vandenbergh H, Schneiderman J. Morphine excretion in breast milk and resultant exposure of a nursing infant. *J Toxicol Clin Toxicol.* 1990;28:365–370

298. Oberlander TF, Robeson P, Ward V, et al. Prenatal and breast milk morphine exposure following maternal intrathecal morphine treatment. *J Hum Lact.* 2000;16:137–142

299. Miller RD, Keegan KA, Thrupp LD, Brann J. Human breast milk concentration of moxalactam. *Am J Obstet Gynecol.* 1984;148:348–349

300. Devlin RG, Duchin KL, Fleiss PM. Nadolol in human serum and breast milk. *Br J Clin Pharmacol.* 1981;12:393–396

301. Belton EM, Jones RV. Haemolytic anaemia due to nalidixic acid. *Lancet.* 1965;2:691

302. Jamali F, Stevens DR. Naproxen excretion in milk and its uptake by the infant. *Drug Intell Clin Pharm.* 1983;17:910–911

303. Liu DT, Savage JM, Donnell D. Nefopam excretion in human milk. *Br J Clin Pharmacol.* 1987;23:99–101

304. Ehrenkranz RA, Ackerman BA, Hulse JD. Nifedipine transfer into human milk. *J Pediatr.* 1989;114:478–480

305. Varsano I, Fischl J, Shochet SB. The excretion of orally ingested nitrofurantoin in human milk. *J Pediatr.* 1973;82:886–887

306. Laumas KR, Malkani PK, Bhatnagar S, Laumas V. Radioactivity in the breast milk of lactating women after oral administration of 3H-norethynodrel. *Am J Obstet Gynecol.* 1967;98:411–413

307. Pincus G, Bialy G, Layne DS, Paniagua M, Williams KI. Radioactivity in the milk of subjects receiving radioactive 19-norsteroids. *Nature.* 1966;212:924–925

308. Olsson B, Bolme P, Dahlstrom B, Marcus C. Excretion of noscapine in human breast milk. *Eur J Clin Pharmacol.* 1986;30:213–215

247

309. Sioufi A, Hillion D, Lumbroso P, et al. Oxprenolol placental transfer, plasma concentrations in newborns and passage into breast milk. *Br J Clin Pharmacol.* 1984;18:453–456

310. Fidler J, Smith V, De Swiet M. Excretion of oxprenolol and timolol in breast milk. *Br J Obstet Gynaecol.* 1983;90:961–965

311. Leuxner E, Pulver R. Verabreichung von irgapyrin bei schwangeren und wochnerinnen. *MMW Munch Med Wochenschr.* 1956;98:84–86

312. Mirkin B. Diphenylhydantoin: placental transport, fetal localization, neonatal metabolism, and possible teratogenic effects. *J Pediatr.* 1971; 78:329–337

313. Ostensen M. Piroxicam in human breast milk. *Eur J Clin Pharmacol.* 1983;25:829–830

314. McKenzie SA, Selley JA, Agnew JE. Secretion of prednisolone into breast milk. *Arch Dis Child.* 1975;50:894–896

315. Greenberger PA, Odeh YK, Frederiksen MC, Atkinson AJ Jr. Pharmacokinetics of prednisolone transfer to breast milk. *Clin Pharmacol Ther.* 1993;53:324–328

316. Katz FH, Duncan BR. Entry of prednisone into human milk. *N Engl J Med.* 1975;293:1154

317. Pittard WB III, Glazier H. Procainamide excretion in human milk. *J Pediatr.* 1983;102:631–633

318. Diaz S, Jackanicz TM, Herreros C, et al. Fertility regulation in nursing women: VIII. Progesterone plasma levels and contraceptive efficacy of a progesterone-releasing vaginal ring. *Contraception.* 1985;32:603–622

319. Kunka RL, Venkataramanan R, Stern RM, Ladik CF. Excretion of propoxyphene and norpropoxyphene in breast milk. *Clin Pharmacol Ther.* 1984;35:675–680

320. Levitan AA, Manion JC. Propranolol therapy during pregnancy and lactation. *Am J Cardiol.* 1973;32:247

321. Karlberg B, Lundberg D, Aberg H. Letter: excretion of propranolol in human breast milk. *Acta Pharmacol Toxicol (Copenh).* 1974;34:222–224

322. Bauer JH, Pape B, Zajicek J, Groshong T. Propranolol in human plasma and breast milk. *Am J Cardiol.* 1979;43:860–862

323. Kampmann JP, Johansen K, Hansen JM, Helweg J. Propylthiouracil in human milk: revision of a dogma. *Lancet.* 1980;1:736–737

324. Findlay JW, Butz RF, Sailstad JM, Warren JT, Welch RM. Pseudoephedrine and triprolidine in plasma and breast milk of nursing mothers. *Br J Clin Pharmacol.* 1984;18:901–906

325. Hardell LI, Lindstrom B, Lonnerholm G, Osterman PO. Pyridostigmine in human breast milk. *Br J Clin Pharmacol.* 1982;14:565–567

326. Clyde DF, Shute GT, Press J. Transfer of pyrimethamine in human milk. *J Trop Med Hyg.* 1956;59:277

327. Hill LM, Malkasian GD Jr. The use of quinidine sulfate throughout pregnancy. *Obstet Gynecol.* 1979;54:366–368

328. Horning MG, Stillwell WG, Nowlin J, Lertratanangkoon K, Stillwell RN, Hill RM. Identification and quantification of drugs and drug metabolites in human breast milk using gas chromatography mass spectrometry computer methods. *Mod Probl Paediatr.* 1975;15:73–79

329. Werthmann MW JR, Krees SV. Quantitative excretion of Senokot in human breast milk. *Med Ann Dist Columbia.* 1973;42:4–5

330. Hackett LP, Wojnar-Horton RE, Dusci LJ, Ilett KF, Roberts MJ. Excretion of sotalol in breast milk. *Br J Clin Pharmacol.* 1990;29:277–278

331. Phelps DL, Karim Z. Spironolactone: relationship between concentrations of dethioacetylated metabolite in human serum milk. *J Pharm Sci.* 1977;66:1203

332. Foulds G, Miller RD, Knirsch AK, Thrupp LD. Sulbactam kinetics and excretion into breast milk in postpartum women. *Clin Pharmacol Ther.* 1985;38:692–696

333. Jarnerot G, Into-Malmberg MB. Sulphasalazine treatment during breast feeding. *Scand J Gastroenterol.* 1979;14:869–871

334. Berlin CM Jr, Yaffe SJ. Disposition of salicylazosulfapyridine (Azulfidine) and metabolites in human breast milk. *Dev Pharmacol Ther.* 1980;1:31–39

335. Kauffman RE, O'Brien C, Gilford P. Sulfisoxazole secretion into human milk. *J Pediatr.* 1980;97:839–841

336. Wojnar-Horton RE, Hackett LP, Yapp P, Dusci LJ, Paech M, Ilett KF. Distribution and excretion of sumatriptan in human milk. *Br J Clin Pharmacol.* 1996;41:217–221

337. Chaiken P, Chasin M, Kennedy B, Silverman BK. Suprofen concentrations in human breast milk. *J Clin Pharmacol.* 1983;23:385–390

338. Lindberberg C, Boreus LO, de Chateau P, Lindstrom B, Lonnerholm G, Nyberg L. Transfer of terbutaline into breast milk. *Eur J Respir Dis Suppl.* 1984;134:87–91

339. Tetracycline in breast milk. *Br Med J.* 1969;4:791

340. Posner AC, Prigot A, Konicoff NG. Further observations on the use of tetracycline hydrochloride in prophylaxis and treatment of obstetric infections. In: Welch H, Marti-Ibanez F, eds. *Antibiotics Annual 1954–1955.* New York, NY: Medical Encyclopedia Inc; 1955:594

341. Yurchak AM, Jusko WJ. Theophylline secretion into breast milk. *Pediatrics.* 1976;57:518–520

342. Andersen LW, Qvist T, Hertz J, Mogensen F. Concentrations of thiopentone in mature breast milk and colostrum following an induction dose. *Acta Anaesthesiol Scand.* 1987;31:30–32

343. Williams RH, Kay GA, Jandorf BJ. Thiouracil: its absorption, distribution, and excretion. *J Clin Invest.* 1944;23:613–627

344. von Kobyletzki D, Dalhoff A, Lindemeyer H, Primavesi CA. Ticarcillin serum and tissue concentrations in gynecology and obstetrics. *Infection.* 1983;11:144–149

345. Moiel RH, Ryan JR. Tolbutamide orinase in human breast milk. *Clin Pediatr.* 1967;6:480

346. Sagranes R, Waller ES, Goehrs HR. Tolmetin in breast milk. *Drug Intell Clin Pharm.* 1985;19:55–56

347. Arnauld R. Etude du passage de la trimethoprime dans le lait maternel. *Ouest Med.* 1972;25:959

348. Miller RD, Salter AJ. The passage of trimethoprim/sulphamethoxazole into breast milk and its significance. Proceedings of the 8th International Congress of Chemotherapy, Athens. *Hellenic Soc Chemother.* 1974;1:687

349. Alexander FW. Sodium valproate and pregnancy. *Arch Dis Child.* 1979;54:240

350. von Unruh GE, Froescher W, Hoffman F, Niesen M. Valproic acid in breast milk: how much is really there? *Ther Drug Monit.* 1984;6:272–276

351. Anderson P, Bondesson U, Mattiasson I, Johansson BW. Verapamil and norverapamil in plasma and breast milk during breast feeding. *Eur J Clin Pharmacol.* 1987;31:625–627

352. Orme ML, Lewis PJ, de Swiet M, et al. May mothers given warfarin breast-feed their infants? *Br Med J.* 1977;1:1564–1565

353. Pons G, Francoual C, Guillet P, et al. Zolpidem excretion in breast milk. *Eur J Clin Pharmacol.* 1989;37:245–248

354. Wild CP, Pionneau FA, Montesano R, Mutiro CF, Chetsanga CJ. Aflatoxin detected in human breast milk by immunoassay. *Int J Cancer.* 1987;40:328–333

355. Maxwell SM, Apeagyei F, de Vries HR, et al. Aflatoxins in breast milk, neonatal cord blood and sera of pregnant women. *J Toxicol Toxin Rev.* 1989;8:19–29

356. Zarba A, Wild CP, Hall AJ, et al. Aflatoxin M1 in human breast milk from The Gambia, west Africa, quantified by combined monoclonal antibody immunoaffinity chromatography HPLC. *Carcinogenesis.* 1992; 13:891–894

357. Stegink LD, Filer LJ Jr, Baker GL. Plasma, erythrocyte human milk levels of free amino acids in lactating women administered aspartame or lactose. *J Nutr.* 1979;109:2173–2181

358. Mangurten HH, Kaye CI. Neonatal bromism secondary to maternal exposure in a photographic laboratory. *J Pediatr.* 1982;100:596–598

359. Radisch B, Luck W, Nau H. Cadmium concentrations in milk and blood of smoking mothers. *Toxicol Lett.* 1987;36:147–152

360. Miyazaki T, Akiyama K, Kaneko S, Horii S, Yamagishi T. Chlordane residues in human milk. *Bull Environ Contam Toxicol.* 1980;25:518–523

361. Resman BH, Blumenthal P, Jusko WJ. Breast milk distribution of theobromine from chocolate. *J Pediatr.* 1977;91:477–480

362. Wolff MS. Occupationally derived chemicals in breast milk. *Am J Ind Med.* 1983;4:259–281

363. Egan H, Goulding R, Roburn J, Tatton JO. Organo-chlorine pesticide residues in human fat and human milk. *Br Med J.* 1965;2:66–69

364. Quinby GE, Armstrong JF, Durham WF. DDT in human milk. *Nature.* 1965;207:726–728

365. Bakken AF, Seip M. Insecticides in human breast milk. *Acta Paediatr Scand.* 1976;65:535–539

366. Adamovic VM, Sokic B, Smiljanski MJ. Some observations concerning the ratio of the intake of organochlorine insecticides through food and amounts excreted in the milk of breast-feeding mothers. *Bull Environ Contam Toxicol.* 1978;20:280–285

367. Savage EP, Keefe TJ, Tessari JD, et al. National study of chlorinated hydrocarbon insecticide residues in human milk, USA. I. Geographic distribution of dieldrin, heptachlor, heptachlor epoxide, chlordane, oxychlordane, and mirex. *Am J Epidemiol.* 1981;113:413–422

368. Wilson DJ, Locker DJ, Ritzen CA, Watson JT, Schaffner W. DDT concentrations in human milk. *Am J Dis Child.* 1973;125:814–817

369. Bouwman H, Becker PJ, Cooppan RM, Reinecke AJ. Transfer of DDT used in malaria control to infants via breast milk. *Bull World Health Organ.* 1992;70:241–250

370. Stevens MF, Ebell GF, Psaila-Savona P. Organochlorine pesticides in Western Australian nursing mothers. *Med J Aust.* 1993;158:238–241

371. Emanuel B, Schoenfeld A. Favism in a nursing infant. *J Pediatr.* 1961; 58:263–266

2. Simpson WJ, Tuba J. An investigation of fluoride concentration in the milk of nursing mothers. *J Oral Med*. 1968;23:104–106

3. Esala S, Vuori E, Helle A. Effect of maternal fluorine intake on breast milk fluorine content. *Br J Nutr*. 1982;48:201–204

4. Dreyfus-See G. Le passage dans le lait des aliments ou medicaments absorbes par denourrices. *Rev Med Interne*. 1934;51:198

5. Ando M, Hirano S, Itoh Y. Transfer of hexachlorobenzene (HCB) from mother to newborn baby through placenta and milk. *Arch Toxicol*. 1985;56:195–200

6. West RW, Wilson DJ, Schaffner W. Hexachlorophene concentrations in human milk. *Bull Environ Contam Toxicol*. 1975;13:167–169

7. Rabinowitz M, Leviton A, Needelman H. Lead in milk and infant blood: a dose-response model. *Arch Environ Health*. 1985;40:283–286

8. Sternowsky JH, Wessolowski R. Lead and cadmium in breast milk. Higher levels in urban vs rural mothers during the first 3 months of lactation. *Arch Toxicol*. 1985;57:41–45

9. Namihira D, Saldivar L, Pustilnik N, Carreon GJ, Salinas ME. Lead in human blood and milk from nursing women living near a smelter in Mexico City. *J Toxicol Environ Health*. 1993;38:225–232

80. Baum CR, Shannon MW. Lead in breast milk. *Pediatrics*. 1996;97:932

81. Koos BJ, Longo LD. Mercury toxicity in the pregnant woman, fetus, and newborn infant. A review. *Am J Obstet Gynecol*. 1976;126:390–409

82. Amin-Zaki L, Elhassani S, Majeed MA, Clarkson TW, Doherty RA, Greenwood MR. Studies of infants postnatally exposed to methylmercury. *J Pediatr*. 1974;85:81–84

83. Pitkin RM, Bahns JA, Filer LJ Jr, Reynolds WA. Mercury in human maternal and cord blood, placenta, and milk. *Proc Soc Exp Biol Med*. 1976;151:565–567

384. Hersh J, Bono JV, Padgett DE, Mancuso CA. Methyl methacrylate levels in the breast milk of a patient after total hip arthroplasty. *J Arthroplasty*. 1995;10:91–92

385. Stegink LD, Filer LJ Jr, Baker GL. Monosodium glutamate: effect on plasma and breast milk amino acid levels in lactating women. *Proc Soc Exp Biol Med*. 1972;140:836–841

386. Miller RW. Pollutants in breast milk: PCBs and cola-colored babies [editorial]. *J Pediatr*. 1977;90:510–511

387. Rogan WJ, Bagniewska A, Damstra T. Pollutants in breast milk. *N Engl J Med*. 1980;302:1450–1453

388. Wickizer TM, Brilliant LB, Copeland R, Tilden R. Polychlorinated biphenyl contamination of nursing mothers' milk in Michigan. *Am J Public Health*. 1981;71:132–137

389. Brilliant LB, Van Amburg G, Isbister J, Bloomer AW, Humphrey H, Price H. Breast-milk monitoring to measure Michigan's contamination with polybrominated biphenyls. *Lancet*. 1978;2:643–646

390. Wickizer TM, Brilliant LB. Testing for polychlorinated biphenyls in human milk. *Pediatrics*. 1981;68:411–415

391. Bagnell PC, Ellenberg HA. Obstructive jaundice due to a chlorinated hydrocarbon in breast milk. *Can Med Assoc J*. 1977;117:1047–1048

392. Higginbottom MC, Sweetman L, Nyhan WL. A syndrome of methylmalonic aciduria, homocystinuria, megaloblastic anemia neurologic abnormalities in a vitamin B12-deficient breast-fed infant of a strict vegetarian. *N Engl J Med*. 1978;299:317–323

ACOG EDUCATIONAL BULLETIN

Number 258, July 2000

Breastfeeding: Maternal and Infant Aspects

Breastfeeding rates decreased significantly in the past half century as formula feeding gained popularity. In 1971, only 24.7% of mothers left the hospital breastfeeding. Recently, breastfeeding initiation rates have been increasing, reaching 64.3% in 1998, according to the Mothers' Survey (Ross Products Division, Abbott Laboratories, Inc., Columbus, Ohio). These increases reflect a growing awareness of the advantages of breast milk over formula. Improvement in breastfeeding initiation rates, however, has been uneven, as women attempt to overcome practical obstacles.

Evidence continues to mount regarding the value of breastfeeding for both women and their infants. Human milk provides developmental, nutritional, and immunologic benefits to the infant that cannot be duplicated by formula feeding. Breastfeeding also provides significant benefits to women. It is critical that women be prepared to make an informed choice in deciding what is best for them, their families, and their babies. Obstetrician-gynecologists and other health professionals caring for pregnant women should regularly impart accurate information about breastfeeding to expectant mothers and be prepared to support them should any problems arise while breastfeeding.

This document will focus primarily on breastfeeding by healthy mothers with healthy infants born at term. Human milk and breastfeeding are recommended for premature newborns and mother–infant pairs with other special needs; however, specific information in this regard is beyond the scope of this document.

This Educational Bulletin was developed under the direction of the Committees on Health Care for Underserved Women and Obstetric Practice of the American College of Obstetricians and Gynecologists. The college wishes to thank John T. Queenan, MD, for his assistance in the development of this bulletin. This document is not to be construed as establishing a standard of practice or dictating an exclusive course of treatment. Rather, it is intended as an educational tool that presents current information on obstetric–gynecologic issues.

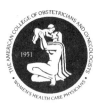

Benefits of Breastfeeding

Research in the United States and throughout the world indicates that breastfeeding and human milk provide benefits to infants, women, families, and society. These studies have been done in a variety of settings, resulting in information derived from culturally and economically diverse populations.

Infants

The benefits of breastfeeding for the infant have been established in the following areas. Human milk provides species-specific and age-specific nutrients for the infant (1). Colostrum, the fluid secreted immediately following e infant's birth, conveys a high level of immune protection, particularly secretory immunoglobulin A (IgA). During the first 4–7 days following delivery, protein and mineral concentrations decrease and water, fat, and lactose increase. Milk composition continues to change to match infant nutritional needs. In addition to the right balance of nutrients and immunologic factors, human milk contains factors that act as biologic signals for promoting cellular growth and differentiation. It also contains multiple substances with antimicrobial properties, which protect against infection (1, 2). Human milk alone, however, may not provide adequate iron for premature newborns, infants whose mothers have low iron stores, and infants older than 6 months.

In 1997, the American Academy of Pediatrics (AAP) published a policy statement, "Breastfeeding and the Use of Human Milk" (3). The statement was developed by the AAP Work Group on Breastfeeding, which evaluated the research literature on relationships between breastfeeding and infant health and development. The statement's summary paragraph (see the box below) on established infant protective effects, as well as positive associations (which require further study), is well referenced. Obstetrician–gynecologists who review these sources of evidence for infant benefit will be better prepared to care for the women in their practices.

Women

The benefits of breastfeeding for women are well documented. During the immediate postpartum period, the oxytocin released during milk let-down causes increased uterine contractions and lessens maternal blood loss (4). Evidence exists that the hormones of lactation (oxytocin and prolactin) contribute to feelings of relaxation and attachment (5). Breastfeeding is associated with a decreased risk of developing ovarian and premenopausal breast cancer (6, 7). Breastfeeding also delays postpartum ovulation, supporting birth spacing (8–10). Although breastfeeding causes some bone demineralization, studies indicate that "catch-up" remineralization occurs following weaning; some studies also show a lower incidence of osteoporosis and hip fracture after menopause (11, 12). The incidence of pregnancy-induced long-term obesity also is reduced (13).

There are psychologic benefits as well. A woman who breastfeeds her baby is able to take advantage of the natural dynamics of nurturing and bonding.

Families and Society

Studies indicate that the breastfed child has fewer illnesses and, therefore, fewer visits to the doctor and hospital (14). This translates into less absenteeism from work for the mother and lower medical expenses. The improvement in work productivity may be significant for society as well, because women now constitute a large portion of the workforce. More than 60% of all women return to outside employment during the first year following birth of a child.

Breastfeeding, while demanding maternal time and attention, can save individual families and society considerable money compared with formula feeding (15). On a national scale, disposal of formula cans, bottles, and bottle liners may be an ecologic consideration.

Research on Established and Potential Protective Effects of Human Milk and Breastfeeding on Infants

Research in the United States, Canada, Europe and other developed countries, among predominantly middle-class populations, provides strong evidence that human milk feeding decreases the incidence and/or severity of diarrhea, lower respiratory infection, otitis media, bacteremia, bacterial meningitis, botulism, urinary tract infection, and necrotizing enterocolitis. There are a number of studies that show a possible protective effect of human milk feeding against sudden infant death syndrome, insulin-dependent diabetes mellitus, Crohn's disease, ulcerative colitis, lymphoma, allergic diseases, and other chronic digestive diseases. Breastfeeding has also been related to possible enhancement of cognitive development.

American Academy of Pediatrics, Work Group on Breastfeeding. Breastfeeding and the use of human milk. Pediatrics 100;1997: 1035–1039 (Paragraph includes 39 citations.)

Obstacles to Breastfeeding

Women need to know that breastfeeding, like other aspects of having a new baby, may be demanding as well as rewarding. They should be assured that they will have support and that there are options for problem solving and for addressing the practical obstacles they may face. Some women will decide the challenges outweigh the benefits for themselves and their babies, given the overall circumstances of their lives. However, physicians and other health professionals should recognize the potential effectiveness of applying their knowledge and skills to encourage and support women in initiating and continuing breastfeeding.

Modern society creates some of the obstacles to breastfeeding. Short hospital stays make the teaching of breastfeeding a challenge. Lack of spousal or partner support and family custom may discourage breastfeeding. Having to return to work is an obstacle, which is being diminished for some women as more employers learn that encouraging breastfeeding as a policy improves employee morale and decreases absenteeism (16, 17). An unfriendly social environment may make it difficult to breastfeed in public. The effect of these obstacles can be mitigated by educating the families, employers, and society. All share in the benefits and, through positive attitudes and workplace and public policies, also can support women who are willing to breastfeed.

Who Can Breastfeed

Breastfeeding is a natural function; nearly every woman can breastfeed her child. Mother and newborn can more easily learn the basics and how to deal with the challenges if they have skilled and experienced support. Mothers who have cesarean deliveries should be reassured that they can breastfeed their newborns as well as those women having vaginal deliveries. Specific infections such as endometritis or mastitis are not contraindications to breastfeeding.

Women with structural problems such as hypoplastic or tubular breasts may have difficulty producing sufficient milk. True inverted nipples are rare but generally preclude nursing; most women with nipples that appear flat or inverted can breastfeed, given appropriate assistance in the early days of lactation. Pumping for a minute or two before offering the breast to the newborn has been shown to facilitate latch-on (1). Lactation is not possible for women who have had breast surgery involving the complete severing of the lactiferous ducts. However, some women may breastfeed after reduction mammoplasty or augmentation mammoplasty with implants, and most women can breastfeed after breast biopsies.

Mothers with premature infants also can breastfeed. A mother's milk has specific properties that match the needs of her premature newborn. However, nutrition requirements for the premature newborn are different and require special attention. Some babies with cleft lips or palate may be able to breastfeed. The soft breast tissue may fill the defect and enable the infant to develop a seal. Sometimes a palatal obturator allows the infant to breastfeed and not aspirate milk. A newborn that is premature or has other special needs may benefit from breastfeeding but requires individual evaluation by appropriate experts.

Who Should Not Breastfeed

Although it is true that most women can breastfeed, there are exceptions. These exceptions should be understood by all clinicians so that a patient's frustration and disappointment can be minimized. The number of contraindications is small (18). Women who should not breastfeed are those who:

- Take street drugs or do not control alcohol use
- Have an infant with galactosemia
- Are infected with the human immunodeficiency virus (HIV)
- Have active, untreated tuberculosis
- Take certain medications
- Are undergoing treatment for breast cancer (1)

Women who use illegal drugs should not breastfeed because it is unknown which agent or how much of the agent the infant will be exposed to. Alcohol is a toxin, so a breastfeeding woman should minimize or avoid it, and a mother who drinks significant amounts of alcohol should not breastfeed (2).

Infants with galactosemia should neither breastfeed, because this will exacerbate the condition, nor consume any formula containing lactose (eg, cows' milk). They need special lactose-free formula.

Some infections contraindicate breastfeeding; others require precautions. Approaches to breastfeeding vary according to the infection and the environment. Comprehensive information about breastfeeding in relation to the following common maternal infections and others is available for further reference (1). Women in the United States who have HIV infections should not breastfeed because breast milk can carry HIV and pass the infection to the infant. In some countries with high infant mortality rates, however, the benefits of breast-feeding in providing nutrition and preventing infections may still outweigh the risks of transmitting HIV.

If a woman has active pulmonary tuberculosis, the repeated and prolonged close contact involved in feeding exposes the infant to risk of airborne infection. Therefore the woman should neither breastfeed nor bottle feed her newborn until she has been appropriately treated for at least 2 weeks and is otherwise considered to be noncontagious. The infant can be given the mother's expressed breast milk because it does not contain *Mycobacterium tuberculosis* (1).

Similarly, if a woman has varicella, she should be isolated from the infant and neither breastfeed nor bottle feed while she is clinically infectious. Once the infant has received varicella-zoster immune globulin (1), the woman can provide expressed breast milk for the infant if there are no skin lesions on the breasts. An immunocompetent woman who develops herpes zoster infection (shingles) can continue breastfeeding if lesions are covered and are not on the breast. Maternal antibodies delivered through the placenta and breast milk will prevent the disease or diminish its severity. An infant may be given varicella-zoster immune globulin in these circumstances as an added precaution (1).

Breastfeeding also is contraindicated in women who have active herpes simplex infections on the breast until the lesion is cleared. In women with cytomegalovirus infection, both the virus and maternal antibodies are present in breast milk. Because of the antibodies, otherwise healthy infants born at term with congenital or acquired cytomegalovirus infections usually do better if they are breastfed. A study of infants who developed infections during breastfeeding found the infants also developed an immune response, did not develop the disease, and rarely manifested symptoms (18).

Hepatitis infections do not preclude breastfeeding. With appropriate immunoprophylaxis, including hepatitis B immune globulin (HBIG) and hepatitis vaccine, breastfeeding of babies born to women positive for hepatitis B surface antigen poses no additional risk for the transmission of hepatitis B virus (19). If a woman has acute hepatitis A infection, her infant can breastfeed after receiving immune serum globulin and vaccine (1). The average rate of hepatitis C virus (HCV) infection reported in infants born to HCV-positive women is 4% for both breastfed and bottle-fed infants. Therefore maternal HCV is not considered a contraindication to breastfeeding (20).

Many medications are compatible with breastfeeding. The AAP Committee on Drugs reviewed the current data on the transfer of drugs and other chemicals in human milk. The committee classified drugs for safety in breastfeeding on a scale of 1 (contraindicated) to 6 (compatible) (21). Generally, breastfeeding is contraindicated for women taking antineoplastic, thyrotoxic, and immunosuppressive agents (Table 1) (19). Medications with relative contraindications may sometimes be used cautiously by timing doses to immediately follow a feeding.

Education on Breastfeeding

Teaching the pregnant woman and her partner about childbirth and breastfeeding is an integral part of good prenatal care. Other family members who could support breastfeeding may be included. Education can occur in the physician's office or clinic. Alternatively, hospitals and other organizations provide education for pregnant women and their partners. The advice and encouragement of the obstetrician–gynecologist are critical in making the decision to breastfeed. Other health professionals such as pediatricians, nurses, and certified lactation specialists play an important role, as do mother-to-mother groups and other lay organizations. The health benefits of breastfeeding warrant efforts in professional cooperation and

Table 1. Medications Contraindicated During Breastfeeding

Medication	Reason
Bromocriptine	Suppresses lactation; may be hazardous to the mother
Cocaine	Cocaine intoxication
Cyclophosphamide	Possible immune suppression; unknown effect on growth or association with carcinogenesis; neutropenia
Cyclosporine	Possible immune suppression; unknown effect on growth or association with carcinogenesis
Doxorubicin*	Possible immune suppression; unknown effect on growth or association with carcinogenesis
Ergotamine	Vomiting, diarrhea, convulsions (at doses used in migraine medications)
Lithium	One third to one half of therapeutic blood concentration in infants
Methotrexate	Possible immune suppression; unknown effect on growth or association with carcinogenesis; neutropenia
Phencyclidine	Potent hallucinogen
Phenindione	Anticoagulant; increased prothrombin and partial thromboplastin time in one infant; not used in United States
Radioactive iodine and other radiolabeled elements	Contraindications to breastfeeding for various periods

*Medication is concentrated in human milk.

American Academy of Pediatrics, American College of Obstetricians and Gynecologists. Guidelines for perinatal care. 4th ed. Elk Grove Village, Illinois: AAP; Washington, DC: ACOG, 1997

coordination among all health care workers to educate and encourage women and their families to choose breastfeeding. Patient education materials can reinforce the message (see the boxes, "Patient Education Materials" and "References for Health Care Workers and Patients Seeking In-depth Information").

Some women who choose to breastfeed were breastfed themselves or had a sibling who was breastfed, which established it as normal behavior in their household. These women would probably benefit from some education and reinforcement concerning breastfeeding. Women whose family and friends have not shared breastfeeding experiences also approach pregnancy with a desire to do what is healthiest for their babies. Guidance and consideration of life situations are important in helping these women and their families make a decision about feeding their infants. Information about the benefits and challenges of breastfeeding compared with the use of formula will help them make good decisions. The obstetrician–gynecologist often

Patient Education Materials

Breast-feeding your baby. Patient Education Pamphlet AP029. Washington, DC: American College of Obstetricians and Gynecologists, 1997

Breastfeeding: loving support for a bright future. Q & A. Physicians' breastfeeding support kit. Tampa, Florida: Best Start Social Marketing, 1998

Working & breastfeeding. Can you do it? Yes, you can! Alexandria, Virginia: National Healthy Mothers, Healthy Babies Coalition, 1997

Ten steps to support parents' choice to breastfeed their baby. American Academy of Pediatrics Task Force on Breastfeeding. Elk Grove Village, Illinois: AAP, 1999

References for Health Care Workers and Patients Seeking In-depth Information

American Academy of Pediatrics and the American College of Obstetricians and Gynecologists. Guidelines for perinatal care. 4th ed. Elk Grove Village, Illinois: AAP, and Washington, DC: ACOG, 1997

American Academy of Pediatrics Committee on Drugs. The transfer of drugs and other chemicals into human milk. Pediatrics 1994;93:137–150.

American Academy of Pediatrics, Work Group on Breastfeeding. Breastfeeding and the use of human milk. Pediatrics 1997;100:1035–1039

ABM News and Views. The Newsletter of The Academy of Breastfeeding Medicine. Lenexa, Kansas: ABM

Lawrence RA. A review of the medical benefits and contraindications to breastfeeding in the United States. Maternal and Child Health Technical Information Bulletin. Arlington, Virginia: National Center for Education in Maternal and Child Health, 1997

Lawrence RA, Lawrence RM. Breastfeeding: a guide for the medical profession. 5th ed. St. Louis, Missouri: Mosby, 1999

U.S. Department of Health and Human Services, Health Resources & Services Administration, Maternal and Child Health Bureau, U.S. Department of Agriculture, Food and Nutrition Service. Physicians' breastfeeding support kit. Tampa, Florida: Best Start Social Marketing, 1998

can allay a woman's anxieties and suggest solutions or resources to make breastfeeding a practical choice for her and her family.

Periodic Gynecologic Examinations

Obstetrician–gynecologists can begin to educate women who have their reproductive lives ahead of them by mentioning breastfeeding during the breast examination portion of routine gynecologic visits, if appropriate. Women whose anatomy appears to be normal can be told that if they decide to have a baby, there are no structural impediments to breastfeeding.

First Obstetric Visit

The initial prenatal visit is the optimal time to encourage or reinforce the decision to breastfeed. It is also an ideal time to let the patient know the advantages of breastfeeding over formula feeding. Most patients seek information and guidance from their doctors. The importance of the physician's recommendation should never be underestimated. If a woman has not yet made a decision to breastfeed, this and subsequent visits may provide an opportunity for her to do so. During the breast examination, the physician can perform a breastfeeding-specific examination and answer any questions about the usual pattern of changes in the breasts during pregnancy and breastfeeding. If there are no structural problems, the woman can be reassured about her ability to breastfeed. If her nipples appear to be inverted, she should know that appearance is not necessarily prognostic and she may be able to breastfeed, but that techniques to assist in nipple eversion are not recommended during pregnancy because of the potential for stimulating contractions.

Antenatal Breastfeeding Instruction

In the past, when hospital stays were longer, women could receive fairly adequate education about breastfeeding before discharge. Today, with shorter hospital stays, it is imperative that pregnant women come to the hospital for delivery with a good foundation of knowledge gained during the antepartum period. Prenatal education groups have been shown to be particularly effective in increasing duration of breastfeeding (22). Education in the hospital can then focus on operational aspects of breastfeeding such as latch-on and feeding techniques.

The woman who is appropriately counseled on breastfeeding options and chooses not to breastfeed should be reassured that her milk production will abate during the first few days after delivery. Hormone treatment to stop milk production is no longer recommended. She should be treated with a well-fitted support bra, analgesics, and ice packs to relieve the pain. She also can be assured that if she changes her mind, she may still be able to initiate breastfeeding within the first few days.

Hospital Stay

Shortened hospital stays for childbirth have made the teaching of breastfeeding difficult. Certain protocols and practices, however, will increase rates of successful breastfeeding (see the box, "Ten Hospital Practices to Encourage and Support Breastfeeding") (23).

Delivery

The immediate postpartum period should allow the woman and her newborn to experience optimal bonding with immediate physical contact, preferably skin to skin. The initial feeding should occur as soon after birth as possible, preferably in the first hour when the baby is awake, alert, and ready to suck. Newborn eye prophylaxis, weighing, measuring, and other such examinations can be done after the feeding. Such procedures usually can be performed later in the woman's room.

Rooming-In

Today, all hospitals should make trained personnel available to provide breastfeeding support and should offer 24-hour rooming-in to maximize the interaction between the woman and her newborn. Separation of a breastfeeding woman and newborn should be avoided whenever possible. Most newborn care and procedures, including bathing, blood drawing, physical examinations, and administration of medication and phototherapy, can be performed in the mother's room. In this way, mother and baby can benefit together from the nursing care available (3).

The rooming-in experience allows a woman and her newborn to start the adjustment to a breastfeeding routine. Normally a newborn will show signs of hunger, such as increased alertness or activity, mouthing, or rooting. Crying is a late sign of hunger. Newborns should be nursed approximately 8–12 times every 24 hours until satiety; time at breast varies but may be 10 to 15 minutes on each breast (3).

Instruction

Hospital personnel should have adequate time allotted to each patient, no matter when the delivery occurs, and provide a specific program on practical aspects of breastfeeding that women master before discharge. Trained staff should assess breastfeeding behavior of the woman and newborn during the first 24–48 hours after birth for correct nursing positions, latch-on, and adequacy of newborn swallowing. They also should ensure that the woman is skilled in the technique of manual expression of milk (3).

Before discharge the woman should be educated about age-appropriate elimination patterns of her newborn during the first week after birth. At least six urinations per day and three to four stools per day are to be expected by 5–7 days of age. She can be shown how to keep simple records for the first few weeks, noting the frequency and length of feedings and the number of stools and wet diapers, for discussion with her care providers. She should understand expected patterns of newborn weight loss and gain (3). Before gaining, the breastfeeding newborn may lose 5–7% of birth weight in the first week. When the loss is greater than 5–7% or reaches that level in the first 3 days, a clinician should evaluate the breastfeeding process to address any problems before they become serious. A loss of up to 10% is the maximum acceptable. Follow-up should confirm that the newborn is beginning to regain weight after the first week (1).

Ten Hospital Practices to Encourage and Support Breastfeeding*

- Maintain a written breastfeeding policy that is communicated to all health care staff.

- Train all pertinent health care staff in skills necessary to implement this policy.

- Inform all pregnant women about the benefits of breastfeeding.

- Offer all mothers the opportunity to initiate breastfeeding within 1 hour of birth.

- Show breastfeeding mothers how to breastfeed and how to maintain lactation even if they are separated from their infants.

- Give breastfeeding infants only breast milk unless medically indicated.

- Facilitate rooming-in; encourage all mothers and infants to remain together during their hospital stay.

- Encourage unrestricted breastfeeding when baby exhibits hunger cues or signals or on request of mother.

- Encourage exclusive suckling at the breast by providing no pacifiers or artificial nipples.

- Refer mothers to established breastfeeding and mother's support groups and services, and foster the establishment of those services when they are not available.

*The 1994 report of the Healthy Mothers, Healthy Babies National Coalition Expert Work Group recommended that the UNICEF-WHO Baby Friendly Hospital Initiative be adapted for use in the United States as the United States Breastfeeding Health Initiative, using the adapted 10 steps above.

Randolph L, Cooper L, Fonseca-Becker F, York M, McIntosh M. Baby Friendly Hospital Initiative feasibility study: final report. Healthy Mothers, Healthy Babies National Coalition Expert Work Group. Alexandria, Virginia: HMHB, 1994

Latch-On

Breastfeeding should not be painful, but minor discomfort is common during the first 2 weeks. Painful breastfeeding almost always results from poor positioning or latch-on, which should be immediately corrected. ACOG's "Breast-feeding Your Baby" pamphlet is an example of a resource that can be used to help women with positioning and latch-on (24). Discomfort may occur temporarily as the woman's milk supply is beginning to be established. Any significant pain or tenderness should be assessed promptly by a physician.

Latch-on is one of the most important steps to successful breastfeeding. There are several helpful approaches, including gently stroking the newborn's lower lip with the nipple to get the baby to open his or her mouth wide, or gently pulling the newborn's chin down. The newborn should take a large amount of breast into his or her mouth, generally an inch or more of the areola with the nipple pointing toward the soft palate. The mother may hold her breast to facilitate this position, using a hand position comfortable for her. The nipple and the areola elongate into a teat, and the baby's tongue should be slightly cupped beneath it. The mother should adopt a comfortable position and draw the baby to the breast. The newborn should be held close, facing the mother, with his chin and the tip of his nose touching but not completely occluded by the breast. Usually, it is wise to alternate the breast used to initiate the feeding and to equalize the time spent at each breast over the day. The mother can break the suction by gently inserting her finger in the newborn's mouth before taking him off the breast.

Home

All breastfeeding women and their babies who are discharged from the hospital in less than 48 hours after delivery should be seen by a pediatrician or other knowledgeable health care practitioner when the baby is 2–4 days old. This is important in order to evaluate health status of the newborn (eg, weight, hydration, and hyperbilirubinemia) at this critical age, as well as to observe the woman and newborn during breastfeeding (3).

Women can be reassured that eating a well-balanced diet generally will provide the nutrients their infants need. On average, it is estimated that women will need approximately 500 kcal per day more than nonpregnant and nonlactating recommended levels, and the additional maternal food intake generally will provide additional needed vitamins and minerals (with the possible exceptions of calcium and zinc). Women of childbearing age need to maintain a calcium intake of 1,000 mg per day at all times, including during pregnancy and lactation

(1,300 for adolescents through 18 years of age). Dietary intake is the preferred source of all needed nutrients. However, many women breastfeed on a lower calorie intake level than suggested, consuming bodily stores instead. This will result in gradual weight loss and is not likely to affect breastfeeding, but further questions may need to be asked about sources of magnesium, vitamin B_6, folate, calcium, and zinc (2, 25, 26). Corrective measures can be suggested for improving nutrient intakes of women with restrictive eating patterns (2). Women should be encouraged to drink plenty of fluids to satisfy their thirst and maintain adequate hydration. They need not avoid certain foods (spicy or strong flavored) because of breastfeeding unless the infant seems to react negatively to specific foods.

The spouse or partner can play a vital support role for the breastfeeding woman by encouraging her, bringing the newborn to her for feeding, changing the newborn, and holding the newborn. Couples may find that caring for a baby can complicate their own relationship, including a desired resumption of sexual intercourse. They may be encouraged to discuss emotional adjustments to their new family status as well as physical problems of soreness, fatigue, and vaginal dryness secondary to lactation. When a woman is ready to resume sexual intercourse, prelubricated latex condoms can be recommended to prevent infection and ease vaginal dryness.

Phone-In Resource

The departure of a woman and her newborn from the hospital can be a joyous but daunting experience. The family is now responsible for the care and feeding of the newborn. Whether or not they have a support system at home, a phone-in resource is needed for ongoing instruction and advice. The obstetrician–gynecologist's office, the place where the woman has received most of her care, should be that resource or at least provide links to other resources in the community, such as lactation specialists and support groups.

Contraception

Women should be encouraged to consider their future plans for additional childbearing during prenatal care and be given information and services that will help them meet their goals. This is especially important for a woman who breastfeeds, because there are fewer variables in her nutrition status if the next pregnancy is delayed until she has completed breastfeeding.

In nonbreastfeeding women, the average time to first ovulation is 45 days (range, 25–72 days) (27). Many women resume intercourse well before they return for their postpartum checkup, thus some women are at risk of becoming pregnant.

For breastfeeding women, however, the situation is different. Exclusive breastfeeding helps prevent pregnancy for the first 6 months after delivery, but should be relied on only temporarily and when it meets carefully observed criteria of the lactational amenorrhea method (LAM) (see "Lactational Amenorrhea Method").

Nonhormonal Methods

If a breastfeeding woman needs or wants more protection from pregnancy, options are available that do not affect breastfeeding or pose even a theoretical risk to the infant. *She should first consider the nonhormonal methods such as copper intrauterine contraceptive devices, condoms, or other barrier methods* (see the box, "ACOG Recommendations for Nonhormonal Contraception for Breastfeeding Women"). Condoms have additional, noncontraceptive advantages. Female sterilization or vasectomy may be considered by couples desiring permanent methods of birth control (27).

Hormonal Methods

Hormonal contraception offers effective protection from becoming pregnant. Several factors should be considered before prescribing hormonal contraception for the lactating woman. Contradictory lines of thought have resulted in conflicting recommendations that have been put forward by generally authoritative sources. The ACOG recommendations represent a more practical approach to the woman's needs, based on relevant research.

Progestin-Only Contraceptives

Progestin-only contraceptives, including progestin-only tablets (minipills), depot medroxyprogesterone acetate

---

ACOG Recommendations for Nonhormonal Contraception for Breastfeeding Women

Exclusive breastfeeding up to 6 months meeting lactational amenorrhea method criteria (see "Lactational Amenorrhea Method")

Additional protection if desired

- Prelubricated latex condoms
- Other barrier methods
- Copper intrauterine contraceptive devices
- Male or female sterilization if permanent contraception is desired

---

(DMPA), and levonorgestrel implants, do not affect the quality of breast milk and may slightly increase the volume of milk and duration of breastfeeding compared with nonhormonal methods (28–32). Accordingly, progestin-only methods are the hormonal contraceptives of choice for breastfeeding women. Nonetheless, some authorities have recommended delays of various lengths before introduction of progestin-only contraceptives on the basis of two sets of theoretical concerns:

- The normal 2–3-day postdelivery decrease of progesterone is part of the process that initiates lactation. There is theoretical concern that giving progestins in the first few days before lactation is established could interfere with optimal lactation. Note that DMPA enters the milk at approximately the same level found in the woman's blood; by contrast norgestrel and norethindrone enter the milk at only one tenth the level in the woman's blood. The injectable route of administration also may result in a comparatively high initial dose (27).

- Progestin methods carry a theoretical risk to the newborn because of exposure to exogenous steroids at a time when the newborn's system is very immature in its ability to metabolize drugs. Because of this concern, research studies presented to the FDA for drug approval investigated only the effects of these methods administered several weeks after birth. Because documentation of experience with earlier initiation was not presented to the FDA, package inserts recommend initiation of progestin-only oral contraceptives at 6 weeks for women who are exclusively breastfeeding and at 3 weeks for those who are breastfeeding with supplementation. Most authorities recommend introduction of long-acting progestin-only injectables or implants 6 weeks after delivery for breastfeeding women (27, 33, 34).

To balance these conservative recommendations, it is important to understand that the few studies that included early administration of progestin-only methods—oral contraceptives at 1 week postpartum (35, 36) and injectable medroxyprogesterone acetate at 2 days (37) and 7 days (38)—found no adverse effects on the newborn or on breastfeeding. In the absence of evidence that earlier introduction of progestin-only contraceptives has adverse effects on the newborn and on breastfeeding, the labeling for progestin-only oral contraceptives focuses instead on what is known about fertility after childbirth. Taking only biologic factors into account, contraception is not needed in the first 3 weeks postpartum because of a delay in return of ovulation in all women. And this delay is extended for women who breastfeed exclusively. An implied prohibition on earlier administration is more in the nature of a pragmatic rather than a scientific resolution of the question. From the perspective of routine clinical practice, it would appear reasonable to apply the same rationale, even though conservative, to the initiation of DMPA and implants in postpartum breastfeeding women. However, the package labeling for these methods has the effect of being even more conservative as noted, outlining a 6-week start for all breastfeeding women, with no flexibility. Sometimes, however, there are practical reasons a breastfeeding woman may consider initiating hormonal contraception while in the hospital or shortly after. For example, there may be uncertainty about opportunities for follow-up visits. The breastfeeding woman and her physician can then weigh the reasons for early use of these contraceptives against potential disadvantages, make an appropriate decision, and continue to evaluate the woman's individual breastfeeding experience if hormonal contraceptives are chosen.

Combination Estrogen–Progestin Contraceptives

The postpartum patient has a hypercoagulable state that predisposes her to venous thrombosis (39). The use of estrogen-containing contraceptives during this phase of approximately 3 weeks after childbirth could contribute to this state. Furthermore, estrogen–progestin contraceptives have been shown to reduce the quantity and quality of breast milk. The World Health Organization recommends that the breastfeeding woman wait at least 6 months after childbirth to start using them (33). Labeling required by the FDA for combined oral contraceptives states, "If possible, the nursing mother should be advised not to use oral contraceptives but to use other forms of contraception until she has completely weaned her child" (34). These conservative approaches emanate for the most part from earlier combination oral contraceptive studies using higher doses of estrogens. Low-dose tablets (35 μg or lower) probably have a lesser effect on quality and quantity of breast milk. Effects are variable and if there are strong reasons the woman wishes to start combined estrogen–progestin contraceptive use earlier, she should understand and weigh the potential disadvantages. If estrogen–progestin contraceptives are prescribed, they should not be started before 6 weeks postpartum, and the physician should continue to evaluate the woman's individual breastfeeding experience.

The summary recommendations given in the box, "ACOG Recommendations for Hormonal Contraception If Used by Breastfeeding Women," with regard to progestin-only methods are based on the conservative timing outlined in labeling. Exceptions may be considered for earlier use on an individual basis. With combined estrogen–progestin contraceptives, a minimum 6-week delay is prudent

because practical obstacles in developing successful breastfeeding techniques are likely to be resolved by 6 weeks. Most women experience reduced milk volume as a result of estrogen ingestion; this may be dealt with more easily after breastfeeding skills and patterns are established, should combined contraceptives be chosen despite this disadvantage. FDA labeling, however, is more conservative than the summary recommendation offered for combined estrogen–progestin contraceptives here. As noted earlier, prelubricated condoms are a good interim contraceptive choice and will address vaginal dryness associated with breastfeeding as well as help prevent infection.

Lactational Amenorrhea Method

Women who breastfeed can make use of the natural contraceptive effect of lactation. The LAM is most appropriate for women who plan to fully breastfeed 6 months or longer. If the baby is fed only mother's milk or is given supplemental nonbreast-milk feedings only to a minor extent and the woman has not experienced her first postpartum menses, then breastfeeding provides more than 98% protection from pregnancy in the first 6 months following delivery (27, 40, 41). Four prospective clinical trials of the contraceptive effect of LAM demonstrated cumulative 6-month life-table, perfect-use pregnancy rates of 0.5%, 0.6%, 1.0%, and 1.5% among women who relied solely on it. Women should be advised that for significant fertility impact, intervals between feedings should not exceed 4 hours during the day or 6 hours at night (Fig. 1). Supplemental feedings should not exceed 5–10% of the total (42–46). For example, more than one supplemental feeding out of every 10 might increase the

---

ACOG Recommendations for Hormonal Contraception If Used by Breastfeeding Women

- Progestin-only oral contraceptives prescribed or dispensed at discharge from the hospital to be started 2–3 weeks postpartum (eg, the first Sunday after the newborn is 2 weeks old)

- Depot medroxyprogesterone acetate initiated at 6 weeks postpartum*

- Hormonal implants inserted at 6 weeks postpartum*

- Combined estrogen–progestin contraceptives, if prescribed, should not be started before 6 weeks postpartum, and only when lactation is well established and the infant's nutritional status well-monitored

*There are certain clinical situations in which earlier initiation might be considered.

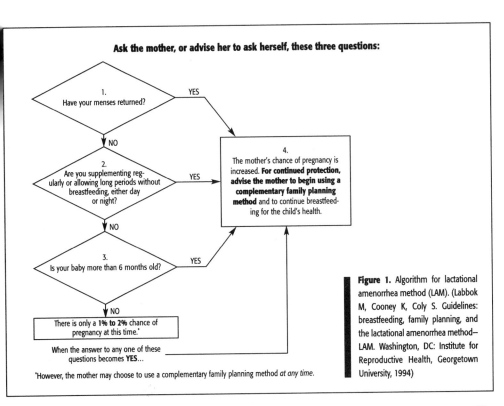

Ask the mother, or advise her to ask herself, these three questions:

1. Have your menses returned? — YES →

NO ↓

2. Are you supplementing regularly or allowing long periods without breastfeeding, either day or night? — YES →

NO ↓

3. Is your baby more than 6 months old? — YES →

NO ↓

4. The mother's chance of pregnancy is increased. **For continued protection, advise the mother to begin using a complementary family planning method** and to continue breastfeeding for the child's health.

There is only a **1% to 2%** chance of pregnancy at this time.*

When the answer to any one of these questions becomes **YES**...

*However, the mother may choose to use a complementary family planning method *at any time.*

Figure 1. Algorithm for lactational amenorrhea method (LAM). (Labbok M, Cooney K, Coly S. Guidelines: breastfeeding, family planning, and the lactational amenorrhea method—LAM. Washington, DC: Institute for Reproductive Health, Georgetown University, 1994)

likelihood of returning fertility. Feeding practices other than direct breastfeeding, insofar as they may reduce the vigor and frequency of suckling and the maternal neuroendocrine response, increase the probability of returning ovulation (47). If there is uncertainty regarding the extent to which a given woman is breastfeeding, it would be prudent to recommend additional contraception.

Maintaining Milk Supply

Regular breastfeeding generally ensures adequate milk supply. As the baby grows and requires more milk, the woman's supply, which is demand driven, increases to accommodate the baby's needs.

Bottle Supplements and Pacifiers

The use of pacifiers and supplemental bottle feeding have been considered deterrents to sustained breastfeeding. Studies do not provide clear evidence that bottle feeding and pacifiers directly interfere with breastfeeding. A recent prospective cohort study indicated that pacifier use in the first 6 weeks was independently associated with declines in the duration of full and overall breastfeeding in the long term, but not short term (during the first 3 months of life). Women who introduced pacifiers early tended to breastfeed fewer times per day. The authors suggested that maternal behavior, such as extending intervals between feedings and decisions to begin weaning, may lead to introduction of pacifiers. They suggested that pacifier use, through an association with infrequent breastfeeding, may mediate (rather than cause) the declines observed in breastfeeding duration (48). It is important to help mothers understand that substituting for or delaying breastfeedings may ultimately reduce milk supply because of the reduction in stimulation of milk production that depends on infant suckling. Another study found that fluid supplements offered by bottle with or without the use of pacifiers during the first 5 days of life were not associated with a lower frequency or shorter duration of breastfeeding during the first 6 months of life (49).

Interruption of Breastfeeding

Separation of mother and infant should be avoided whenever possible, especially during the early establishment of lactation (first 3 weeks). If it is known in advance that hospitalization or a trip, for example, will require the mother to be separated from the infant for more than a day, careful planning can ensure that the ability to breastfeed will be preserved and breast milk will be available for the infant. During the separation, regular pumping of the breasts should be sufficient to maintain the milk supply. The milk may be saved for feeding the infant. When the separation is because of hospitalization, the milk should be discarded if it is judged to contain anesthetic or contraindicated medications. When the mother and infant are reunited, the reestablishment of normal breastfeeding generally progresses well.

Sore Nipples

Having sore nipples is a common problem for the breastfeeding woman. It usually results from poor positioning or latch-on (see box, "Positioning and Latch-On for Breastfeeding"). The first-line treatment should be counseling about these basic techniques (24). Purified lanolin cream and breast shells (to protect the nipples from friction between feedings) may be initiated to facilitate healing (50).

Mastitis

Mastitis occurs in 1–2% of breastfeeding women (51). It most commonly occurs between the first and fifth weeks postpartum but may be seen any time throughout the first year (52). Mastitis is manifested by a sore, reddened area on one breast and often is accompanied by chills, fever, and malaise. A segment of the breast becomes hard and erythematous, the fever can be as high as 40°C, and the mother feels ill.

The differential diagnosis includes clogged milk duct, marked engorgement, and a rare condition, inflammatory breast carcinoma. Clogged milk ducts present as localized tender masses. They respond to warm wet compresses and manually massaging the loculated milk towards the nipple. Breast engorgement is always bilateral with generalized involvement. It occurs most commonly in the first 2 weeks postpartum. The major feature that differentiates it from inflammatory breast cancer is the knowledge of previous negative breast examination results during the pregnancy. If examination results have been normal, breast engorgement is the more likely diagnosis (51). Inflammatory breast cancer is a lethal form of breast cancer. It presents as unilateral erythema, heat, and induration that is more diffuse and recurrent (53).

Positioning and Latch-On for Breastfeeding

When observing an infant being breastfed, take note of the following:

- Position of mother, body language, and tension. Pillows may provide support for arms or infant.
- Position of infant. Ventral surface should be to mother's ventral surface, with lower arm, if not swaddled, around mother's thorax. Infant cannot swallow if head has to turn to breast, and grasp of areola will be poor. Infant's head should be in crook of arm and moved toward breast by arm movement.
- Position of mother's hand on breast not in way of proper grasp by infant
- Position of infant's lips on areola about 1–1½ inches (2.5–3.7 cm) from base of nipple
- Lower lip not folded in so that infant does not suck it; lips flanged
- Actual events around presenting breast and assisting infant to latch on
- Response of infant to lower lip stimulus by opening mouth wide
- Motion of masseter muscle during suckling and sounds of swallowing
- Mother comfortable with no breast pain

Lawrence RA, Lawrence R. Breastfeeding: a guide for the medical profession. 5th ed. St. Louis, Missouri: Mosby, 1999

The most common causative agent in mastitis is *Staphylococcus aureus*, occurring in 40% of cases (54). It is also the most common cause of abscess. Other common organisms in mastitis are *Hemophilus influenzae* and *H parainfluenzae*, *Escherichia coli*, *Enterococcus faecalis*, *Klebsiella pneumoniae*, *Enterobacter cloacae*, *Serratia marcescens*, and *Pseudomonas pickettii* (53).

The condition usually can be treated successfully with narrow-spectrum antibiotic therapy (first choice for women who are not allergic is dicloxacillin, 500 mg four times daily), hydration, bedrest, and acetaminophen. The mother should continue to breastfeed or express the milk from both breasts because it is important to empty the affected breast. In some cases, the woman may be advised to discard the milk until she has been treated for 24 hours.

If mastitis is not treated aggressively, an abscess may develop. Treatment is successful in curing mastitis if started early; the most common cause of recurrent mastitis is inadequate treatment. Delayed administration of antibiotics is associated with an increased incidence of breast abscess. Many staphylococcal infections are caused by organisms sensitive to penicillin or a cephalosporin. Dicloxacillin may be started empirically (55). Women who are allergic to penicillin may be given erythromycin. If the infection is caused by resistant, penicillinase-producing staphylococci, an antibiotic such as vancomycin or cefotetan should be given and continued until 2 days after the infection subsides, a minimum of 10–14 days.

Abscess

Abscess is diagnosed by a palpable mass or failure to defervesce within 48–72 hours of antibiotic therapy. Generally, abscesses are treated with incision and drainage. Multiple abscesses may require multiple incisions, with a finger inserted to break down the locules. Breast milk should be discarded for the first 24 hours after surgery, with breastfeeding resuming thereafter if there is no drainage into the breast milk (1). Recently, ultrasonographically guided needle aspiration was shown to be successful in treating abscesses in 18 of 19 women (56).

Working Mothers and Time Away

Over half of mothers are employed outside the home. In some situations, the mother is able to feed her infant at work, but this is not common. Health professionals can help the mother consider the method by which she plans to feed her infant when she returns to work. Employers are increasingly supportive of accommodating the needs of their breastfeeding employees (16). If a woman wants to continue to breastfeed or breast-milk feed, she should plan to pump her breasts to maintain her milk supply and to provide stored milk for the caregiver to feed the infant in her absence. A mother can be reassured that continuing breastfeeding and use of breast milk to whatever degree she finds possible will benefit her infant.

Expressing Milk

Several methods are available to collect milk. Health professionals should ensure that breastfeeding women can successfully express milk by hand. Because use of a breast pump is more efficient, rental or purchase of a pump can be considered. In general, electric pumps are more efficient than hand pumps. Pumping both breasts simultaneously is more effective and saves time.

On occasion, women have to educate employers about the necessity of time and location to pump breasts during the workday. The influence of the physician in creating a better environment should not be underestimated. A physician's letter or phone call to the employer explaining how simple but vital the breastfeeding employee's needs are can be effective.

Storage of Milk

Breast milk can be stored in the refrigerator or on ice in glass or plastic containers. The use of refrigerated milk within 2 days is recommended, which is well before appreciable bacterial growth usually occurs. Breast milk intended for longer storage should be frozen as soon as possible and kept at the lowest and most constant temperatures available; for example, a deep freezer is preferable to a refrigerator freezer with a self-defrost cycle. Milk should be dated and used in date order to avoid loss of beneficial properties over time. Frozen milk can be thawed quickly under running water or gradually in the refrigerator. It should not be left out at room temperature for more than 4–8 hours, exposed to very hot water, or put in the microwave. Once the milk has thawed, it can be kept in the refrigerator for 24 hours (1, 57).

Breastfeeding Expectations in Daily Life

Despite sporadic instances of authorities forbidding breastfeeding in public, there is an increased level of acceptance of breastfeeding nationally. Supportive laws and policies are becoming the trend. Recently, breastfeeding mothers have had increasing success in leading active lives. Couples commonly take their babies with them to meetings, outings, restaurants, and while traveling. Women can be skillful at unobtrusively feeding their babies in public. There are many baby-friendly restaurants that welcome families and have a positive approach to breastfeeding.

Physicians' offices and other health facilities should welcome and encourage breastfeeding by providing educational material and an atmosphere receptive to breastfeeding women. All staff members should be aware of the value and importance of breastfeeding and understand that their contacts with patients can help them decide to breastfeed and encourage them to continue (see the box, "Office Tips").

Formula companies try to attract the interest of pregnant women with gift packs. Care providers should be aware that the giving of gift packs with formula to breastfeeding women is commonly a deterrent to continuation of breastfeeding (58, 59). A professional recommendation of the care and feeding products in the gift pack is implied. Physicians may conclude that noncommercial educational alternatives or gift packs without health-related items are preferable.

How Long to Breastfeed

During the first 6 months of life, exclusive breastfeeding is the preferred feeding approach for the healthy infant born at term. It provides optimal nutrients for growth and development of the infant. The ACOG recommends that exclusive breastfeeding be continued until the infant is about 6 months old. A longer breastfeeding experience is, of course, beneficial. The professional objectives are to encourage and enable as many women as possible to breastfeed and to help them continue as long as possible.

Gradual introduction of iron-enriched solid foods in the second half of the first year should complement the breast milk diet (3). The AAP recommends that breastfeeding continue for at least 12 months, and thereafter for as long as is mutually desired (3). "Vitamin D and iron may need to be given before 6 months of age in selected groups of infants (vitamin D for infants whose mothers are vitamin D-deficient or those infants not exposed to adequate sunlight, iron for those who have low iron stores or anemia)" (3).

Weaning

The weaning process should be gradual. Eliminating a feeding every 2–3 days will achieve a comfortable transition for the infant and prevent engorgement in the mother. An infant weaned before 12 months should receive iron-fortified infant formula rather than cows' milk (3). If an infant is less than 9 months, weaning can be accomplished by substituting a bottle or cup for a breastfeeding. If an infant is 9 months or older, he or she may use a cup and substitute other foods for breastfeeding.

Abrupt weaning can be difficult for the mother and the baby. When this is necessary, certain measures can be helpful. The mother should wear a support bra. She does not need to restrict fluids. She may manually express sufficient milk to relieve the engorgement, but not so much that more milk production is stimulated. Cool compresses will reduce engorgement. Hormonal therapy is not recommended.

Weaning creates a hormonal milieu conducive to remineralization of bone and maternal replenishment. This may be a consideration favoring delay of the next pregnancy until the mother has completed breastfeeding.

Breast Cancer Detection

Because of normal changes in the breasts during pregnancy and lactation, cancer detection by palpation becomes more difficult. Breast self-examination is recommended, as it is for all women; however, in general, significant changes are difficult to distinguish from the normal changes in the breast during breastfeeding. Any suspicious lesion should be investigated. Studies indicate there are delays in diagnosis of breast cancer during pregnancy and lactation, including greater intervals between palpation of a lesion and diagnosis. These delays result in an increased risk of metastatic disease at diagnosis and a reduced chance of diagnosis at stage I (60). If a mass or other abnormality is detected during lactation, it should be fully evaluated, including biopsy, if indicated. Breastfeeding can continue during the evaluation. During lactation, mammograms are less reliable because of the associated increase in breast tissue density, which may make the test more difficult to interpret (53).

With these difficulties in detection during pregnancy and lactation as a backdrop, clinical breast examinations of women who may become pregnant are especially important. In addition, increasing age is one of many risk factors for breast cancer. Women are having babies in their late 30s and early 40s, and screening may be difficult during a 1- or 2-year period of pregnancy and lactation. This may influence some women who would not otherwise be candidates for mammography to consider it with their physicians as part of the total clinical evaluation before pregnancy.

Healthy People 2010

The goal set by the U.S. Public Health Service for *Healthy People 2010* is to "increase the proportion of mothers who breastfeed their babies" with specific targets for breastfeeding of 75% in the early postpartum period, 50% at 6 months, and 25% at 12 months (61). These are basically the same levels that were called for in *Healthy People 2000* except that the 12-month target has been added. Significant progress has been made from the rates of the early 90s. By 1998, the most recent year for which data are available, the proportion of mothers choosing to breastfeed reached a high of 64.3% after a concerted effort on the part of health professionals and support people. The highest breastfeeding rates are among college-educated women, those older than the age of 30, those living in the Mountain or Pacific census regions, and those not enrolled in WIC (Special Supplemental Nutrition Program for Women, Infants, and Children). Breastfeeding initiation rates are lowest among black women, women younger than 20 years old, women enrolled in WIC, those who did not complete high school, and those living in the East South Central census region (Mothers' Survey, Ross Products Division, Abbott Laboratories, Inc., Columbus, Ohio).

Some concentrated educational efforts also have had a statistical impact in specific populations (62). Women enrolled in WIC, because of increased breastfeeding support, are among those with the most rapid increases in rates of breastfeeding, although their rates remain well below national averages. Between 1990 and 1998, the most rapidly increasing initiation rate was among black women, the demographic group with the lowest breastfeeding rate (44.9% in-hospital compared with 64.3% nationally) in 1998 despite this increase (Mothers' Survey).

In 1998, the breastfeeding rate at 6 months reached 28.6%, the highest rate in the nearly 30 years such data have been collected. The highest 6-month rates are among mothers with the same demographic and socioeconomic characteristics as those who have the highest in-hospital breastfeeding rates. Younger women, black women, WIC participants, women in the East South Central census region, and women who are employed full time outside the home have the lowest 6-month breastfeeding rates (Mothers' Survey).

With the cooperation of many dedicated caregivers, it appears that the 2010 goals may be achievable. However, even if 75% of women initiate breastfeeding, two thirds of them will need to continue breastfeeding, to reach the proposed 6-month target of 50% of all women breastfeeding. Obstetrician–gynecologists should ensure that women have the correct information to make an informed decision and, together with pediatricians, they should ensure that each woman has the help and support necessary to continue to breastfeed successfully (63). The combined efforts of all health care providers will be necessary to meet this goal.

References

1. Lawrence RA, Lawrence RM. Breastfeeding: a guide for the medical profession. 5th ed. St. Louis, Missouri: Mosby, 1999

2. Institute of Medicine. Subcommittee on Nutrition During Lactation, Committee on Nutritional Status During Pregnancy and Lactation, Food and Nutrition Board. Nutrition during lactation. Washington, DC: National Academy Press, 1991

3. American Academy of Pediatrics, Work Group on Breastfeeding. Breastfeeding and the use of human milk. Pediatrics 1997;100:1035–1039

4. Chua S, Arulkumaran S, Lim I, Selamat N, Ratham SS. Influence of breastfeeding and nipple stimulation on postpartum uterine activity. Br J Obstet Gynaecol 1994;101: 804–805

5. Carter CS, Altemus M. Integrative functions of lactational hormones in social behavior and stress management. Ann N Y Acad Sci 1997;807:164–174

6. Rosenblatt KA, Thomas DB. Lactation and the risk of epithelial ovarian cancer. The WHO Collaborative Study of Neoplasia and Steroid Contraceptives. Int J Epidemiol 1993;22:192–197

7. Newcomb PA, Storer BE, Longnecker MP, Mittendorf R, Greenberg ER, Clapp RW, et al. Lactation and a reduced risk of premenopausal breast cancer. N Engl J Med 1994; 330:81–87

8. Kennedy KI, Visness CM. Contraceptive efficacy of lactational amenorrhoea. Lancet 1992;339:227–230

9. Gray RH, Campbell OM, Apelo R, Eslami SS, Zacur H, Ramos RM, et al. Risk of ovulation during lactation. Lancet 1990;335:25–29

10. Labbok MH, Colie C. Puerperium and breast-feeding. Curr Opin Obstet Gynecol 1992;4:818–825

11. Melton LJ 3d, Bryant SC, Wahner HW, O'Fallon WM, Malkasian GD, Judd HL, et al. Influence of breastfeeding and other reproductive factors on bone mass later in life. Osteoporos Int 1993;3:76–83

12. Cumming RG, Klineberg RJ. Breastfeeding and other reproductive factors and the risk of hip fractures in elderly women. Int J Epidemiol 1993;22:684–691

13. Dewey KG, Heinig MJ, Nommsen LA. Maternal weight-loss patterns during prolonged lactation. Am J Clin Nutr 1993;58:162–166

14. Ball TM, Wright AL. Health care costs of formula-feeding in the first year of life. Pediatrics 1999;103:870–876

15. Montgomery DL, Splett PL. Economic benefit of breast-feeding infants enrolled in WIC. J Am Diet Assoc 1997; 97:379–385

16. Jacobson M, Kolarek MH, Newton B. Business, babies and the bottom line: corporate innovations and best practices in maternal and child health. Washington, DC: Washington Business Group on Health, 1996

17. Cohen R, Mrtek MB, Mrtek RG. Comparison of maternal absenteeism and infant illness rates among breast-feeding and formula-feeding women in two corporations. Am J Health Promot 1995;10:148–153

18. Lawrence RA. A review of the medical benefits and contraindications to breastfeeding in the United States. Maternal and Child Health Technical Information Bulletin. Arlington, Virginia: National Center for Education in Maternal and Child Health, 1997

19. American Academy of Pediatrics, American College of Obstetricians and Gynecologists. Guidelines for perinatal care. 4th ed. Elk Grove Village, Illinois: AAP; Washington, DC: ACOG, 1997

20. Recommendations for prevention and control of hepatitis C virus (HCV) infection and HCV-related chronic disease. Centers for Disease Control and Prevention. MMWR Morb Mortal Wkly Rep 1998;47(RR-19):1–39

21. American Academy of Pediatrics Committee on Drugs. The transfer of drugs and other chemicals into human milk. Pediatrics 1994;93:137–150

22. Pugin E, Valdes V, Labbok MH, Perez A, Aravena R. Does prenatal breastfeeding skills group education increase the effectiveness of a comprehensive breastfeeding promotion program? J Hum Lact 1996;12(1):15–19

23. Randolph L, Cooper L, Fonseca-Becker F, York M, McIntosh M. Baby friendly hospital initiative feasibility study: final report. Healthy Mothers Healthy Babies National Coalition Expert Work Group. Alexandria, Virginia: HMHB, 1994

24. American College of Obstetricians and Gynecologists. Breast-feeding your baby. ACOG Patient Education Pamphlet AP029. Washington, DC: ACOG, 1997

25. Institute of Medicine. Standing Committee on the Scientific Evaluation of Dietary Reference Intakes, Food and Nutrition Board. Dietary reference intakes for calcium, phosphorus, magnesium, vitamin D, and fluoride. Washington, DC: National Academy Press, 1997

26. Institute of Medicine. Committee on Nutritional Status During Pregnancy and Lactation, Food and Nutrition Board. Nutrition services in perinatal care. 2nd ed. Washington, DC: National Academy Press, 1992

27. Hatcher RA, Trussell J, Stewart F, Cates W Jr, Stewart GK, Guest F, et al. Contraceptive technology. 17th rev. ed. New York: Ardent Media, Inc, 1998

28. Tankeyoon M, Dusitsin N, Chalapati S, Koetsawang S, Saibiang S, Sas M, et al. Effects of hormonal contraceptives on milk volume and infant growth. WHO Special Programme of Research, Development, and Research Training in Human Reproduction, Task Force on Oral Contraceptives. Contraception 1984;30:505–522

29. World Health Organization (WHO) Task Force on Oral Contraceptives. Effects of hormonal contraceptives on milk composition and infant growth. Stud Fam Plann 1988;19:361–369

30. Speroff L, Darney P. A clinical guide for contraception. 2nd ed. Baltimore, Maryland: Williams & Wilkins, 1996

31. Abdulla KA, Elwan SI, Salem HS, Shaaban MM. Effect of early postpartum use of the contraceptive implants, NOR-PLANT, on the serum levels of immunoglobulins of the mothers and their breastfed infants. Contraception 1985; 32:261–266

32. Shaaban MM, Salem HT, Abdullah KA. Influence of levonorgestrel contraceptive implants, NORPLANT, initiated early postpartum upon lactation and infant growth. Contraception 1985;32:623–635

33. World Health Organization. Division of Family and Reproductive Health. Improving access to quality care in family planning: medical eligibility criteria for contraceptive use. Geneva: WHO, 1996

34. Physicians' Desk Reference. 53rd ed. Montvale, New Jersey: Medical Economics, Inc, 1999

35. McCann MF, Moggia AV, Higgins JE, Potts M, Becker C. The effects of a progestin-only oral contraceptive (levonorgestrel 0.03 mg) on breast-feeding. Contraception 1989;40:635–648

36. Moggia AV, Harris GS, Dunson TR, Diaz R, Moggia MS, Ferrer MA, et al. A comparative study of a progestin-only oral contraceptive versus non-hormonal methods in lactating women in Buenos Aires, Argentina. Contraception 1991;44:31–43

37. Guiloff E, Ibarra-Polo A, Zañartu J, Toscanini C, Mischler TW, Gómez-Rogers C. Effect of contraception on lactation. Am J Obstet Gynecol 1974;118:42–45

38. Karim M, Ammar R, el Mahgoub S, el Ganzoury B, Fikri F, Abdou I. Injected progestogen and lactation. BMJ 1971; 1:200–203

39. WHO Task Force on Oral Contraceptives. Contraception during the postpartum period and during lactation: the effects on women's health. Int J Gynaecol Obstet 1987;25 (suppl):13–26

40. Kennedy KI, Rivera R, McNeilly AS. Consensus statement on the use of breastfeeding as a family planning method. Contraception 1989;39:477–496

41. World Health Organization. Task Force on Methods for the Natural Regulation of Fertility. The WHO multinational study of breast-feeding and lactational amenorrhea. III. Pregnancy during breast-feeding. Fertil Steril 1999;72;431–440

42. Perez A, Labbok MH, Queenan JT. Clinical study of the lactational amenorrhoea method for family planning. Lancet 1992;339:968–970

43. Ramos R, Kennedy KI, Visness CM. Effectiveness of lactational amenorrhea in prevention of pregnancy in Manila, the Philippines: non-comparative prospective trial. BMJ 1996;313:909–912

44. Labbok MH, Hight-Laukaran V, Peterson AE, Fletcher V, von Hertzen H, Van Look PF. Multicenter study of the Lactational Amenorrhea Method (LAM): I. Efficacy, duration and implications for clinical application. Contraception 1997;55:327–336

45. Kazi A, Kennedy KI, Visness CM, Khan T. Effectiveness of the lactational amenorrhea method in Pakistan. Fertil Steril 1995;64:717–723

46. Labbok M, Cooney K, Coly S. Guidelines: breastfeeding, family planning, and the lactational amenorrhea method—LAM. Washington, DC: Institute for Reproductive Health, Georgetown University, 1994

47. Campbell OM, Gray RH. Characteristics and determinants of postpartum ovarian function in women in the United States. Am J Obstet Gynecol 1993;169:55–60

48. Howard CR, Howard FM, Lanphear B, deBlieck EA, Eberly S, Lawrence RA. The effects of early pacifier use on breastfeeding duration. Pediatrics 1999;103:E33

49. Schubiger G, Schwarz U, Tonz O. UNICEF/WHO baby-friendly hospital initiative: does the use of bottles and pacifiers in the neonatal nursery prevent successful breastfeeding? Neonatal Study Group. Eur J Pediatr 1997;156:874–877

50. Brent N, Rudy SJ, Redd B, Rudy TE, Roth LA. Sore nipples in breast-feeding women: a clinical trial of wound dressings vs conventional care. Arch Pediatr Adolesc Med 1998;152:1077–1082

51. Stehman FB. Infections and inflammations of the breast. In: Hindle WH, ed. Breast disease for gynecologists. Norwalk, Connecticut: Appleton & Lange, 1990:151

52. Niebyl JR, Spence MR, Parmley TH. Sporadic (nonepidemic) puerperal mastitis. J Reprod Med 1978;20: 97–100

53. Hankins GD, Clark SL, Cunningham FG, Gilstrap LC III. Breast disease during pregnancy and lactation. In: Hankins GD, Clark SL, Cunningham FG, Gilstrap LC III, eds. Operative obstetrics. Norwalk, Connecticut: Appleton & Lange, 1995:667–694

54. Matheson I, Aursnes I, Horgen M, Aabo O, Melby K. Bacteriological findings and clinical symptoms in relation to clinical outcome in puerperal mastitis. Acta Obstet Gynecol Scand 1988;67:723–726

55. Hindle WH. Other benign breast problems. Clin Obstet Gynecol 1994;37:916–924

56. Karstrup S, Solvig J, Nolsoe CP, Nilsson P, Khattar S, Loren I, et al. Acute puerperal breast abscesses: US-guided drainage. Radiology 1993;188:807–809

57. Arnold LDW. Recommendations for collection, storage and handling of a mother's milk for her own infant in the hospital setting. 3rd ed. Denver: Human Milk Banking Association of North America, 1999

58. Howard C, Howard F, Lawrence R, Andresen E, DeBlieck E, Weitzman M. Office prenatal formula advertising and its effect on breast-feeding patterns. Obstet Gynecol 2000;95:296–303

59. Pérez-Escamilla R, Pollitt E, Lönnerdal B, Dewey KG. Infant feeding policies in maternity wards and their effect on breast-feeding success: an analytical overview. Am J Public Health 1994;84:89–97

60. Zemlickis D, Lishner M, Degendorfer P, Panzarella T, Burke B, Sutcliffe SB, et al. Maternal and fetal outcome after breast cancer in pregnancy. Am J Obstet Gynecol 1992;166:781–787

61. Healthy people 2010, volume II. Washington, DC: U.S. Department of Health and Human Services, 2000: 16-46–16-48

62. Ryan AS. The resurgence of breastfeeding in the United States. Pediatrics 1997;99:E12

63. Freed GL, Clark SJ, Cefalo RC, Sorenson JR. Breast-feeding education of obstetrics-gynecology residents and practitioners. Am J Obstet Gynecol 1995;173:1607–1613

Index*

*Page numbers followed by f indicate figures; t, tables.

Dental health, 115
Depression, 176. *See also* Antidepressants; Postpartum blues/depression
Desipramine, 239t
Dexbrompheniramine maleate, 240t
DHA, 23
Diabetes, 31
Diabetes therapy, 177–178
Diagnostic mammography, 147
Diatrizoate, 240t
Diazepam, 177, 239t
Dicumarol, 240t
Dieldrin, 242t
Digoxin, 240t
Diltiazem, 179, 240t
Dipyrone, 240t
Discharge planning, 96–99, 199–200
Disopyramide, 240t
Diuretics, 179
DMPA, 189
Docosahexaenoic acid (DHA), 23
Doctor appointments. *See* Office visits; Physician's office
Domperidone, 240t
Donor human milk, 170
Dothiepin, 239t
Double pumping system, 162, 162f
Down syndrome, 203, 204t
Doxepin, 239t
Doxorubicin, 238t
Drugs. *See* Medications and breastfeeding
Drugs of abuse, 175, 238t
Ductal ectasia, 147
Dyphylline, 240t

E
Early breastfeeding, 198
Education. *See* Breastfeeding education
EGF, 27
Electric breast pump, 160, 170
Electronic baby scale, 167
Elimination patterns, 90–91
Embryogenesis, 46
Enalapril, 240t
Enriched formula, 200
Enteromammary immune system, 27–28
Environmental agents, 185, 242t
Epidermal growth factor (EGF), 27
Epidural anesthesia, 74
Ergotamine, 239t

Ergotamine family of drugs, 182
Erythromycin, 139, 240t
Estradiol, 240t
Ethambutol, 240t
Ethanol, 240t
Ethics, 11–13
Ethosuximide, 241t
Exclusive breastfeeding, 2t, 113
Exhaustion, 76
Expressing milk, 154, 157–162, 195, 261

F
FABM, 11
Famotidine, 178
Father, 62
Fatty acids, 23
Fava beans, 242t
Feedback inhibitor of lactation, 51
Feeding methods
  bottle-feeding, 92–93, 154–155, 259
  breastfeeding. *See* Breastfeeding
  cup feeding, 164–166
  donor human milk, 170
  feeding-tube devices, 164, 165t
  syringe/medicine dropper, 166
  tube feeding, 166–167
Feeding on cue, 78
Fentanyl, 75, 241t
Fexofenadine, 241t
First newborn visit, 118–119t, 214
Fish lips, 89
5-Aminosalicylic acid, 239t
Flecainide, 241t
Fleroxacin, 241t
Fluconazole, 181, 241t
Flufenamic acid, 241t
Fluorescein, 241t
Fluoride supplementation, 113
Fluorides, 242t
Fluoroquinolone, 180
Fluoxetine, 177, 239t
Fluvoxamine, 239t
Folic acid, 241t
Follow-up, 98. *See also* Office visits
Football hold, 70, 70f
Foremilk, 195, 196
Formula marketing, 13
Free amino acids, 26
Freezing milk, 169
Fussy/unsettled infants, 87

Index

Milk composition, *Continued*
 nitrogen, 19, 22
 nucleotides, 27
 nutritional components, 19–25
 vitamins, 20–21t, 24–25
Milk duct, 47f
Milk ejection, 45, 52
Milk expression, 154, 157–162, 195, 261
Milk fat content, 24, 195
Milk leakage, 141
Milk let-down reflex, 72
Milk stasis, 137
Milk storage, 168–170, 261
Milk storage containers, 169–170
Milk supply, 84t, 259
Minerals, 21t, 24
Minipills, 189
Minoxidil, 241t
Mixed breastfeeding, 2t
Monosodium glutamate, 242t
Montgomery tubercles, 48
Morphine, 73t, 74, 75, 241t
Mother
 benefits of breastfeeding, 31–34
 bloody nipple discharge, 147
 breast abscess, 140–141, 261
 breast cancer, 148, 260, 262–263
 breast engorgement, 95, 96t, 136, 137t, 260
 breast self-examination, 148, 262
 breastfeeding education, 212–213
 contraception, 187–191, 256–259
 contradictions to breastfeeding, 39–42
 diseases, 31–34, 134–142, 260
 long-term illness, 142–144
 mastitis, 137t, 138–140, 260–261
 milk leakage, 141
 nipple pain, 93–94, 134–136
 nutrition, 144–146
 office visits. *See* Office visits
 plugged ducts, 137–138, 260
 post-birth surgery, 143–144, 152–154
 postpartum blues/depression, 141–142
 postpartum period, 93–96
 relactation, 206
 return to work, 98, 134, 149–151, 152–153t
 risk factors, 56t, 81–83
 sleep pattern, 114
 weight loss, 146
Mother-in-residence, 152
Mother-infant separation, 149–155

ACOG educational bulletin, 260
 bottle-feeding, 154–155
 maternal illness/surgery, 143–144, 152–154
 milk expression, 154, 157–162
 newborn/infant illness, 151–152
 return to work/school, 149–151, 152–153t
Mother-led weaning, 117
Moxalactam, 241t
Multiple births, 205
Multivitamin supplementation, 200
Multivitamins, 112
Myoepithelial cells, 47

N
Nadolol, 241t
Nalbuphine, 73t, 74
Nalidixic acid, 180, 181, 241t
Naproxen, 181, 182, 241t
Naratriptan, 182
Necrotizing enterocolitis (NEC), 30
Nefopam, 241t
Nerve growth factor, 27
Never breastfed, 2t
Newborn. *See* Infant
Nicotine patches, 174
Nifedipine, 241t
Nipple, 47f
Nipple *Candida* infections, 134–136
Nipple pain, 93–94, 134–136
Nipple shields, 163
Nitrofurantoin, 241t
Nitrogen, 19, 22
Non-governmental organizations, 10–11
Non-protein nitrogen (NPN), 19, 22
Nonsteroidal anti-inflammatory drugs (NSAIDs), 74, 75, 181, 182
Norethynodrel, 241t
Normeperidine, 74
Norsteroids, 241t
Nortriptyline, 176, 239t
Noscapine, 241t
NPN, 19, 22
NSAIDs, 74, 75, 181, 182
Nucleotides, 27
Nurse-midwives, 9–10
Nursing strike, 108–109
Nystatin, 135

O
Obesity, 31

274

Office visits. *See also* Physician's office
  ACOG educational bulletin, 254
  breast evaluation while nursing, 146–148
  day 3 to 5 follow-up visit, 118–119t, 214
  first newborn visit, 118–119t, 214
  initial prenatal visit, 55–57, 60t, 254
  1-month visit, 120–121t
  2-month visit, 122–123t
  4-month visit, 124–125t
  6-month visit, 126–127t
  9-month visit, 128–129t
  12-month visit, 130t
  physical examination, 57–59
  post-Cesarean delivery, 134
  prenatal visits, 60–61t
  routine obstetrics visit, 133–134
  visit to pediatric care professional, 62, 63t
Ofloxacin, 180, 241t
Oligosaccharides, 23, 26
Olsalazine, 178
On-site child care, 149
Oral fluconazole, 136
Oral hypoglycemics, 177
Oral narcotics, 75
Otitis media, 28, 30
Oxacillin, 139
Oxazepam, 177
Oxprenolol, 241t
Oxytocin, 33, 49, 50
Oxytocin spray, 184
Oxytocin stimulation, 52

P
Pacifiers, 79, 93, 197, 259
Pain management, 182
  cesarean delivery, 75–76
  labor and delivery, 73–75
Palmitic acid, 23
Paroxetine, 239t
Partial breastfeeding, 2t
Patient education, 212–213
Peer counseling services, 213
Penicillin, 139
Perphenazine, 239t
Pharmacologic principles, 173–174
Phencyclidine, 238t
Phenindione, 239t
Phenobarbital, 182, 239t
Phenylbutazone, 241t

Phenylketonuria, 42
Phenytoin, 182, 241t
Phone-in resource, 256
Phosphorus, 24
Physician education, 8, 211
Physician's Desk Reference, 173
Physician's office, 209–215
  breastfeeding-friendly environment, 209–210
  lactation specialists, 212
  meeting with patients. *See* Office visits
  staff education, 210–212
Physiology of lactation, 49–53
Pierced nipples, 39
Pierre Robin sequence, 202–203
Piroxicam, 241t
Piston/cylinder breast pump, 157
Plugged ducts, 137–138, 137t, 260
Policy statement (AAP), 225–235
Polybrominated biphenyls, 242t
Polychlorinated biphenyls, 242t
Positioning, 69–70, 260
Postpartum blues/depression, 141–142
Postpartum pain relief, 74
Postsurgical pain relief, 75
Prazepam, 239t
Prednisone, 241t
Prednisolone, 241t
Prematurity, 193. *See also* Special-needs infants
Prenatal classes, 212
Prenatal visits, 60–61t
Primary insufficient milk syndrome, 42
Primidone, 239t
Procainamide, 242t
Progesterone, 48, 242t
Progestin-only contraceptives, 188–189, 257–258
Prolactin, 45, 48, 49
Prolactin secretion, 51
Propanolol, 181
Propoxyphene, 75, 242t
Propranolol, 242t
Propylthiouracil, 183, 242t
Pseudoephedrine, 242t
Psychological stress, 53
Psychotropic drugs, 176–177, 236, 239t
Puberty, 46
Publications, 213, 217–220
Pyridostigmine, 242t
Pyridoxine, 240t
Pyrimethamine, 242t